INVITATION TO HOLISTIC HEALTH: A GUIDE TO LIVING A BALANCED LIFE

Charlotte Eliopoulos RN, MPH, ND, PhD
Specialist in Holistic Chronic Care

Past President, American Holistic Nurses'
Association

JONES AND BARTLETT PUBLISHERS
Sudbury, Massachusetts
BOSTON   TORONTO   LONDON   SINGAPORE

World Headquarters
Jones and Bartlett Publishers
40 Tall Pine Drive
Sudbury, MA 01776
978-443-5000
info@jbpub.com
www.jbpub.com

Jones and Bartlett Publishers
Canada
6339 Ormindale Way
Mississauga, ON L5V 1J2
CANADA

Jones and Bartlett Publishers
International
Barb House, Barb Mews London
W6 7PA
UK

Library of Congress Cataloging-in-Publication Data

Eliopoulos, Charlotte.
    Invitation to holistic heath : a guide to living a balanced life / Charlotte Eliopoulos.—
1st ed.
        p. cm.
Includes bibliographical references and index.
    ISBN 0-7637-4562-6 (Paperback)
    1. Holistic medicine. 2. Medicine, Chinese. I. American Holistic
Nurses' Association. II. Title.
    R733.E425 2004
    613—dc22
                            2003020603

The authors, editor, and publisher have made every effort to provide accurate information. However, they are not responsible for errors, omissions, or for any outcomes related to the use of the contents of this book and take no responsibility for the use of the products described herein. Research, clinical practice, and government regulations often change the accepted standards in this field. When consideration is being given to use of any drug, herbal treatment, or health supplement, the health care provider or reader is responsible for determining FDA status of the product, reading the package insert, and prescribing information for the most up-to-date recommendations on dose, precautions, and contraindications and determining the appropriate usage for the product. This is especially important in the case of drugs or supplements that are new or seldom used.

Production Credits
Acquisitions Editor: Kevin Sullivan
Production Manager: Amy Rose
Editorial Assistant: Amy Sibley
Production Assistant: Tracey Chapman
Marketing Manager: Ed McKenna
Cover Design: Bret Kerr
Manufacturing Buyer: Amy Bacus
Composition: Dartmouth Publishing, Inc.
Printing and Binding: Malloy, Inc.
Cover Printing: Malloy, Inc.

Printed in the United States of America
08 07 06 05   10 9 8 7 6 5 4 3 2

TABLE OF CONTENTS

PART II

Developing Healthy Lifestyle Practices 113

PART III

Taking Charge of Challenges to the Mind, Body, and Spirit

PREFACE

If the bulging bookstore shelves on health topics, record sales of nutritional supplements, and growing memberships in health clubs are any indication, Americans are becoming increasingly health conscious. Rather than seeking help after an illness has developed, we are being proactive in reducing our health risks and preventing disease. We are taking responsibility for our health and demanding partnership relationships with our health care providers. Technology has enabled us to become informed not only of new medical advancements, but also, natural and complementary therapies popular in remote parts of the world—and we're using them, often independent of our physicians' advice or knowledge. In fact, nearly one half of all Americans are using some type of complementary and alternative therapy, and paying for it out of pocket. Further, we have become acutely aware that the state of our bodies, minds, and spirits are interrelated and interdependent, and we are concerned with the care of each of these elements of our total beings.

Health Care Is Changing

The growing health consciousness of Americans has been accompanied by changes in the approach to health care. Actually, *health care* is a misnomer as Western medicine has functioned under a sick care model that we have come to know as the biomedical model. The biomedical model was built upon certain tenets, highly valued by scientific minds, that include:

- *Mechanism*: This belief advanced the concept that the human body is much like a machine, explainable in terms of physics and chemistry. Health is determined by physical structure and function, and disease is a malfunction of the physical part. Malfunctions and malformations are undesirable. Disease is treated by repairing the malformed or malfunctioning organ or system with physical or chemical interventions (e.g., drugs, surgery). Nonphysical influences on health status are not considered, and healing, and dysfunction and deformity serve no purpose.

- *Materialism*: This thinking considers the human body and its state of health as being influenced only by what is seen and measurable. Physical malfunction is the cause of illness, therefore illness is addressed by concrete treatments. Emotional and spiritual states have no impact on health and healing.
- *Reductionism*: This thinking reduces the human body to isolated parts rather than a unified whole. Treatment of a health condition focuses on the individual organ or system rather than the whole being. Good health is judged as having body systems that function well, despite one's feelings or spiritual state.

The first major challenge to the biomedical model occurred in the 1960s when the relationship of body and mind began to be discussed. In retrospect, it is difficult to believe that the medical community was skeptical that the mind could cause illness, yet the resistance to accepting the body-mind connection was real. Similarly, recognition of the role of the spirit in the cause and treatment of illness has met similar skepticism. As the dust settles, however, health care practitioners are understanding the profound, dynamic relationship of body, mind, and spirit to health and healing and moving toward a holistic model of health care.

The Meaning of Holism

It would do us well to define holistic health before going any farther. The term holism refers to a whole that is greater than the sum of its parts. In other words, 1+1+1=3 or 5 or more. When applied to health, holism implies that the health and harmony of the body, mind, and spirit create a higher, richer state of health than would be achieved with attention to just one part, such as physical functioning. Although some people equate it with the use of complementary and alternative therapies, holistic health is a philosophy of care in which a wide range of approaches are used to establish and maintain balance within an individual. Complementary and alternative therapies may be part of the approach to holistic health promotion, but so can healthy lifestyle choices, counseling, prayer, conventional (Western) medical treatments, and other interventions.

About This Book

This book offers guidance to you in your journey to holistic health. There are no special formulas provided that guarantee eternal youth and freedom from illness. There is no revolutionary diet or plan that will change your life in 30 days or less. No exotic substances that you can use to develop a new you will be found among the pages of this book. Instead, solid principles for building a strong foundation for optimal health are presented with practical advice that you can easily adopt and integrate into your life.

The book is divided into three parts. In the first part, **Strengthening Your Inner Resources,** practices are discussed that can build your body's reserves and help it to function optimally. You will be guided through a self-assessment of your health habits so that you can determine areas that may need special attention. The realities of good nutrition are examined along with an in-depth look at dietary supplements. Exercise is approached from a body, mind, spirit perspective. Likewise the important activity of enhancing your immune system is considered from a mind-body framework. Methods to flow with the inescapable reality of stress are discussed.

Developing Healthy Lifestyle Practices is the theme of the second part of this book. The many complex factors that influence your health status as you interact with the world beyond your body are addressed in chapters on topics such as growing healthy relationships, family survival skills, spirituality, humor, touch, and the environment. Chapters are also dedicated to recognizing the significant impact of work and money on one's total being, chapters are dedicated to each of these topics.

The third part of this book, **Taking Charge of Challenges to the Mind, Body, and Spirit,** offers information to equip you to be proactive in keeping yourself in balance. The hidden meaning of symptoms is explored to help you learn about the factors behind your health conditions. Practical advice is offered on how you can work in partnership with your health care provider to assure you get the best care possible. Transitions associated with menopause are examined, along with a wide range of approaches to manage the symptoms that may be experienced. Interesting insights into gambling, drugs, overeating, and other addictions are shared. With the growing use of complementary therapies, a chapter describing their purpose, benefits, and related precautions provides valuable information for sensible use of these products and practices. In addition, chapters focusing on herbs, aromatherapy, and homeopathic remedies offer practical insights into these popular therapies. Skills for being an effective caregiver are presented, along with a chapter outlining resources that can aid you in being an informed health care consumer.

A useful approach to using this book is to give it an initial fast read from cover to cover. You then can focus on chapters that address your specific interests and needs. Although some of the chapters may not pertain to you directly (for instance, if you're not a caregiver you may not have a keen interest in the Surviving Caregiving chapter), you may find that a quick review of the chapter could acquaint you with its content so that you'll recall it in the future if you or people who know are faced with this issue. You'll probably find that the rich facts and resources provided make this book a great reference for your personal library.

Why Nurses Wrote This Book

This book was completely written by holistic nurses. These nurses work in a variety of settings, ranging from private practice to acute hospitals. The thread that weaves them together is their support of a holistic philosophy of care.

In an era when many health books are written by physicians and celebrities, you may wonder why nurses wrote this book. Actually, nurses are ideal people to teach and guide people on holistic health care. Nurses have long enjoyed closer relationships with clients than any other health care professional, and they are highly respected by the public. When people need assistance with their most intimate care needs, seek comfort, and want answers to questions that they're uncomfortable asking their doctors, they most often look to nurses. In their caring, practical ways, nurses provide skills, tools, information, and support to assist clients on their journey toward health. Further, nurses are educated to offer mind, body, spirit care. Since Florence Nightingale's time, nurses have understood and quietly practiced holistic care. In this book, their dedication to empowering clients to achieve optimal health is demonstrated. They invite you to use this resource and empower yourself to achieve your highest possible state of health.

About the American Holistic Nurses' Association

The American Holistic Nurses' Association (AHNA) is a professional nursing organization dedicated to the promotion of holism and healing. The AHNA believes that holistic nurses engage in therapeutic partnerships with clients, their families, and their communities to serve as facilitators in the healing process. The holistic caring process supported by AHNA is one exemplified by nurses:

- Recognizing each person as a whole comprised of body, mind, and spirit
- Assessing clients holistically, using appropriate traditional and holistic methods
- Creating a plan of care in collaboration with clients and their significant others consistent with cultural background, health beliefs, sexual orientation, values, and preferences that focuses on health promotion, recovery or restoration, or peaceful dying so that the person obtains the highest level of independence
- Providing care and guidance to individuals through nursing interventions and therapies consistent with research findings and other sound evidence
- Acquiring and maintaining current knowledge and competencies in holistic nursing practice, including the integration of selected complementary therapies within that practice
- Preserving the wholeness and dignity of self and others
- Engaging in self-care

AHNA is involved in various activities to promote holistic nursing, which include sponsorship of an annual conference, publication of the *Journal of Holistic Nursing*, scholarships, research grants, and an endorsement process for educational programs related to holistic nursing practice. The AHNA in partnership with Jones and Bartlett Publishers also produces a leading reference guide for nurses: Holistic Nursing: A Handbook for Practice, 4th ed (0-7637-3183-8). This title can be ordered from Jones and Bartlett at 800-832-0034 or *www. jbpub.com*. More information on AHNA can be obtained by visiting their website at *www.AHNA.org*, or contacting their headquarters at P.O. Box 2130, Flagstaff, AZ, 86003.

Contributors:

Foreword:
Barbara Dossey, RN, PhD, FAAN
Director, Holistic Nursing Consultants
Santa Fe, NM

Ch 1: Assessing Health Habits
Anneke Young, RN, CNAT
Former dean of School for Holistic Nursing at
    New York College of Health Professions
Syosset, NY

Ch 2: Healthful Nutrition
Ann M. McKay, RN, C, MA, HNC
Health and Wellness Consultant
Providence, RI

Ch 3: Dietary Supplements
Ann M. McKay, RN, C, MA, HNC
Health and Wellness Consultant
Providence, RI

Ch 4: Exercise: Mindfulness in Movement
Barbara Starke, MSN, FNP, HNC
Western Michigan University School
    of Nursing
Kalamazoo, MI

Ch 5: Immune Enhancement:
    Mind/Body Considerations
Barbara Starke, MSN, FNP, HNC
Western Michigan University School
    of Nursing
Kalamazoo, MI

Ch 6: Flowing with the Reality of Stress
Linda S. Weaver, RN, MSN
University of Colorado—Beth El College
    of Nursing
Colorado Springs, CO

Ch 7: Growing Healthy Relationships
Irene Wade Belcher, RN, CNS, HNC, CNMT
Instructor, Holistic Nursing Institute
Tucker, GA

Ch 8: Survival Skills for Families
Joyce Oetinger Murphy, RN, HNC
Holistic Nurse Consultant, The Northwood
    Nurse
Strong, ME

Ch 9: The Spiritual Connection
Carole Ann Drick, DNS, RN
Conscious Living Center
Atglen, PA

Ch 10: Balancing Work and Life
Genevieve Bartol, RN, EdD, HNC
Professor Emeritus, University of North
    Carolina at Greensboro
Greensboro, NC

Ch 11: Creative Financial Health
Marilee Tolen, RN, HNC
President, Marilee Tolen, Inc.
Mt. Laurel, NJ

**Ch 12: Environmental Effects on
the Immune System**
Natalie Pavlovich, PhD, RN, DiHt, CNHP
Duquesne University School of Nursing
Pittsburgh, PA

Ch 13: Promoting a Healthy Environment
Katherine Young, RN
Founder, Essentials of Life,
Wilmot, NH

Ch 14: The Power of Touch
Charlene Christiano, MSN, CS,
ARNP-BC, CHTP
Jackson Memorial Hospital
Miami, FL

**Ch 15: Taking Life Lightly:
Humor, the Great Alternative**
Julia Balzer Riley, RN, MN, HNC
President, Constant Source Seminars
Ellenton, FL

**Ch 16: Understanding the
Hidden Meaning of Symptoms**
Marsha McGovern, MSN, FNP, RN, CS
King College School of Nursing
Bristol, TN

**Ch 17: Working in Partnership with
Your Health Practitioner**
Marie Fasano-Ramos, RN
Holistic Nurse, Private Practice

Ch 18: Menopause: Time of the Wise Woman
Cynthia Aspromonte, RNC, NP, HNC, HTP-I
Nurse Practitioner, Holistic Women's
Healthcare

**Ch 19: Addiction: Diseases of Fear,
Shame, and Guilt**
Joan Elfinger, DNSc, RN, CS, HNC
Research and Holistic Healing Consultant
Franklin, NC
Consultant, Nancy L. Maldonado, PhD

Ch 20: Symptoms and Chakras
Charlene Christiano, MSN, CS,
ARNP-BC, CHTP
Jackson Memorial Hospital
Miami, FL

Ch 21: Safe Use of Complementary Therapies
Betty L. Stadler, RN, MSN, CFNP, HNC
President, Health in Harmony
Family Nurse Practitioner
Brentwood, TN

Ch 22: Herbal Remedies
Linda A. Coulston, RN
Vitas Hospice
Blue Bell, PA
Sue H. Fisher-Mustalish, RN, HNC
Herbal Therapies Consultant
East Fallowfield, PA

Ch 23: Aromatherapy: Common Scents
Jane Buckle, PhD
RN Director, RJ Buckle Associates
Hunter, NY

**Ch 24: Effective Use of Homeopathic
Remedies**
Natalie Pavlovich, PhD RN, DiHt, CNHP
Duquesne University School of Nursing
Pittsburgh, PA

Ch 25: Medication Wisdom
Carol M. Patton, DrPH, RN, CRNP
Duquesne University School of Nursing
Pittsburgh, PA

Ch 26: Surviving Caregiving
Joyce V. Deane, MS, RN, CCM, CMC, CALA
NJ Department of Health & Senior Services
Toms River, NJ
Eve Karpinski, RNC, HNP, HNC
Holistic Nurse Practitioner

Resources:
Myra Darwish, RN, MSN, CS, HNC
St. Mary's Medical Center
West Palm Beach, FL

FOREWORD

Throughout history, the nursing profession has been one of the most dynamic of our social institutions. Nurses always have been in the midst of healthcare change, as they are currently. Today, members of the American Holistic Nurses' Association (AHNA) represent leaders in understanding and interpreting the important changes occurring in healthcare. But more importantly, holistic nurses also are vanguard of the quickening of the currents as consumers seek increased health information and insights about healthy living.

Invitation to Holistic Health offers the first book for the promotion of holistic health that has been entirely written by nurses. The intent of this book is to help educate and inform health care providers and those they serve about health care information and options; expand and shape new perceptions, attitudes, and behaviors about health and healing; and explore caring-healing interventions for a healthier, balanced life.

Holistic living is enhanced with the integration of daily self-care and complementary and alternative therapies. Living a healthy and balanced life requires that each person address his or her own body-mind-spirit needs and nurture the spiritual qualities of life.

How are consumers responding to these aspects of honoring the human spirit when faced with a major illness. Surveys of hospitalized patients found that 75 percent believed their physicians should be concerned with their spiritual welfare, and 50 percent desired that their physicians not just *pray* for them, but *with* them. Currently, three-fourths of family physicians believe spiritual issues are a major factor in their patients' health. Another survey found that 40 percent of working scientists in the United States believe in God. These findings suggest that the "spiritual" has never really disappeared from healing, and that the chasm between science and spirituality is not as wide as we have thought.

In the last century we believed that all the major illnesses and chronic conditions would yield to the progressive insights of science with more effective drugs and surgical procedures. The focus has been on the physical causes, such as with heart disease's recognized risk factors: smoking, cholesterol, diabetes, high blood pressure. But all of these factors are influenced by the way we choose to *be* which must be among the risk factors, as well.

Today, despite majestic accomplishments of modern medicine, there is a gnawing realization that something has been omitted—something vital, something that concerns not the physical function of our bodies but our very *being*. Something unforeseen and magnificent is happening. Healthcare, having in our time entered its dark night of the soul, shows signs of emerging, transformed.

Being is not a concept that has been valued in our society. *Being* may sound too esoteric to have a place in the health care system, but it is exceedingly practical and relevant. In fact, our decisions as to how we choose to *be* constitute life and death. Consider, for example, that more individuals have fatal heart attacks on Monday morning, 8 to 9 AM, than at any other time of the week (this has been labeled the Black Monday Syndrome) and that job dissatisfaction has been found to be a potent predictor of first heart attacks.

Invitation to Holistic Health assists you in how to choose to be in the world—your priorities, your choices, your relationships—which are life and death factors; and unless individuals consider the *being* aspects of their lives, they will *be* incomplete. We are rediscovering a central fact about healing that we have forgotten: health care, to be complete, must focus on more than *doing*; it also must address matters of *being*.

It is important to understand that holistic nurses honor science and traditional medical care and medications when needed, but they also value the importance of self-care and prevention of illness. Their mission is to teach and to co-participate with consumers to develop a system of living that honors both self-care and complementary therapies and medicine when needed. The pearls within this book must become embedded in the everyday. There is science to support these ideas for healthy living.

This book guides individuals in the art and science of holistic living and healing. Further, it provides guidance in evaluating therapies that capitalize dramatically on body-mind and complementary and alternative therapies. Increasingly, more research findings are revealing that these therapies not only work and are extremely safe, but they are cost-effective as well. Among these therapies are relaxation, imagery, biofeedback, hypnosis, touch therapies, expressive therapies (art, music, dance), and spiritual healing (prayer, meditation). At the present time these therapies should, in general, be considered complements to orthodox medical treatments and not a replacement for them. The AHNA advocates a "both/and" instead of an "either/or" approach in integrating these healing modalities with contemporary medical and surgical therapies.

Living a healthy and balanced life must address many aspects of healing. This book challenges readers to explore the following three questions:

- What do you know about living a healthy and balanced life?
- What do you know about the meaning of healing?
- What can you do each day to facilitate self-care and healing in yourself?

Healing is a lifelong journey into understanding the wholeness of human existence. It is not just about curing symptoms or getting through a crisis. Rather, it is the exquisite blending of caring, love, compassion, and creativity in our lives. Along this journey, our lives mesh with families, friends, and various communities where moments of new meaning and insight emerge in the midst of all aspects of daily life, such as relationships, work, health challenges, and crisis.

Healing occurs when we embrace what is feared most. It occurs when we seek harmony and balance. Healing is learning how to open what has been closed so that we can expand our inner potentials. It is accessing what we have forgotten about connections, unity, and interdependence. With a new awareness of these interrelationships, healing becomes possible, and the experience of living a healthy, balanced life can become a daily reality.

Invitation to Holistic Health can help you explore new meanings of healing in your work and life. The many diverse nuggets of wisdom that have been interwoven in this book can create a more vivid, dynamic, and diverse understanding about the nature of holism, healing, and its implications for living healthy and inspired lives. It challenges you to explore the inward journey toward self-transformation and to learn and identify steps to begin the growing capacity for change and healing. Best wishes to you in your healing work and life.

Barbara M. Dossey , RN, PhD, HNC, FAAN

PART I

Strengthening Your Inner Resources

CHAPTER I

ASSESSING YOUR HEALTH HABITS

Objectives

This chapter should enable you to:

- List at least six features of an ideal health profile
- Describe at least four questions that need to be considered in evaluating nutritional status
- Identify at least eight major areas to consider when taking stock of stress patterns
- Describe four areas involved in acquiring relaxation skills

Self-care is a term used to describe the active role a person takes in maintaining or improving his or her health. It is an aspect of health that is often overlooked when health care is discussed. Even in the arena of preventive medicine, which comes the closest to the idea of self-care in modern medicine, the emphasis is more on the early detection of disease than the active promotion of health. Although there is a focus on health screening, there is less attention given to educating people about healthy living habits, such as exercise, stress management, and nutrition.

You will find that making minor adjustments in your health practices to prevent diseases is easier than caring for diseases after they've developed. Prevention starts with taking stock of your health habits and comparing them to those consistent with optimum health. By confronting the behaviors in yourself that lead to ill health, you can identify unhealthy practices and sources of imbalance, and begin taking steps to change.

KEY POINT

In the United States we have come to accept the World Health Organization (WHO) definition of *health* as a state of physical and mental well being, and not just the absence of disease. However, in Traditional Chinese Medicine (TCM), health is seen as the sufficient amount of energy circulating freely in the organism. TCM believes that the human being is comprised of and surrounded by an energy system or field. This energy system is understood to resemble an electromagnetic field, expressed on the minute level as the behavior of electrons and neurons and on the gross level as the experience of vitality. The energy system is made up of energy pathways, often referred to as *meridians*. The pathways are believed to carry energy and information throughout the human organism, to unite body, mind, and spirit.

Self-Assessment

An overall evaluation of health begins with a review of the current health status and health practices. An ideal health profile is one in which an individual:

- Consumes an appropriate amount of quality food
- Exercises regularly
- Maintains weight within an ideal range
- Has good stress coping mechanisms
- Balances work and play
- Looks forward to activities with energy and enthusiasm
- Falls asleep easily and sleeps well
- Eliminates waste with ease
- Enjoys a satisfying sex life
- Feels a sense of purpose
- Is free from pain and other symptoms

When the ideal is not being met, there needs to be an exploration into the reasons so that strategies to improve health habits can be identified and implemented.

Physical Self-Assessment

Nutrition

In order to assess how your nutritional habits impact health, a person's eating habits need to be evaluated for a certain period of time. Factors to consider include not just the type of foods consumed, but also:

- The time of day that the food is consumed, for example, eating late at night
- What is being done when the person eats, such as watching TV or having a heated discussion
- The amount of food consumed at meal time and the amount eaten between meals
- The amount of food eaten compared to the person's unique nutritional needs

When Food Is Consumed Late night eating puts extra stress on the digestive system. According to TCM, at night the *Yin* (which is associated with rest, darkness, and stillness) predominates, and consequently, the digestive system slows down. The circulation slows down as well, conserving the amount of blood circulating to all the digestive organs. Clearly, nighttime—when the body is supposed to be resting and preparing for restoring and repairing tissues—is not a good time to offer the body the challenge of digesting a big meal. Viewed from within the context of TCM, this behavior can lead to a condition called Stomach Yin Deficiency, which is a condition where the fluids of the stomach diminish, causing a sensation of heat in the stomach, manifesting as heartburn and indigestion. When this condition is allowed to persist, more serious stomach problems, such as a hiatal hernia, ulcer, or even cancer may develop.

KEY POINT

Late night eating stresses the digestive system.

What One Does While Eating When there is emotional tension while eating there is less energy available for digestion. This emphasizes the importance of relaxing during mealtime so there will be sufficient resources for digestion. When stressed by heated conversations or upsetting news on the television, a person's energy is drawn away from the digestive system, causing indigestion. For optimum digestion adequate supplies of enzymes, co-enzymes, and hormones are needed, and in order for these substances to be available, adequate amounts of blood must be circulating. Free flowing energy or *Qi* promotes blood flow.

KEY POINT

In Traditional Chinese Medicine, *Qi* is considered the vital life force or energy that circulates throughout the body.

The Amount That Is Consumed   When too much food is consumed during a meal the stomach gets stressed. This kind of behavior not only leads to indigestion, but also creates an energy deficit as energy is pulled from other areas to meet the demands of digestion. Between meal nibbling creates the same kind of energy deficit as energy is constantly required by the digestive organs to digest and not enough energy is available for other activities. Each time food is being consumed, blood is routed to the digestive organs and less is available for other physiological activities, creating an imbalance in the body. In addition, the many muscle layers of the stomach need to rest for a certain amount of time.

Reflection   Consider what, when, and how you eat. Is your pattern conducive to having optimal energy available for other activities?

Identifying Patterns   Daily food journals that record food consumed, when it is consumed, and how one feels during food consumption can be beneficial in identifying patterns. Everything that enters the mouth, be it a piece of candy or a few sips of juice should be recorded. Keeping this type of food diary increases self-awareness, which in turn can become the catalyst for positive changes in nutritional habits. After keeping a food journal for a couple of weeks, sufficient data will be available to determine the pattern and content of nutritional habits. Are meals being eaten on a regular basis? How much snacking is taking place? Are the foods chosen basically nutritious? Is one kind of food eaten in excess? Are some nutrients missing from the diet?

What kinds of beverages are consumed? Is caffeine consumed from coffee and carbonated beverages, and if so, how much? Carbonated beverages are high in sugar or artificial sweetener, neither of which have any nutritional value. Caffeine is addictive, a mild stimulant to the central nervous system, and a diuretic (fluid loss through urine). There have been mixed scientific reports as to the role caffeine plays in health and wellness. Because caffeine affects many body systems and can interfere with certain drugs it is best taken in moderation—no more than one or two cups of caffeinated beverages per day.

What is the alcohol intake on an average day? Alcohol supplies no nutrients, but it does supply calories. High levels of alcohol intake increase the risk of stroke, heart disease, certain cancers, high blood pressure, birth defects, and accidents. Women should drink no more than one alcoholic beverage per day, and men should drink no more than two alcoholic beverages per day.

A deeper examination of nutritional patterns and habits can be done by examining a person's childhood relationship with food. What were his or her habits and patterns of nutrition and diet during childhood? Does the individual continue to carry these patterns and habits? How does the childhood experience with food and eating affect current nutritional choices and lifestyle?

Reflection Do you believe if you make sensible nutrition choices that you will live a healthier, more energetic life and reduce your risk of disease? Or, do you think that you can deviate from sound nutritional habits without consequences? What has influenced your beliefs? If your beliefs do not support good nutritional habits what can you do to change them?

It could be that small actions are all that are needed to realize significant change. This can be explored by evaluating daily lifestyle. The way lifestyle impacts eating habits, food preferences, and food choices can be determined in a few short minutes by answering some basic questions. The answers will help in determining if there are nutritional imbalances (excesses or deficiencies). Decisions can then be made as to which foods need to be added and/or removed from the daily diet to improve nutrition.

The Nutritional Lifestyle Survey (Table 1–1) is a short questionnaire designed to help a person evaluate these areas. The individual should set aside 10 to 15 minutes of quiet time to complete this assessment. Writing the answers is important so that there will be a baseline to use for comparison after changes have been made.

Maintaining weight within an ideal range is important to general health. Obesity has been on the rise for the last two decades, and approximately 35 percent of women and 31 percent of men aged 20 and older are obese. Obesity increases the risk of hypertension; heart disease; diabetes; arthritis; and uterine, breast, colon, and gall bladder cancers. People should be taught to use a weight chart to learn where their weight is in respect to their height (Figure 1–1). The higher the weight for a specific height the greater the risk of health problems. Obese individuals need to be encouraged and assisted in implementing a reduction program; at minimum, they should commit to not gain any additional weight. Being underweight for height or having a recent unexplained weight loss may be a sign of other health problems, and warrants further diagnostic evaluation.

The next step is to begin the process of eliminating or replacing foods that lead to ill health. Foods that are laden with artificial colorings, sweeteners, and preservatives should be cut in half for the first few weeks and eventually reduced to virtually none. Other foods that lead to ill health when consumed in excess are foods high in fat, refined sugar, salt, and dairy products.

TABLE 1–1   NUTRITIONAL LIFESTYLE SURVEY

- What is your general health?
- What is your height and weight? Do they fall within normal limits?
- What health conditions do you presently have?
- Do you have any problems with your blood sugar?
- Do you have elevated cholesterol or triglyceride levels?
- Do you have high blood pressure?
- Are you aware of any food intolerances or allergies?
- What is your pattern of eating? How many meals do you eat per day?
- Do you snack regularly throughout the day or evening? During the night?
- How many snacks do you have per day? What do they consist of?
- What is your energy pattern? Do you have any slumps during the day?
- How much caffeine in coffee, tea, carbonated drinks do you drink per day?
- What is your alcohol intake?
- What is your coping style when under stress? Do you use food to calm or excite you? Do you choose comfort foods to make you feel better if you are down, or to calm you when you are anxious?
- When you are making food choices do you pick healing foods?

Developed by Ann McKay

KEY POINT

Paying attention to your diet and nutritional habits does not mean that you need to become obsessed with your eating to the point that you become stressed when you have an occasional slip from good eating. This type of stress may also create an emotional imbalance, which has a negative effect on your general health.

Fat Eating high-fat foods such as ice cream, sour cream, cream cheese, hard cheese, heavy butter sauces, red meat, pork, duck, oil, and whole milk is a contributing factor in conditions such as atherosclerosis, heart disease, and cancer. Besides the studies that have been done from within a reductionistic framework (ones where answers are sought by breaking substances down into their smallest particles), there is also an understanding in energy medicine, such as TCM, that fatty foods create heat in the

Figure 1–1: Weight Gauge Guide

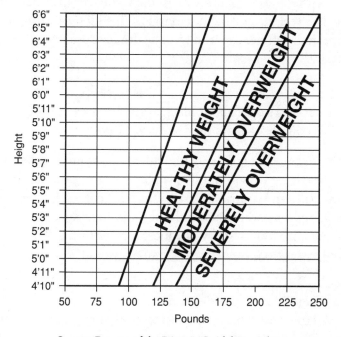

Source: Report of the Dietary Guidelines Advisory Committee on the Dietary Guidelines for Americans, 1995, pages 23–24. In FDA Consumer Publication No. 98-127.

system, which exceeds our needs given our ecological situation. Eskimos eat large amounts of fat because their bodies need to produce high amounts of heat. When average Americans eat the same amount of fat as Eskimos they most likely will develop severe cholesterol problems. Further, too much heat in the system creates an imbalance between hot and cold, or *Yin* and *Yang,* according to TCM. When this balance is thrown off, problems in the bio-energy system begin to manifest.

Sugars Like saturated fats, refined sugars cause imbalances in your system when eaten in excess. Refined sugars are the simple sugars such as white, raw, brown, or turbinado sugar, as well as honey, corn syrup, corn sweeteners, dextrose, and fructose. Although a sweet flavor has a strengthening effect on the digestive system, according to TCM, it must come from complex carbohydrates, such as grains, fruits, and beans. Unlike the refined carbohydrates, these foods provide a more lasting energy, facilitating a more balanced physical, emotional, and intellectual experience every day. Foods filled with refined sugars create an excess in the system as they overstimulate the endocrine system in the production of enzymes and hormones to deal with the sudden onslaught of glucose into the cells. When cookies, cakes, candies, ice cream, and other foods laden with refined sugars are consumed, you feel an initial burst of energy, but shortly thereafter feel fatigued and lethargic. This kind of eating pattern, when continued for a period of time, can lead to ill health because it stresses the endocrine system unnecessarily.

KEY POINT

Fresh fruit, the use of malt barley, rice syrup, or blackstrap molasses are good to use as sweeteners because as complex sugars they stress your body less.

Dairy The next food group to consider is dairy. Although milk is touted as the complete food by the dairy industry, it is not without its problems. Dairy products negatively affect the mucous membranes and contribute to digestive difficulties. Humankind is the only species that drinks milk as adults and milk of a different species no less. According to TCM, excess consumption of dairy produces a condition called *dampness,* displayed as abdominal distention, edema, cysts, and allergies.

Energetic Quality of Food

A quality of food that is generally not considered during the assessment of nutritional needs is that of energy. However, when it is considered that the human organism is an aggregate of physical and chemical components that has been given form by an energy system, it can be understood that the living substance of food also has energetic properties. For example, the energetic quality of a hot red pepper is obviously different from that of a green cucumber, the former being hot and producing a diaphoretic effect (inducing perspiration) on the system, while the latter is wet and cool and producing a diuretic (need to urinate) effect. The more people note cravings of particular foods and the effects of foods on their bodies, the more they will become aware of the subtle qualities of foods and how these foods affect digestion and general level of energy. The ultimate aim is to eat only those foods that facilitate good health, which will vary at different times. For instance, in the winter when they are suffering cold symptoms it is useful for people to consume hot or warming foods, such as foods spiced with ginger and cayenne pepper, whereas in the middle of a hot, sticky summer the consumption of cold foods, such as lettuce, cucumbers, and fruits such as watermelon are preferred.

A Healthy Diet

Recognizing that each individual is unique, some general recommendations can be followed to promote health and well being. First, it is important to consider the times of day that food is eaten. It is generally not a good idea to skip breakfast, as it provides the foundation for the day. Eating a hot breakfast such as oatmeal or any other warm cereal or toast in the morning creates a warming and nourishing effect and supplies necessary energy to sustain daily activities. It is best to eat the heaviest meal in the middle of the day when the digestive energies are the strongest. Eating while in a rush or while conducting business is not a good idea; taking the time to eat in a relaxed manner without being engaged in any other activity is more healthful. In general, fresh organic foods (foods not treated with pesticides, hormones, and antibiotics) are preferred. A basic food guide is provided in Table 1–2. Natural vitamins and food supplements can provide additional benefits (see the chapter on Nutritional Supplements for more information about this).

Exercise

Reviewing the type and frequency of exercise is a significant component of the assessment of health habits. It is important to evaluate if the right kind of exercise for your

---

TABLE 1–2   BASIC DAILY FOOD PLAN

Breakfast
- Warm cereals, whole-grain muffin, or toast
- Fresh fruit
- Herbal tea or a grain beverage such as Postum, Cafix, or Bambu (one cup of coffee a day is fine.)

Lunch
- Fresh organic salads
- Homemade soup or a sandwich made with organic turkey, chicken, hard-boiled organic eggs, or nutbutter on whole-grain bread
- Fresh fruit

Dinner
- Protein, such as organic poultry, fish, beef (not more than once a month), or beans
- A complex carbohydrate, such as a vegetable, whole grains, peas, and beans
- Organic vegetables (meaning they are free of contaminants, synthetic pesticides and herbicides, hormones, preservatives, and artificial coloring)
- Fresh fruit

body is being done on a regular basis. The proper quantity and quality of exercise are essential for good health. Exercise needs to be part of the daily routine to offer maximum benefit. A good exercise program is one that is well rounded and contains components that will develop the body's musculature, improve and increase metabolic rate, and establish a balanced, uninterrupted flow of energy. A combination of aerobic exercise, weight training, and energy-based exercises, such as Hatha Yoga and T'ai Chi Kung are preferred. (For more information on exercise, see Chapter 4, Exercise: Mindfulness in Movement.)

KEY POINT

Lack of exercise results in weakness and atrophy of muscles, skeletal misalignment, reduced circulation of blood and energy, and poor metabolism.

Stress Patterns and Coping Mechanisms

Stress, a phenomenon associated with tension and a sense of urgency, is experienced by more and more people every day in response to an extremely complex social and economic world. Even children are not exempt from this experience as evidenced by the increasing numbers of children with Attention Deficit Disorder (ADD), Attention Deficit Hyperactive Disorder (ADHD), asthma, and other stress-related conditions.

To gain some insight into their stress level, people should be advised to take a few minutes to self-evaluate, using a tool such as that shown in Table 1–3. As these questions are answered, people should be encouraged to reflect on their answers to gain insight into their level of tension and its effect on overall health and well being. It is essential to understand the motivation behind behaviors in order to be able to change. For instance, does a person speak loudly because he or she feels angry and requires that people give their full attention, or because he or she is anxious and the tension in the chest and throat is such that it manifests as a loud and forceful voice? Once the behavior is recognized, its causes can be explored. The more information people have about their behavior and its underlying motivations, the more ammunition they have for change and attaining optimum health.

The person who becomes irritable while standing in a slow line or being stuck in traffic may be seeing only the negative aspects of waiting. Waiting provides a wonderful opportunity to practice relaxation techniques such as being present in the moment, which is a concept found in ancient Eastern teachings. To be present in the moment, one has to put aside worries and anxieties for the sake of the experience of a calmer state. The level of stress is directly proportional to the way one perceives the world.

TABLE 1–3   TAKING STOCK OF YOUR STRESS PATTERNS

- How do you talk? Do you tend to talk fast and/or loud?
- How do you make decisions? Do you make them in a slow and deliberate way, or quickly to get them done with?
- Do you let people finish what they are saying before you speak (especially people close to you, such as family and friends)?
- Do you consider sitting alone quietly to think or practice a relaxation or meditation exercise a waste of time?
- Do you feel that you have enough time to finish your work when expected?
- Do you tend to feel impatient when doing routine tasks, such as writing checks, filling out forms, or washing dishes?
- Do you skip meals to have more time to get things done?
- Do you feel satisfied with your current position and status at your job?
- Do you feel satisfied with your relationships?
- Do you become irritable when waiting in line or stuck in traffic?
- Do you enjoy a challenging competition?
- Do you react to most problems in an easy-going manner?

If it is perceived that there is not enough time a person will feel harried, whereas when there is the belief that there is ample time to accomplish a task, one is relaxed. Table 1–4 offers some pointers for acquiring relaxation skills.

Chapter Summary

Self-care refers to the active role individuals assume in maintaining and improving their health. In Western medicine, self-care primarily implies preventing illness and recognizing symptoms early; however, Traditional Chinese Medicine (TCM) views health in terms of sufficient free-flowing energy circulating freely within a person. An ideal health profile is one in which a person consumes an appropriate quality and quantity of food, exercises regularly, maintains weight within an ideal range, has good stress coping skills, balances work and play, looks forward to activities with energy and enthusiasm, falls asleep easily and sleeps well, eliminates waste with ease, enjoys a satisfying sex life, feels a sense of purpose, and is free of pain and other symptoms.

TABLE 1–4　LEARNING TO RELAX

In addition to becoming aware of attitudes that color your perceptions, you also can benefit by developing relaxation skills. There are four areas involved with acquiring relaxation skills:

1. Place and time of practice.　Relaxation exercises are best done in a quiet environment at the same time each day. This helps to make the exercise part of the daily routine.

2. Posture.　The idea is that your body becomes as relaxed as possible without falling asleep. When you sit, it is important that the head and neck are aligned with the rest of the spine to ensure the proper flow of energy.

3. Cultivation of the right attitude.　Having the proper attitude is very important. When you first make an intentional effort to relax you may feel anxious, and you need to conscientiously try to put aside your worries and anxiety while you practice the relaxation technique. It is understandable that an untrained mind will wander, but as you return your attention to the exercise you are engaged in, you will gain control over your mind more and more.

4. Directing attention.　The practice of relaxation is impossible without directing your attention. This means that as you make the effort to concentrate and return your wandering mind to the object of concentration, you are developing the ability to focus on any object or activity or idea without being sidetracked by passing thoughts or external events.

Reflection　In taking stock of your overall personal health habits, what specific actions can you take to improve your health?

Assessment entails more than identifying abnormalities. Factors impacting health state also must be explored, which include eating patterns, factors related to eating, and quality and quantity of food intake, type and frequency of exercise, decision-making, speech pattern, ability to relax, satisfaction with work and relationships, and reactions to circumstances. People need to understand underlying factors affecting their health state so that they can develop individualized plans that address their unique situations.

Suggested Readings

Callaghan, D. M. (2003). Health-promoting self-care behaviors, self-care self-efficacy, and self-care. *Nursing Science Quarterly, 16*(3):247–54.

Clark, C. C. (2003). *American Holistic Nurses' Association Guide to Common Chronic Conditions. Self-Care Options to Complement Your Doctor's Advice.* Hoboken, NJ: John Wiley and Sons.

Forkner-Dunn, J. (2003). Internet-based patient self-care: The next generation of health care delivery. *Journal of Medical Internet Research, 5*(2):e8.

Funnell, M. M. and Anderson, R.M. (2003). Patient empowerment: A look back, a look ahead. *Diabetes Education, 29*(3):454–8, 460, 462.

Hertz, J. E. and Anschutz, C. A. (2002). Relationships among perceived enactment of autonomy, self-care, and holistic health in community-dwelling older adults. *Journal of Holistic Nursing, 20*(2):166–185.

Maciocia, G. (1989). *The Foundations of Chinese Medicine.* New York: Churchill Livingstone.

Murray, R. B. and Zentner, J. P. (2000). *Health Promotion Strategies through the Lifespan.* 7th ed. New York: Prentice Hall.

Sohn, T. and Rockwell, R. C. (1996). *AMMA Therapy: A Complete Textbook of Oriental Bodywork and Medical Principles.* Rochester, VT: Healing Arts Press.

Sutherland, J. A. (2000). Getting to the point. *American Journal of Nursing, 100*(9):40–45.

Spero, D. (2002). *The Art of Getting Well: A Five Step Plan for Maximizing Health When You Have a Chronic Illness.* Alameda, CA: Hunter House.

CHAPTER 2

HEALTHFUL NUTRITION

Objectives

This chapter should enable you to:

- Define nutrition
- Discuss factors related to the emotional, psychological, cultural, and traditional aspects of food
- Outline a sample, one-month plan to change eating habits
- List the components of a food journal
- Describe a healthy style for meal intake
- Outline recommended dietary intake according to the Food Guide Pyramid
- Give at least two examples of equivalent servings from the bread, vegetable, fruit, dairy, meat, and fat groups
- Describe the information that can be found on Nutrition Facts labels
- Define macronutrients and micronutrients
- List at least six tips for good nutrition

Sensible nutrition is a primary factor in leading a life that will allow for ample energy, productivity, and overall health. The old common sense adage "you are what you eat" is now regarded as definitive, scientific-based knowledge. In fact, the last decade has seen an explosion of data, information, and scientific research in the areas of nutrition and nutritional supplementation. The results continue to demonstrate that the foods we eat determine health, well being, and longevity, and that some foods offer medicinal qualities; something our foremothers and forefathers knew hundreds, even thousands of years ago!

Consumers are increasingly aware of the importance of nutrition to their health. A survey by the American Dietetic Association found that 4 out of 10 Americans know nutrition to be a significant factor in health and are working to improve this area of their lives (1). Yet, many people believe eating nutritiously will mean sacrifices. This was reinforced by a national survey of nearly 3,000 adults, which found that consumers believed they would have to invest more time and money and forfeit good taste in order to eat healthfully (2). The overload of nutrition information from the media is leading many people to simply give up thinking about their nutrition and diet altogether. Moreover, food companies run 60-second commercials that promote 60-second meals. The focus keeps us eating certain foods for their taste, texture, and quick preparation time rather than their nutritive value. Americans have lowered their fat and salt intakes yet continue to have a considerable gap between recommended dietary patterns and what they actually eat. Our diets have improved since the 1980s yet they have essentially remained the same since 1996 (3).

KEY POINT

The idea that balanced nutrition is directly related to health, wellness, longevity, and the ability to heal the body is ageless. During the Stone Age plants were used for medicinal purposes; the Chinese have used food for prevention and cures for centuries. Hippocrates was at the forefront of holistic health and wellness by suggesting diet and nature be taken into account when treating illness. Florence Nightingale also believed that "selecting and preparing healing foods, in addition to fresh air, quiet, and 'punctuality and care in administration of diet'" were necessary to keep the body working properly and for healing in times of injury or illness (4). Samuel Hahnemann, the father of homeopathy, believed diet, including foods that were least/most medicinal, were integral to health and wellness (5). These great minds had an innate understanding that nutrition was directly related to health, wellness, and healing.

What is Nutrition?

Nutrition refers to the ingestion of foods and their relationship to human health. Sensible nutrition requires the intake of nutrients from good quality, wholesome foods that support and maintain health throughout the lifespan. The need for sensible nutrition is essential throughout life because all humans require the same basic nutrients no matter what their stage of life. What varies is the amount of nutrients needed at each growth stage. There are also special needs due to growth and development, pregnancy and lactation, age, and disease or injury.

Proper nutrition works primarily through food choices. In order for proper digestion, absorption, metabolism, and elimination to take place you must have high quality food that contains optimum nutrients.

KEY POINT

Nutrients are substances the body needs to provide you with energy, allow you to maintain your health, and repair and regenerate your tissues and cells.

Nutrients are not immediately available as you eat your food but must be broken down by the digestive process, taken by the blood and lymph to be utilized as needed, and finally their waste must be eliminated. The food you put on your plate must be worked into proper condition and shape for use by the body. In other words it must be digested. This begins the process; then it must be further assimilated, metabolized, and finally eliminated.

Eating slowly and with few distractions, masticating (chewing) the food thoroughly, and drinking (any beverage) minimally during meals, will allow the gastric juices to accomplish their proper function, and healthy digestion can occur. If food is swallowed nearly whole, not only will a longer time be required for its digestion and assimilation, but also it ferments in the stomach, not allowing the nutrients to be released to do their work.

KEY POINT

Imagine the body as a group of workmen who are building a house. Each substance (food) like pieces of wood must be cut to just the right size (chewing) and prepared for use (digestion). Next, these pieces (nutrients), after due preparation in the workshop, must be taken by the different groups of workmen (blood and lymph) to its appropriate locality in the house (muscles, organs, tissues, and cells), and there it is fitted into its proper place; this is assimilation.

Refuel, Reload, Rejuvenate

Energy is the most important reason to keep the body nutritionally sound. Each day you must refuel the body so that it can move and work. Your body is continually undergoing changes; worn-out tissues and cells are constantly being repaired and renewed. The elimination of digestive waste continually requires new supplies of energy, vitamins, minerals, and other nutrients that are derived from our food. Other reasons for proper diet and nutrition include: fighting infection, balancing hormones, assisting in better quality sleep, and keeping the body running smoothly in times of stress. Sensible and proper nutrition is important to fulfill these demands.

Paramount to the value of nutrition in your life are the emotional, psychological, spiritual, cultural, and traditional aspects of food. How food is presented, its smell, taste, the emotional climate as a meal is eaten—all have a connection to how food is digested. Many people use food to help ward off anxiety, tension, depression, or boredom. Certain negative feelings can cause a physiological (bodily) response, where the hypothalamus (the brain's appetite control center) sets up a chain reaction in the autonomic (self-controlling) nervous system. Additionally, the meaning food has for each individual, from early childhood experiences to the present, and how that impacts nutritional and digestive habits must also be considered.

Reflection   How do your food preferences and eating patterns relate to your childhood experiences?

All of the senses are stimulated when you eat through:

- The visual presentation of the food
- The surroundings in which the food is consumed
- The aroma or odor associated with the food
- The texture and taste of the food
- The conversation and environmental sounds that are present while the food is being consumed

The chemical reactions that take place in the body differ according to the combination of experiences. A delicious meal with friends, filled with beautiful sights and sounds, will elicit calmness and ease of the digestive process. Relaxing, enjoyable meals are a goal to work toward for health and wellness.

Consistency in your life, whether positive or negative, usually reigns. If food is consistently eaten quickly, poorly, and under stressful conditions, then the body, mind, and spirit will be quickly depleted, lack energy, and eventually become stressed, unhappy, uncomfortable, and diseased.

The gathering, preparing, eating, and sharing of food offers more than just nutritional value. Food and diet have social and cultural aspects. Traditions, family gatherings, and religious ceremonies that include food probably have been part of your life on a regular basis. These activities help you to carry on tradition, culture, and values. Food is considered an expression of your individuality, history, values, and beliefs. Nutrition then is much more than what food group is eaten on any particular day at any particular meal.

KEY POINT

From June Cleaver to Micky D's

As late as the 1950s many people were consuming food that was grown locally, bought fresh, and eaten in a mindful, respectful, and unstressed atmosphere. Today, you may find yourself eating in your car, on a bench at a sporting event, standing at the kitchen counter or refrigerator, or as you are walking from one meeting to the next. The demand for convenience in eating has skyrocketed to the point that nearly 40% of our food is consumed outside the home (6).

Small Changes Can Make Big Differences

The adage, "it's never too late" applies well to changing nutrition habits. Some small changes, in increments, can make a huge difference. The goal is to develop a pattern of healthier eating, using varied foods, in a relaxed manner. You can begin with 2–3 new actions that are easy to implement and repeat them over a week or so. The following week add another 2–3 new, small actions that will be added to the first week's changes. This helps make these small changes easy to adapt and a routine part of everyday eating. Make a one-month plan that incorporates the ideas shown in the following example.

A Nutritional Evaluation

Keeping a food journal for a week or two is a great help. It can be simple—carrying a small pocket-sized notebook and jotting down:

- What you eat
- The time
- Where you are
- Who you are with
- What feelings you were having related to the food

A food journal can be of great assistance in finding established patterns that are occurring in your nutritional lifestyle. (See Chapter 1 on Assessing Health Habits for more discussion of nutritional assessment.)

EXAMPLE OF A ONE-MONTH PLAN TO CHANGE YOUR EATING HABITS

Week 1. Cut down on portion size and begin paying attention to what you are eating.

Week 2. Eat less fat—switch to skim milk if you drink 1%; or to 1% if you drink 2%. Use reduced fat or nonfat salad dressings. Cut back on cheese using 1 oz. amounts on sandwiches, or use lower fat and fat-free cheeses (1 percent cottage cheese, nonfat hard cheese, or part-skim mozzarella).

Week 3. Add more vegetables in an array of colors, use the salad bar at your local supermarket if time is a factor. Eat one or two more fruits from a different color group than usual. Keep a small fruit bowl with small packs of applesauce, raisins, or other dried fruit on the kitchen counter, table, or on your desk in the office.

Week 4. Plan what small changes you will make for next month. If you followed all the steps for these four weeks then continue by using the Nutritional Lifestyle Survey (Chapter 1, Table 1–1). If you did not incorporate all the ideas for this month, then implement those you missed this week.

The Tune-Up

Good general health requires that you have balance in all areas of life— mind, body, spirit, family, and community. Physically it means that you eat healthful foods that provide energy and balance, without the problems of overeating, indigestion, or food intolerances. Psychologically and spiritually it means that you enjoy meals in peace, cherish and respect your food and those you share it with, and practice intention (belief and faith that all is right and as is should be) to a higher power. Family and community are areas where tradition and events usually occur around food and eating. Family get-togethers and social events are ways for us to feel connected to others. However, if you have established patterns of eating that are not beneficial to your general health at these times, some changes may be necessary. If your general health is not quite right, eating healthful foods will allow for a better flow in all areas.

A Nutritional Lifestyle for the Ages

The holistic approach to nutrition and diet considers self-care, healthful food selection, moderate intake, and balance. It suggests listening to one's own inner wisdom, being present (paying attention to what is happening at the present), following a healthful lifestyle, and a diet that includes foods that work in synergy (together) with other aspects of life.

Nutritional Intake

A varied, balanced diet from wholesome, quality foods will provide much of what is needed to live a healthy, productive, longer life. Varying colors, tastes, textures, and temperatures from good quality, organic food will yield best results.

Time should be taken at meals to enjoy food, masticate (chew) it, and allow the action of the digestive powers to be fully utilized. Relaxation, enjoyable company, tranquility of mind, and pleasant conversation while eating help to fulfill the psychological, social, and cultural needs associated with food intake. The spiritual aspects of eating can be addressed through rituals and family traditions that are incorporated into each day's meals.

Reflection Do you have rituals—such as prayer, candle-lighting, or sharing time—that you incorporate into your main meals with significant others in your life? If not, how could you incorporate at least one?

Regular Meals

Consistency of regular meals is important. The body must have intervals of rest from eating or its energies are soon exhausted, resulting in impaired function and dyspepsia (stomach upset), and other problems. Constant munching, whether on pastries and candy or apples and carrots, will lead to a digestive tract that is almost constantly at work, and poor and weak digestion will follow, causing nutritional imbalances. Six small meals, beginning with a good breakfast is best. Approach your meals with an attitude of self-caring that will allow the mind, body, and spirit a much needed respite from your regular schedule.

Eating Too Much or Too Late

People generally eat too much rather than too little. It is an excellent plan to rise from the table before the desire for food is quite satisfied. Your body's nutrition does not depend upon the *amount* eaten, but on the *quality* of food consumed (Exhibit 2–1). Eating too much is nearly as bad as swallowing food before it is properly chewed. The stomach is unable to digest food that is not masticated; it ferments and gives rise to unpleasant results. Those who dine late should eat two or three hours before retiring. Late evening meals usually lead to a poor night's rest, with organs such as the liver, for example, being unable to detoxify properly.

EXHIBIT 2–1 SMART SNACKING	
Instead of	*Try*
Potato chips or pretzels	Mini bagels or breadsticks
A candy bar	A piece of fruit or a glass of juice
Cookies	Graham crackers or raisins
Fried meats	Baked or grilled meats
Whole milk	Skim or 1% or 2% milk
Butter or syrup on pancakes	Fresh fruit
Ice cream	Frozen lowfat or light yogurt
French fries or home fries	Baked potato with herbs
Sour cream on baked potato	Nonfat yogurt and chives
Butter or cheese on vegetables	Lemon juice or herbs

The Food Guide Pyramid and Other Helpers

The Food Guide Pyramid (Figure 2–1), Nutrition Facts label (Figure 2–2), and Dietary Guidelines (Figure 2–3), are set forth by the Food and Nutrition Board of the National Academies of Science and serve as tools to put sensible nutrition and

Figure 2–1: Food Guide Pyramid

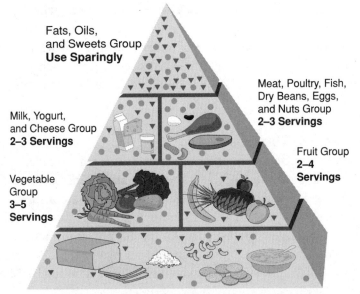

Fats, Oils, and Sweets Group **Use Sparingly**

Meat, Poultry, Fish, Dry Beans, Eggs, and Nuts Group **2–3 Servings**

Milk, Yogurt, and Cheese Group **2–3 Servings**

Fruit Group **2–4 Servings**

Vegetable Group **3–5 Servings**

Bread, Cereal, Rice, and Pasta Group **6–11 Servings**

Figure 2–2: Nutrition Facts Label

Nutrition Facts

Serving Size ½ cup (114g)
Servings Per Container 4

Amount Per Serving

Calories 90   Calories from Fat 30

	% Daily Value*
Total Fat 3g	**5%**
Saturated Fat 0g	**0%**
Cholesterol 0mg	**0%**
Sodium 300mg	**13%**
Total Carbohydrate 13g	**4%**
Dietary Fiber 3g	**12%**
Sugars 3g	
Protein 3g	

Vitamin A 80%	•	Vitamin C 60%
Calcium 4%	•	Iron 4%

* Percent Daily Values are based on a 2,000 calorie diet. Your daily values may be higher or lower depending on your calorie needs.

	Calories:	2,000	2,500
Total Fat	Less than	65g	80g
Sat Fat	Less than	20g	25g
Cholesterol	Less than	300mg	300mg
Sodium	Less than	2,400mg	2,400mg
Total Carbohydrate		300g	375g
Dietary Fiber		25g	30g

Calories per gram:
Fat 9 • Carbohydrate 4 • Protein 4

Source: U.S. Food and Drug Administration, FDA Backgrounder, May 1999.

diet choices into practice. These guidelines offer a way to eat less fat and consume a diet high in plant foods and low in animal foods. Becoming familiar with the Food Guide Pyramid, looking at the labels of the food you buy, and understanding the Dietary Guidelines is simple yet empowering. The key is to choose the foods from each group that will provide an individualized, tasty, nutrient balance and at the same time fit your lifestyle, food preferences, and cultural needs.

Figure 2–3: Dietary Guidelines

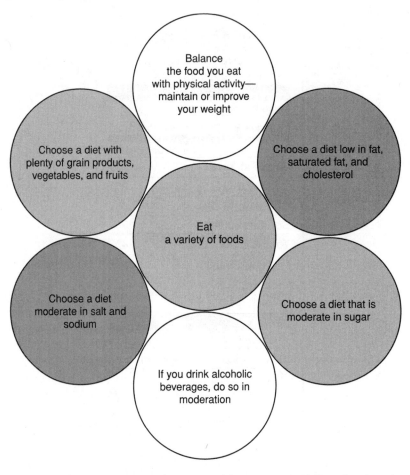

Balance
the food you eat
with physical activity—
maintain or improve
your weight

Choose a diet with
plenty of grain products,
vegetables, and fruits

Choose a diet low in fat,
saturated fat, and
cholesterol

Eat
a variety of foods

Choose a diet
moderate in salt and
sodium

Choose a diet that is
moderate in sugar

If you drink alcoholic
beverages, do so in
moderation

Adapted from Nutrition and Your Health: Dietary Guidelines for Americans. U.S. Department of Agriculture & U.S. Department of Health and Human Services, 1995. House and Garden Bulletin number 232.
Computer designed by KAM

The Food Guide Pyramid translates the RDAs (Recommended Dietary Allowances) and Dietary Guidelines for Americans into the kinds and number of servings of food to eat each day. The Food Guide Pyramid can be used to help you make food choices from the five food groups. It is an excellent way to begin looking at your eating and nutrition habits, and can be a starting point to making necessary changes in diet and eating for a healthier life. With the help of the pyramid you can meet your nutrient needs while selecting foods that satisfy your taste preferences. Balance, variety, and moderation are the key to these guidelines.

The shape of the pyramid illustrates the importance of balance and variety among the food groups. It is a visual presentation of the daily servings of food that should be selected with the amount of servings to be taken from each group.

Beginning at the base of the pyramid there is the *bread group*, which are the foods that form the foundation of the diet. This group includes bread, cereals, rice, and pasta. There should be 6–11 servings per day from this group, chosen from whole-grain products whenever possible.

ONE SERVING OF BREAD COUNTS AS

1 slice of bread

1/2 cup of rice or pasta

1/2 cup cooked cereal

1 ounce of ready-to-eat cereal

These should be in the form of complex carbohydrates from whole grains: wheat, oats, rye, bulgur, millet, or barley.

Whole-grain and enriched breads, rolls, potatoes, rice, corn, and pasta.

This group also includes bagels, pancakes, biscuits, and crackers, which are not as nutrient rich as the whole grains. The poorest selections in this group are muffins, granola, fried grains or dough, and pastries. The important point to remember is to choose foods from this group that are not refined or processed and have little or no added fats and sugars.

Next, are the *vegetables,* which should occupy second place in amount in our daily food choices, with a minimum of 3–5 servings per day. Fresh vegetables are best; frozen, steamed, or baked should be your second choice. A variety of colors should be chosen from this group from green leafy to orange, red, and yellow.

ONE SERVING OF VEGETABLES COUNTS AS

3/4 cup of vegetable juice

1 cup raw leafy vegetables

1/2 cup of other vegetables, cooked or chopped raw

Fruits make up the right half of the second tier of the Food Guide Pyramid. You should consume 2–4 servings per day of this group, with fresh fruit being the primary choice, then frozen or canned in water or juice. Color and preference again should vary in this group.

Grains, vegetables, and fruits comprise more than two-thirds of the pyramid, reflecting that they should make up the major portion of the daily diet.

ONE SERVING OF FRUIT COUNTS AS
One medium whole fresh fruit
1/4 cup dried fruit
1/2 cup chopped, cooked, or canned fruit
3/4 cup of fruit juice

Moving up the pyramid you'll find the *milk group* from which there should be 2–3 servings per day. Because caloric intake will depend on whether whole milk or low-fat products are used, it is best to use low fat unless you have high caloric needs.

ONE SERVING OF MILK COUNTS AS
1 cup of milk or yogurt
1-1/2 to 2 ounces of natural cheese
Process cheese is least desired

The *meat group* includes red meats, poultry, fish, eggs, dried beans, and nuts. A hamburger bun or a deck of cards is the size of an average meat serving. Meat that is broiled or baked with all excess fat trimmed and the skin removed is best.

ONE SERVING OF MEAT COUNTS AS
2–3 ounces of cooked lean meat, fish, or poultry
1/2 cup of cooked beans
one egg
1/3 cup of nuts
2 tablespoons of peanut butter is equal to 1 ounce or 1/3 serving of meat

Only two servings daily from the milk and meat groups are suggested because of the high level of fats and calories that these foods tend to have. They are important to the diet for B12, phosphorus, calcium, and other important nutrients, but are needed in lesser amounts than other foods.

Finally, *fats, oils, and sugars,* which are at the tip of the pyramid, should be used sparingly and on an occasional basis. This group provides few nutrients and is high in fat and simple sugar content. If you are trying to lose weight or wish to maintain your present weight, these foods should be limited.

Fats consumed in foods such as french fries or other fried foods count also, as do fats and oils used in cooking. Vegetable oils are preferable because they are low in saturated fat. A diet providing no more than 30% of total calories from fat is suggested: 10% from saturated fat, 10% from monounsaturated fats, and 10% from polyunsaturated fats. Because fat contains more than twice the calories of an equal serving of carbohydrates or protein, reducing fat intake will help you take in fewer calories.

FATS		
butter	margarine	cream
cream cheese	mayonnaise	oils
salad dressings	gravy	sauces

TYPICAL SUGARS		
table sugar (sucrose)	brown sugar	honey
molasses	raw sugar	syrup
corn sweetener	corn syrup	glucose
high-fructose corn syrup	fructose	lactose (milk sugar)

KEY POINT

One way to calculate calories from fat is to use this simple formula:

1. Take the number of calories eaten daily

2. Multiply by 30% (the suggested percentage of calories from fat)

3. Divide the answer by 9 (the amount of calories in one gram of fat)
   For example, if you eat 1,500 calories per day, the equation would look like this:

$$1,500 \times .30 = 450 \text{ then divide by } 9 = 50$$

50 grams of unsaturated fat would be your daily intake.

The taste of sugar is appealing. Sugars are used in many processed foods that you eat, such as bakery goods, cereals, and thickeners. Sugars are also used as natural preservatives. The sugar you consume should be naturally present in fruits, grains, some vegetables, and dairy.

Exhibit 2–2 describes nutritional strategies for the Food Guide Pyramid.

Nutrition Facts Label

The regulation of food dates back to the beginning of the last century. Under regulations from the Food and Drug Administration (FDA) of the Department of Health and Human Services (DHHS) and the Food Safety and Inspection Service (FSIS) of the U.S. Department of Agriculture (USDA), the food label was designed to give more information about nutrition. By law, nearly all food labels must contain a Nutrition Facts panel that contains information as to how the food can fit into an overall daily diet.

Nutrition Panel Format

The Nutrition Facts label (Figure 2–2), on the side or back of a package states the amount of saturated fat, cholesterol, fiber, and other nutrients each serving contains. By checking the serving size on several products you can compare the nutritional qualities of similar foods.

The % Daily Values on the panel is based on a 2,000-calorie diet and shows the percentage of a nutrient provided in one portion. The aim is to meet 100% of the Daily Value for total carbohydrate, fiber, vitamin, and minerals listed. The percent for fat,

---

EXHIBIT 2–2 NUTRITION STRATEGIES FOR THE FOOD GUIDE PYRAMID

- Consume different foods from each group to improve your chances of receiving all the nutrients that your body needs in the proper balance.

- As you head to the checkout at the supermarket, look over your choices. If there is a Food Guide Pyramid on one of the products use it to determine if you have a good representation of all the foods groups in your cart. Cereal, bread, rice, and pasta in good number; next a variety of types and colors of vegetables and fruit, enough for five servings per day per person; then some dairy (low fat), fish, poultry, or meat/meat alternatives; and finally a limited number of candy, cookies, cakes, pies, or other rich desserts, chips, or salty snacks.

- Use the Nutrition Facts label on food packages to guide you in meeting 100% of the RDA nutrients.

sodium (salt), and cholesterol can add up to less than 100. The amount of fat, cholesterol, sodium, carbohydrates, and protein (in grams or milligrams) are listed to the immediate right of these nutrients.

Nutrition at Different Life Stages

The Dietary Guidelines for Americans, the Food Guide Pyramid, and Nutrition Facts labels are meant to be used by the average adult who is healthy, active, and within the guidelines for height and weight. There are other factors that affect the amount and type of food needed daily.

Children from birth to five years require more vitamins, calcium, and other nutrients for growth and development. Dietary Guidelines generally are not meant to be used for children under two. In childhood these guidelines can be applied, using smaller portions for younger children and increasing portions as they get older. *Adolescents, pregnant adolescents, and pregnant and lactating women* need more breads, fruit, vegetables, milk, and meat due to higher nutrient needs.

Good nutrition for those *50 years of age and older* can decrease the effects of health problems that are prevalent among older Americans. It also can improve the quality of life for people who have chronic disease. Older people are likely to have poor appetites, experience health problems, be taking medications, and have sedentary lifestyles. They may also limit beneficial foods due to chewing, digestive, or intestinal health problems. This may lead to poor dietary intake and nutritional imbalances.

Diversity in Nutritional Lifestyles

Ethnic cuisine is becoming more and more popular in the U.S., with the Mediterranean Diet perhaps the best-known and used alternative diet. It includes bread and pasta, vegetables, legumes, fresh fruit, breads, and some unsaturated oils (olive), a few red meats and fish, and more eggs and poultry than the U.S. Food Guide Pyramid. Garlic is usually a staple, and the food is cooked fresh with the use of other herbs for flavor. Diet Pyramids have emerged for Asian, Latin American, and Vegan diets, representing what epidemiological (development of a particular issue within a certain population) studies have associated with optimum health (7).

Interest in vegetarianism is increasing and leading the way for Asian, specifically Japanese, Chinese, and Native American (hunter–gatherer) diets. The Japanese diet is one of the healthiest in the world, while other Asian cuisines offer low-fat diets with various selections from plant and some animal (fish) foods. Some studies have suggested that these diets lower risk factors for heart disease and some cancers (8).

Nutrients are elements of our food that make up macronutrients and micronutrients. Macronutrients are consumed in large amounts, tens and hundreds of grams (ounces and pounds). Micronutrients, minerals, and trace elements, are ingested in thousandths and millionths of a gram (milligrams and micrograms). Fiber and water, although not classified as nutrients, are essential to proper nutrition, digestion, assimilation, and elimination. Although each nutrient has its own job, all nutrients function together to help the body function at optimal levels. The combined action is far greater than if taken separately (synergy).

The Macronutrients

Macronutrients include *water, fiber, carbohydrates, protein, and fats*. These are essential for the body and mind to *work efficiently, function properly, and maintain and repair itself.*

Water

Water, not truly a macronutrient, is fundamental for life. It has a role in every major bodily function, and is the substance that allows chemical reactions to occur from the nutrients we ingest. This makes it essential to proper diet and nutrition. Water maintains the body's proper temperature, transports nutrients to and toxins from the cells, lubricates our joints, transports oxygen through the blood and lymphatic systems, and comprises from one-half to two-thirds of our body. Without water death is imminent within days. Your body requires between 9 and 12 cups of pure drinking water daily, in addition to water obtained through soups, fruits, and other foods. Caffeinated, carbonated, and alcoholic beverages are not counted as part of the fluid intake.

Tap water quality varies by locale in the United States. Various processes are used to purify water and remove major contaminants from water supplies. These processes are filtration, distillation, and reverse osmosis. The results of all water testing done by your local water supply board are part of the public record and you can request copies of recent monitoring reports as part of the Freedom of Information Act. If you have a private well you can have the water tested by a certified lab. (Refer to the Resources section at the end of this chapter for information about safe water sources.)

Fiber

Like water, fiber is not a true macrontrient although it is another important element in the nutrition equation. A diet containing a minimum of 20–30 grams of fiber per day is recommended. The typical American is said to eat only about 11 grams of fiber per day.

Vegetables, fruits, peas, beans, and whole grains contain fiber. Proper bowel elimination can be attained by eating fiber because it adds bulk and hastens the course of food and waste through the intestinal system. Fiber, in conjunction with a low (saturated) fat, low cholesterol diet has been found to reduce the risk for heart disease, digestive disorders, certain cancers, and diabetes. The sustained absence of fiber in the diet can lead to problems of the gastrointestinal tract including, diverticular disease and constipation.

KEY POINT

Following the suggestions of the USDA's Food Guide Pyramid, eating 2–4 servings of fruit (fresh, unpeeled) and 5 servings of vegetables (some raw and unpeeled) will allow for an average of 20–30 grams of fiber in the diet—the recommended daily intake.

Carbohydrates

Carbohydrates provide the body with energy and are made up of two classes—complex and simple carbohydrates. Foods that contain starches and fiber are called complex carbohydrates; sugars are simple carbohydrates. Fruits, vegetables, and grain products (breads, cereals, and pasta) are complex carbohydrates. Avoiding simple carbohydrates—foods containing added sugar such as candy, soft drinks, cookies, cakes, ice cream, and pies—will increase your energy and lower your risks for health problems. The body cannot differentiate between complex and simple carbohydrates, therefore, the body will metabolize candy, which has a high added sugar content (and is high in saturated fat), and a piece of fruit, which has natural sugar, the same way. The candy bar, however, contains few nutrients, and the excess sugar will be immediately stored as fat in the body. The fruit contains many required nutrients as well as fiber, and will be utilized for energy more quickly than the candy.

Carbohydrates are necessary for protein to be digested. They provide the blood with glucose, which is formed during the digestive process and is needed by the body and brain to give energy to muscles, tissues, and organs. When carbohydrates are present in the system the body is able to use protein for regeneration and repair.

Protein

Protein is the body's secondary energy source and has many functions. Protein must be present for the body to grow, repair damaged or injured tissue, create new tissue, and regulate water balance. It is the component that lays the foundation for major organs, blood and blood clotting, muscles, skin, hair, nails, hormones, enzymes, and antibodies. It maintains a proper balance of acid and alkaline in the blood.

> ### KEY POINT
>
> There are 22 amino acids, 8 of which are called essential "amino acids" and must be consumed in the diet because the body is unable to manufacture them.

The essential elements in protein are amino acids. Foods that consist of all the essential amino acids are considered complete proteins. These usually come from meat, fish, fowl, eggs, and dairy. Those that come from vegetable sources such as beans, grain, and peas are considered incomplete protein because they supply the body with only some of the essential amino acids.

Fats

Lipids (fats) are another source of energy for the body. The lipid group of macronutrients is vital for health, but is needed in small amounts. Fats supply essential fatty acids (EFAs), such as linoleic (Omega-6) and linolenic acid (Omega-3). They also help maintain healthy skin; regulate cholesterol metabolism; are precursors to prostaglandin (a hormone-like substance that regulates some body processes); carry fat-soluble vitamins A, D, E, and K, and aid in their absorption from the intestine; act as a cushion and stabilizer for our internal organs; and supply a protective layer that helps regulate body temperature and maintain heat. (The section on Diabetes in Chapter 3, has further discussion of EFAs.)

Fats supply greater energy than carbohydrates or protein. Fat has nine calories per gram, while carbohydrates and protein contain only four calories per gram. One molecule of fat can be broken down into three molecules of fatty acids and one molecule of glycerol. This structure is known chemically as triglycerides, which make up approximately 90% of all dietary fat.

Fatty acids are generally classified as saturated, monounsaturated, and polyunsaturated. In general, fats that contain a majority of saturated fatty acids are solid at room temperature. Fats containing mostly unsaturated fatty acids are usually liquid at room temperature and are called oils. *Saturated fatty acids* are found in meats, cream, whole milk, butter, cheese, coconut oil, palm kernel oil, and vegetable shortening. *Monounsaturated fatty acids* are found in olive and canola oils. *Polyunsaturated fatty acids* (PUFA) are found in other vegetable oils, nuts, and some fish. Both types of fatty acids, when used to replace saturated fats, reduce the level of cholesterol in blood (9).

Cholesterol is not fat, but rather a fat-like substance classified as a *lipid*. Cholesterol is vital to life and is found in all cell membranes. It is necessary for the production of bile acids and steroid hormones. Dietary cholesterol is found only in animal foods and is abundant in organ meats, egg yolks, meats, and poultry. Low-density lipoprotein (LDL), bad cholesterol, and high-density lipoprotein (HDL), good cholesterol, are the two types. LDLs are those that increase the risk of cardiovascular disease.

Because all fats contain different amounts of the three fatty acids, the ratio of polyunsaturated to saturated fats in what is eaten is important. The recommendation from the National Institutes of Health is that overall intake should be in the highest ratio of mono and polyunsaturated fats with no more than 30% of daily calories from fat sources in the diet and reducing saturated fat to less than 10% of calories.

KEY POINT

When buying foods that contain fat be sure to read the labels. Some foods say low cholesterol but are still high in fat.

The Micronutrients

Vitamins and minerals are the micronutrients (elements) in food that allow the body to function properly. They are needed in trace or small amounts, and occur naturally in food.

Vitamins and minerals work in synergy. This word comes from Greek *synergos,* meaning *work*. Synergism is the working together of all the nutrients that are in food, in the needed ratio, for the optimal functioning of the body/mind.

Vitamins and minerals should be taken in whole foods as much as possible because foods contain hundreds of compounds that assist the body to utilize these nutrients.

Vitamins

Vitamins do not have any calories and cannot be used as a food source, but are necessary for life. They are needed for the body to grow, develop, maintain its metabolic processes, and assist in digestion and assimilation. Vitamins are assisted in the body by enzymes. Table 2–1 lists signs of deficiency, functions, signs of toxicity, and food sources for each vitamin.

There are two types of vitamins: *water-soluble* and *fat-soluble*. Water-soluble vitamins are those that dissolve in water and are excreted through our skin (perspiration), lungs (breathing), intestines (bowel), and mainly through the kidneys (urine) if not needed or used by the body. They include the B complex group: B1 (thiamin), B2 (riboflavin), B3 (niacin), B6 (pyridoxine), folic acid (folacin, folate, or PGA), B12 (cobalamin or cyanocobalamin), biotin, pantothenic acid, and vitamin C. (See Table 2–1.)

Each vitamin has its own function. The *B complex* group's functions are many. They range from normal neurological (nervous) system functioning; synthesizing (linking) nonessential amino acids; helping oxidize (burn) glucose; assisting in the digestion of carbohydrates; promoting protein metabolism; and assisting in the production of various hormones, red blood cells, and genetic materials (such as RNA and DNA).

TABLE 2–1 VITAMINS

Vitamin	Lack of May Cause	How It Works	Excess May Cause	Best Foods to Eat
A	Night blindness; skin problems; dry, inflamed eyes	Bone & teeth growth; vision; keeps cells, skin; & tissues working properly	Birth defects; bone fragility, vision & liver problems	Eggs; dark green & deep orange fruits & vegetables; liver; whole milk
B1 Thiamin	Tiredness, weakness, loss of appetite, emotional upset, nerve damage to legs (late sign)	Helps release food nutrients and energy, appetite control, helps nervous system and digestive tract	Headache, rapid pulse, irritability, trembling, insomnia, interferes with B2, B6	Whole grains & enriched breads, cereals, dried beans, pork, most vegetables, nuts, peas
B2 Riboflavin	Cracks at corners of mouth, sensitivity to light, eye problems, inflamed mouth	Helps enzymes in releasing energy from cells, promotes growth, cell oxidation	No known toxic effects. Some antibiotics can interfere with B2 being absorbed	Whole grains; enriched bread & cereals; leafy, green vegetables; dairy; eggs; yogurt
Niacin	General fatigue, digestive disorders, irritability, loss of appetite, skin disorders	Fat, carbohydrate, & protein metabolism; good skin; tongue & digestive system; circulation	Flushing, stomach pain, nausea, eye damage, can lead to heart & liver damage	Whole wheat, poultry, milk, cheese, nuts, potatoes, tuna, eggs
B6 Pyridoxine	Dermatitis, weakness, convulsions in infants, insomnia, poor immune response, sore tongue, confusion, irritability	Necessary protein metabolism, nervous system functions, formation of red blood cells, immune system function	Reversible nerve injury, difficulty walking, numbness, impaired senses	Wheat & rice, bran, fish, lean meats, whole grains, sunflower seeds, corn, spinach, bananas
Biotin	Rarely seen since it can be made in body if not consumed. Flaky skin, loss of appetite, nausea	Cofactor with enzymes for metabolism of macronutrients, formation of fatty acids, helps other B vitamins be utilized	Symptoms similar to vitamin B1 overdose	Egg yolks, organ meats, vegetables, fish, nuts, seeds. Also made in intestine by normal bacteria there
Folic Acid	Anemia, diarrhea, digestive upset, bleeding gums	Red blood cell formation, healthy pregnancy, metabolism of proteins	Excessive intake can mask B12 deficiency and interfere with zinc absorption	Green, leafy vegetables; organ meats; dried beans
B12 Cobalamin	Elderly, vegetarians, or those with malabsorption disorder are at risk of deficiency-pernicious anemia, nerve damage	Necessary to form blood cells, proper nerve function, metabolism of carbohydrates and fats, builds genetic material	None known except those born with defect to absorb	Liver, salmon, fish, lean meats, milk, all animal products
Panto-thenic Acid	Not usually seen; vomiting, cramps, diarrhea, fatigue, tingling hands & feet, difficult coordination	Needed for many processes in body, converts nutrients into energy, formation of some fats, vitamin utilization, making hormones	Rare	Lean meats, whole grains, legumes
C Ascorbic Acid	Bleeding gums, slow healing, poor immune response, aching joints, nose bleeds, anemia	Helps heal wounds, collagen maintenance, resistance to infection, formation of brain chemicals	Diarrhea, kidney stones, blood problems, urinary problems	Most fruits, especially citrus fruits, melon, berries, & vegetables
D	Poor bone growth, rickets, osteoporosis, bone softening, muscle twitches	Calcium & phosphorus metabolism & absorption, bone & teeth formation	Headache, fragile bones, high blood pressure, increased cholesterol, calcium deposits	Egg yolks, organ meats, fortified milk, also made in skin when exposed to sun
E	Not usually seen, after prolonged impairment of fat absorption, neurological abnormalities	Maintains cell membranes, assists as antioxidant, red blood cell formation		Vegetable oils & margarine, wheat germ, nuts, dark green vegetables, whole grains
K	Tendency to hemorrhage, liver damage	Needed for prothrombin, blood clotting, works with vitamin D in bone growth	Jaundice (yellow skin) with synthetic form-flushing & sweating	Green vegetables, oats, rye, dairy, made in intestinal tract

Vitamin C (ascorbic acid) has its best-known source in citrus fruits, but can also be found in most *fresh* fruits and vegetables, especially, tomatoes, broccoli, and potatoes. It is essential for the formation of collagen, the protein that helps form skin, bone, and ligaments. It is also needed for iron to be absorbed, to prevent hemorrhaging, for wounds to heal, and to help with allergic reactions.

Fat-soluble vitamins attach to protein and are carried throughout the body by the blood. Unlike water-soluble vitamins, fat-soluble vitamins can be stored in the liver and adipose (fatty) tissues of the body if taken in excess. Fat-soluble vitamins include vitamins A, D, E, and K.

KEY POINT

The opportunity for toxicity is greater with fat-soluble vitamins because they are stored in the body.

Small amounts of vitamin D and K can be made by the body. The sources for these vitamins are green/deep yellow/orange vegetables, deep yellow/orange fruits, whole grains, low-fat dairy, vegetable oil, seeds, nuts, eggs, and liver. Their functions include preventing night blindness; helping vision; promoting healthy skin, hair, teeth, and nails; boosting the immune system; assisting the absorption of calcium; maintaining mucous membranes; and blood clotting.

Minerals

Minerals (Table 2–2) are further broken down into groups: *macrominerals,* those required in milligrams (larger amounts) by the body; *trace minerals,* required in micrograms (smaller amounts) by the body; and *other trace minerals or elements.* The body is unable to synthesize minerals so they must be taken in through diet on a regular basis.

The macrominerals are calcium, magnesium, phosphorus, sodium, and potassium. The trace minerals include iron, iodine, manganese, chromium, selenium, copper, fluoride, molybdenum, boron, and zinc. It is important to note that these are only needed in the body in minute amounts, but if a deficiency or imbalance exists it can lead to serious health problems and, if left unchecked, sometimes even death.

Calcium and phosphorus are the two most abundant minerals, and work together in the body. *Calcium* is found predominately in the bones where it is needed for structure. The bones store calcium for its release into the blood as needed. It assists in blood clotting, transmitting of nerve conduction, and helping with muscle contractions.

Phosphorus is found in nearly all cells of the body. It is used for energy production, metabolizing some vitamins and minerals, and building and renewing tissue and cells. The best source of phosphorus is animal protein, although milk and legumes also contain this mineral. Deficiencies of phosphorus are not usually seen because of its abundance in foods used by most Americans.

TABLE 2–2 MINERALS

Minerals	Lack of May Cause	How It Works	Excess May Cause	Best Foods to Eat
Calcium	Rickets, soft bones, osteoporosis, cramps, numbness & tingling arms & legs	Strong bones, teeth, muscle & nerve function, blood clotting	Confusion, lethargy, blocks iron absorption, deposits in body	Dairy, salmon and small bony fish, tofu
Phosphorus	Weakness & bone pain, otherwise rare	Works with calcium, helps with nerve, muscle, & heart function	Proper balance needed with calcium	Meat, poultry, fish, eggs, dairy, dried beans, whole grains
Magnesium	Muscle weakness, twitching, cardiac problems, tremors, confusion, formation of blood clots	Needed for other minerals & enzymes to work, helps bone growth, muscle contraction	Proper balance needed with calcium, phosphorus, & vitamin D	Nuts, soybeans, dried beans, green vegetables
Potassium	Lethargy, weakness, abnormal heart rhythm, nervous disorders	Fluid balance, controls heart, muscle, nerve, & digestive function	Vomiting, muscle weakness	Vegetables, fruits, dried beans, milk
Iron	Anemia, weakness, fatigue, pallor, poor immune response	Forms of hemoglobin & myoglobin—supplies oxygen to cells muscles	Increased need for antioxidants, heart disorders	Red meats, fish, poultry, dried beans, eggs, leafy vegetables
Iodine	Goiter, weight gain, increased risk of breast cancer	Helps metabolize fat, thyroid function	Thyroid-decreased activity, enlargement	Seafood, iodized salt, kelp, lima beans
Zinc	Poor growth, poor wound healing, loss of taste, poor sexual development	Works with many enzymes for metabolism & digestion, immune support, wound healing, reproductive development	Digestive problems, fever, dizziness, anemia, kidney problems	Lean meats, fish, poultry, yogurt
Manganese	Nerve damage, dizziness, hearing problems	Enzyme cofactor for metabolism, control blood sugar, nervous & immune system functions	High doses affect iron absorption	Nuts, whole grains, avocados
Copper	Rare, but can cause anemia and growth problems in children	Enzyme activation, skin pigment, needed to form nerve & muscle fibers, red blood cells	Liver problems, diarrhea (most excess due to taking supplements, not dietary intake alone)	Nuts, organ meats, seafood
Chromium	Impaired glucose tolerance in low blood sugar and diabetes	Glucose metabolism	Most Americans have low intakes	Brewer's yeast, whole grains, peanuts, clams
Selenium	Heart muscle abnormalities, infections, digestive disturbances	Antioxidant with vitamin E, protects against cancer, helps maintain healthy heart	Nail, hair, & digestive problems, fatigue, garlic odor of breath	Meat & grains, dependent on soil in which they were raised
Molybdenium	Unknown	Element of enzymes needed for metabolism, helps body store iron	Gout, joint pains, copper deficiency	Beans, grains, peas, dark green vegetables

Magnesium is stored in bone where it can be utilized by the body as needed. It is important for calcium, potassium, and vitamin D assimilation, and is necessary for the relaxation phase of muscle contraction. Magnesium also assists in the proper functioning of the heart, liver, and other soft tissue.

Potassium, sodium, and chloride are the three minerals that are sometimes called electrolytes. *Potassium* is essential for life and necessary for heart, nerve, muscle, and digestive functioning. *Sodium* is necessary for the balance of fluid outside the cells and is important in maintaining nerve and muscle conduction. Because sodium is abundant in food, there rarely is a chance of deficiency. *Chloride* mainly occurs with salt in foods, and is needed by the body with sodium for fluid balance of the cells and also to digest proteins. Sodium and chloride are found together in common table salt.

The microminerals (trace elements) include iron, iodine, zinc, copper, manganese, molybdenum, selenium, fluoride, chromium, and silicon. *Iron* is a most essential mineral because it is needed to carry oxygen from the lungs to all the cells. Vitamin C helps with iron absorption from food, while calcium and phosphorus have been found to inhibit it. When there is too much iron in the body it can cause liver and oxidative damage and lead to iron toxicity. Low iron levels can cause iron-deficiency anemia.

Iodine is needed in miniscule amounts in the body to maintain the thyroid gland. Deficiency is rare, but if it occurs it leads to goiter (enlargement of the thyroid gland). Seafood and salt are high in iodine.

Every organ in the body utilizes *zinc*. Zinc has an effect on immune function, healing wounds, digestion, and converting vitamin A to a usable form. A zinc deficiency can lead to many problems, such as poor immune function, digestive problems, and poor growth and development. Although rare zinc toxicity can interfere with iron absorption and alter cholesterol metabolism (10).

Selenium has been found to work together with vitamin E as an antioxidant (see Dietary Supplement chapter). Because it is found in the soil, deficiencies are rare because any plant that has been grown in selenium-rich soil provides selenium. Toxicity may occur when too much selenium is added to the diet through supplementation.

Chromium has recently been linked to insulin in controlling blood glucose levels. The American diet often is deficient in chromium (11); the reasons include diets high in sugar, refined foods, and diminished soil and water supplies. Deficiencies in this vital mineral can lead to severe health problems.

The idea that what you eat will impact your health and longevity has been gaining momentum for decades. Scientific research seems to have finally caught up with it. The best nutritional strategy for reducing the risk of chronic disease and living a healthy productive life is to follow a basic, sensible nutritional plan, as outlined in Exhibit 2–3.

Some basic tips for good nutrition are also listed in Exhibit 2–3. Even with good intake, however, there are many factors suggesting that diet alone cannot meet the total nutritional needs for some individuals. The next chapter offers information on vitamin and mineral supplementation.

Exhibit 2–3 Ten Tips for Good Nutrition

1. Use the Food Guide Pyramid as a guideline for what to eat every day.
2. Read the labels on everything you consume.
3. Choose plenty of whole-grain products (bread, pasta, and cereals).
4. Eat at least five fruits and vegetables per day.
5. Choose foods low in fat, added sugars, and salt.
6. Enjoy meals (this helps them digest better).
7. Have dinner in a quiet atmosphere (eating mostly complex carbohydrates will help ease you into the evening and promote better sleep).
8. If you take dietary supplements, take them with meals.
9. Keep coffee, tea, alcohol, and carbonated beverages to a minimum.
10. Drink at least eight glasses of water per day.

Chapter Summary

Nutrition refers to the ingestion of foods and their relationship to human health. All humans require the same basic nutrients although the amount and type can vary based on age, diseases, and special needs.

Changes to nutritional habits can begin with just a few new actions that are achievable. A food journal can be a useful tool for assessing nutritional status and could include what is eaten, time consumed, with whom, and feelings associated with food consumption.

Six small meals, beginning with a good breakfast, provide a regularity of intake that helps maintain good energy. The Food Guide Pyramid, which promotes a diet high in plant foods and low in animal foods and fat, is a guide for the types of foods to include in the diet. When planning dietary intake, consideration should be given to the macronutrients, which include water, carbohydrates, protein and fat, and the micronutrients, which consist of vitamins and minerals.

References

1. The American Dietetic Association Nutrition Trends Survey, 1997.
2. Glanz, K. (1998). Why Americans Eat What They Do: Taste, Nutrition, Cost, Convenience, and Weight Control Concerns as Influences on Food Consumption. *Journal of the American Dietetic Association, 98*(10):1118–1126.

3. The American Dietetic Association 1997 Nutrition Trends Survey, Executive Summary.

4. Light, K. (1997). Florence Nightingale and Holistic Philosophy. *Journal of Holistic Nursing 15*(1):25–38.

5. Hahnemann, S. (1982). Organon of Medicine. In Kunzli, J., Alain, N., Pendleton, P.: *The First Integral English Translation of the Definitive Sixth Edition of the Original Work on Homoeopathic Medicine.* Blaine, Washington: Cooper Publishing, p. 110.

6. Food Marketing Institute. (1997). Trends in the United States: Consumer Attitudes and the Supermarket.

7. McMahon, K. E. and Cameron, M. A. (1998). Nutrition/Behavior/Performance Consumers and Key Nutrition Trends for 1998. *Nutrition Today, 33*(1):20.

8. Escobar, A. (1997). *Nutrition Insights: Are All Food Pyramids Created Equal?* Washington, DC: USDA Center for Nutritional Policy and Promotion.

9. Minsink, R. P. and Katan, M. B. (1990). Effect of Dietary Trans-Fatty Acids on High-Density and Low-Density Lipoprotein Cholesterol Levels in Healthy Subjects. *New England Journal of Medicine*, 323:439–445.

10. Whittaker, P. (1998). Iron on Zinc Absorption—Iron and Zinc Interactions in Humans. *American Journal of Clinical Nutrition*, 68S:442–446S.

11. McBride, J. (1991). Chromium Supplementation Helps Keep Blood Glucose Levels in Check. *Journal of the American Dietetic Association*, 91:178.

Suggested Readings

Atkins, R. C. (2003). *Atkins for Life: The Complete Controlled Carb Program for Weight Loss and Good Health.* New York: St. Martin's Press.

Balch, P. A. and Balch, J. F. (2000). *Prescription for Nutritional Healing*, 3rd ed. New York: Avery Press.

Mahan, K. and Escott-Stump, S. (2000). *Krause's Food, Nutrition, and Diet Therapy*, 10th ed. Philadelphia: W.B. Saunders.

Willett, W. C. (2001). *Eat, Drink, and Be Healthy: The Harvard Medical School Guide to Healthy Eating.* New York: Fireside, Simon and Schuster.

U.S. Department of Agriculture and U.S. Department of Health and Human Services. (2000). *Nutrition and Your Health: Dietary Guidelines for Americans*, 5th ed. [Brochure]. Washington, DC: U.S. Government Printing Office.

Resources

American Diabetes Association
505 8th Ave.
New York, NY 10018
212-947-9707
www.diabetes.org
Offers education, information, and referrals regarding diabetes.

The American Dietetic Association (ADA)
216 West Jackson Blvd.
Chicago, IL 60606-6995
800-366-1655
Chicago Area
312-899-0040 x4653
www.eatright.org/ncnd.html
Provides information about a variety of nutrition resources and programs; includes "tip of the day," as well as numerous areas for reading.

American Heart Association
7320 Greenville Ave.
Dallas, TX 75231
214-750-5300
www.americanheart.org
Excellent site with areas called "Healthy Tools" and "Healthy Lifestyle" particularly geared to nutrition.

American Institute for Cancer Research (AICR)
1759 R Street, NW
Washington, DC 20009
800-843-8114
Washington, DC Metropolitan area
202-328-7744
www.aicr.org
Gives a variety of nutrition information relating to cancer.

Anorexia Nervosa and Related Eating Disorders
P.O. Box 5102

Eugene, OR 97405
503-344-1144
http://www.anred.com
Offers referrals and information on treatment of eating disorders.

Center for Science in the Public Interest (CSPI)
1875 Connecticut Ave., NW, Suite 300
Washington, DC 20009-5728
202-332-9110
www.cspinet.org/
The *Nutrition Action Healthletter* is an excellent source of nutrition information
for just $15.00 per year. Offers quizzes on nutrition and health.

Food & Drug Administration
Center for Food Safety & Applied Nutrition
1500 Paint Branch Parkway
College Park, MD 20740-3835
http://vm.cfsan.fda.gov
FDA's Web site of the Center for Food Safety & Applied Nutrition. Provides information on food, foodborne illness, food labeling, food safety, special interest areas,
and FDA documents; links to FDA home and other government sites.

Food and Nutrition Information Center
National Agricultural Library, Agricultural Research Service, USDA
10301 Baltimore Ave. Room 304
Beltsville, MD 20705-2351
www.nal.usda.gov/fnic
This resource offers a way to search any food-related topic on their Web site.
Various information on nutrition with links to other sites; updated daily.

International Food Information Council
Publications Department IFIC Foundation
1100 Connecticut Ave., NW, Suite 430
Washington, DC 20036
www.wheatfoods.org
Devoted to help increase awareness of dietary grains as an essential component to a
healthy diet.

Iowa State University, University Extension
Food Science and Human Nutrition Extension
1127 Human Nutritional Sciences Bldg.
Iowa State University
Ames, IA 50011-1120
http://www.extension.iastate.edu/nutrition/
User-friendly site devoted entirely to nutrition and health with various calculators.

National Institute of Diabetes and Digestive and Kidney Diseases (NIDDK)
Weight Control Information Network
1 WIN Way
Bethesda, MD 20892-3665
800-WIN-8098
www.niddk.nih.gov/health/nutrit/win.htm
Nicely laid out Web site with information on nutrition and obesity.

National Women Health Resource Center
2425 L Street, NW 3rd Floor
Washington, DC 20037
800-944-WOMAN (9662)
www.4woman.gov
U.S. Department of Health and Human Services site offering various information on women's health, nutrition, and many links to important resources.

Nutrient Data Laboratory USDA Agricultural Research Service
Beltsville Human Nutrition Research Center
4700 River Rd., Unit 89
Riverdale, MD 20737
301-734-8491
www.nal.usda.gov/fnic/foodcomp/
This USDA Nutrient Database gives facts about the composition of food, a glossary of terms, and links to other agencies.

Suburban Water Testing Labs
4600 Kutztown Rd.
Temple, PA 19560-1548
800-433-6595
http://www.h2otest.com/
Sells testing kits online; various kits to test different problems.

Tufts University Health and Nutrition Letter
6 Beacon St., Suite 1110
Boston, MA 02108
617-557-4994
www.healthletter.tufts.edu/
Excellent subscription newsletter with a bonus for online subscribers. Web site rates and links to other sites.

U.S. Department of Agriculture
Center for Nutrition Policy and Promotion
1120 20th Street, NW
Suite 200, North Lobby
Washington, DC 20036
202-418-2312
www.usda.gov/fcs/cnpp.htm
The Food Guide Pyramid and Dietary Guidelines can be downloaded by clicking the CNPP button from this Web site.

U.S. Department of Health and Human Services
Consumer Information Center
Department WWW
P.O. Box 100
Pueblo, CO 81009
www.pueblo.gsa.gov/food.htm
Booklets on food and nutrition can be downloaded (free) or ordered through this site.

U.S. Food and Drug Administration,
Center for Food Safety and Applied Nutrition Food Labeling
5600 Fishers Ln. (HFE-88)
Room 1685
Rockville, MD 20847
301-443-9767
www.vm.cfsan.fda.gov/label.html
The FDA Consumer Magazine is accessible through this Web site as well as a plethora of information about health, nutrition, and dietary choices.

University of Maryland, Cooperative Extension Service
Extension Publications On-Line
Publications Office

Symons Hall
University of Maryland at College Park
College Park, MD 20742
www.agnr.umd.edu/CES/Pubs/newsletters.html#nut
Contains a summary of articles in recent editions of their extension publications.
The Nutrition button at this Web site will allow you to view nutrition articles with
many interesting topics from weight control to Food Guide Pyramid choices.

University of Minnesota, Department of Food Science and Nutrition
Nutritionist's Tool Box
1334 Eckles Ave.
Saint Paul, MN 55108
612-624-1290
www.fsci.umn.edu/tools.htm
This site offers a calorie calculator and a Nutrition Analysis Tool to analyze the
foods you eat for a variety of nutrients.

Watersafe Test Kits
Silver Lake Research Corporation
P.O. Box 686
Monrovia, CA 91017
888-438-1942
www.watersafetestkits.com
This site offers test kits for sale and also provides information on buying their kits
in retail stores.

CHAPTER 3

DIETARY SUPPLEMENTS

Objectives

This chapter should enable you to:

- Describe the difference between Recommended Daily Allowances (RDAs) and Dietary Reference Intakes (DRIs)
- Discuss the development of the nutritional supplement industry
- List factors to consider in assessing the need for supplements
- Describe facts that are listed on supplement labels
- List the antioxidants and their sources
- Define the term *phytochemical*
- Discuss health conditions for which nutritional supplements can be beneficial

The importance of proper and sensible nutrition, as stated in the previous chapter, cannot be emphasized enough. The Healthy People 2000 Report states that what adults eat, especially adults who do not smoke and/or drink excessively, is the most significant controllable risk factor affecting their long-term health (1). The best way to feel good and maintain optimum health is to:

- Eat a wide variety of foods that provide adequate nutrients, including plenty of fresh fruits and vegetables, complex carbohydrates, plant protein, and fiber.
- Keep consumption of sugary foods, caffeine beverages, and alcohol to a minimum.

- Eat only a small amount of animal protein and fat.
- Drink plenty of water.
- Exercise at least 30 minutes daily.

It has long been held that anyone who followed this plan was considered properly nourished and did not need supplementation. However, as Americans continue their adherence to the Standard American Diet (SAD), they remain overweight and undernourished.

Views on Vitamin Supplementation

There has been much debate regarding vitamins and minerals as nutritional supplements and how (or if) they should be taken daily. The early 1900s focused largely on deficiencies of vitamins and minerals that caused diseases such as scurvy and beriberi. Then vitamins were added to our food; this process is called *fortification*. The 1950s and 1960s were replete with such examples, especially fortifying breads, cereals, and milk. Recent fortification of food includes the addition of calcium to many food products.

However, by the mid-1970s the focus was less on vitamin deficiency and more on the value of vitamin and mineral supplementation for the prevention of illness and disease. Vitamin C was thought to alleviate symptoms and prevent the common cold. Vitamin E was said to help keep the heart healthy. A low-fat, high-fiber diet was the order of the decade. The late 1970s saw the response of the U.S. Senate Select Committee on Nutrition that listed the number one public health problem in this country as poor nutrition. Experts believed Americans consumed too much food of too little nutritive value and that this was a contributing factor to poor quality of life and increased disease (2).

KEY POINT

Over the past decade there has been an explosion in the use of nutritional supplements, which has caused the government to begin to regulate the supplement industry.

How the Government Is Involved

Recommended Dietary Allowances

Since the 1940s the Food and Nutrition Board of the National Academy of Sciences has made recommendations for nutrient intake. These recommendations have been termed Recommended Dietary Allowances (RDAs) and represent the standards that should meet the needs of most healthy people in the United States. The RDAs addressed energy, protein, and most vitamins and minerals. Fats and carbohydrates standards were set in 2002 (3); they had never been set prior to that time because the experts assumed that if the average person met the energy requirements for protein, then the demand for fats and carbohydrates would also be met.

There has been much confusion surrounding RDAs. Most consumers have had some misunderstanding of how to use RDAs and what food choices best meet these recommendations. The idea that RDAs are optimum daily requirements rather than recommended minimum intakes as a standard for healthy individuals is rampant. The development of Daily Values (DV) and Dietary Reference Intakes (DRIs) are phasing out RDAs.

> ### KEY POINT
>
> The RDAs reflect the *minimum*, not *optimum* daily requirements for nutrients.

Dietary Reference Intakes (DRIs)

In an attempt to continue focusing on the benefits of healthy eating, DRIs were developed to update RDAs. These new guidelines represent the latest understanding of nutrient requirements for optimum health. The first set focused on nutrients related to bone health and fluoride (4); in 1998, folate, the B vitamins, and choline were added (5). Vitamin C, vitamin E, selenium, and carotenoids came in 2000 (6); in 2001 recommendations were published for vitamin A, vitamin K, arsenic, boron, chromium, copper, iodine, iron, manganese, molybdenum, nickel, silicon, vanadium, and zinc (micronutrients) (7). Slated for the future: macronutrients [dietary fat, individual fatty acids (omega-3 and omega-6, trans fatty acids)], electrolytes (sodium, potassium, chloride, and sulfate) and water; bioactive compounds, e.g., phytoestrogens and other phytochemicals, carnitine; and the role of alcohol in health and disease in 2005 (8).

The need to update and change the standards for intake of nutrients remains a challenge. The Food and Nutrition Board of the National Academy of Sciences is updating these standards on a regular basis. The newest work through these agencies is called Daily Values (DVs). DVs are divided into two groups: Reference Daily Intakes (RDIs) and Daily Reference Values (DRVs). RDIs are to be used in reference to vitamins, minerals, and proteins.

DRIs are divided into four subcategories:

1. Estimated Average Requirements (EARs)

2. RDAs, continued from 1989

3. Adequate Intakes (AIs)

4. Tolerable Upper Intake Levels (TULs)

EARs would satisfy 50% of requirements for men and women for specific age groups and are intended for use by nutritional professionals. If calculations of EARs are not available, AIs are used instead of RDAs. RDAs continue to be considered as sufficient amounts of nutrients to meet nearly all needs. TULs indicate the largest amount of a nutrient that someone can ingest without adverse affect (9).

KEY POINT

In 1994, an office was created within the National Institutes of Health for overseeing research on dietary supplements through the Dietary Supplement Health and Education Act (DSHEA). This requires manufacturers to include the words *dietary supplement* on product labels.

The FDA describes acceptable claims that can be made for relationships between a nutrient and the risk of a disease or health-related condition. These claims must be clear as to the relationship of the nutrient to the disease and be understandable by the general public. The claims can be made in several ways: through third-party references (such as the National Cancer Institute), symbols (such as a heart), and vignettes or descriptions. (See Exhibit 3–1.)

The FDA does not allow claims for healing, treatment, or cure of specific medical conditions on the labels or advertisements of nutritional supplements. This would put supplements in the category of drugs. The DSHEA allows only three types of claims to be used with supplements: nutrient content, disease, and nutrition support claims. The nutrient content explains how much of a nutrient is in a supplement. Claims regarding disease must have a basis in scientific evidence and refer to health-related conditions or diseases and a particular nutrient. Nutrition support claims (which may be used without FDA approval, but not without notification to that agency) is set up to explain how a deficiency could develop if the diet was deficient in that nutrient. These claims are accompanied by an FDA disclaimer on the label of the supplement and are therefore easy to determine. In March 1999, the DSHEA required that all nutritional supplements carry a "Supplement Facts" panel (Figure 3–1).

Reflection What motivates you to use supplements? Do you carefully evaluate claims about them?

A Supplement Extravaganza

Vitamins and minerals were what traditionally made up typical nutritional supplements. Today the definition of nutritional supplements is expanded to include "vitamins,

---

EXHIBIT 3–1 STATUS OF HEALTH CLAIMS

Approved Health Claims for Dietary Supplements and Conventional Foods

Calcium and osteoporosis

Folate and neural tube defects

Soluble fiber from whole oats and coronary heart disease

Soluble fiber from psyllium husks and coronary heart disease

Sugar alcohols and dental caries

Approved Health Claims for Conventional Foods Only

Dietary lipids and cancer

Dietary saturated fat and cholesterol and coronary heart disease

Fiber-containing grain products, fruits, and vegetables and cancer

Fruits and vegetables and cancer (for foods that are naturally a "good source" of vitamin A, vitamin C, or dietary fiber)

Fruits, vegetables, and grain products that contain fiber, particularly soluble fiber, and coronary heart disease

Sodium and hypertension

Health Claims Not Authorized

Antioxidant vitamins and cancer

Dietary fiber and cancer

Dietary fiber and cardiovascular disease

Omega-3 fatty acids and coronary heart disease

Zinc and immune function in the elderly

Source: The Commission on Dietary Supplementation, November 24, 1997.

---

minerals, herbs, botanicals, and other plant-derived substances; and amino acids, concentrates, metabolites, constituents, and extracts of these substances." (10)

The burgeoning of scientific studies on nutrients, the immediate release of single studies relating to nutrition, diet, and health, and supplement advertisements that use health claims to increase sales, have thrown the consumer into confusion. In many cases one report contradicts another—what was good yesterday is harmful today.

Figure 3–1: Supplement Label

Serving Size is the manufacturer's suggested serving. It can be stated per tablet, capsule, softgel, packet, or teaspoonful.

Amount Per Serving identifies the nutrients contained in the supplement, followed by the quantity present in each serving.

International Unit (I.U.) is a unit of measurement for vitamins A, D, and E.

Milligrams (mg) and micrograms (mcg) are units of measurement for B complex and C vitamins and minerals.

A list of all ingredients used in the product may appear outside the Nutrition Facts box. The nutrients are listed in decreasing order by weight.

BRAND NAME Tablets USP

USP means that product meets U.S. Pharmacopeia standards for quality, strength, purity, packaging, and labeling.

Nutrition Facts

Serving Size 1 tablet

Amount Per Serving	% Daily Value
Vitamin A 6000 I.U.	100%
50% as Beta–Carotene	
Vitamin C 80 mg.	100%
Vitamin D 100 I.U.	100%
Vitamin E 90 I.U.	100%
Thiamin 1.5 mg.	100%
Riboflavin 1.7 mg.	100%
Niacin 20 mg.	100%
Vitamin B_6 2 mg.	100%
Folate D .4 mg.	100%
Vitamin B_{12} 5 mcg.	100%
Calcium 120 mg.	10%
Iron 15 mg.	100%
Iodine 150 mcg.	100%
Magnesium 100 mg.	120%
Zinc 15 mg.	100%
Boron 5 mg.	*
Copper 2 mg.	100%

*Daily Value not established

Daily Value (D.V.) is a label reference term to indicate the percent of the recommended daily amount of each nutrient that serving provides.

INGREDIENTS: vitamin A acetate, betacarotene, lactose, magnesium stearate, talc, starch, ascorbic acid, ergocalciferol, di-alpha tocopherol acetate, thiamine hydrochloride, riboflavin, niacinamide, pyridoxine hydrochloride, folic acid, vitamin B_{12}, calcium gluconate, ferrous sulfate, sodium iodide, magnesium sulfate, zinc chloride, sodium metabolate, copper

DIRECTIONS: Take one tablet daily with a meal.

STORAGE: Keep tightly closed in a dry place; do not expose to excessive heat.

Storage information for the product.

All dietary supplements (especially those containing iron) should be kept out of the reach of children.

This is the manufacturer's batch number for the product.

KEEP OUT OF REACH OF CHILDREN
LOT # B7QF
EXPIRATION DATE: DECEMBER 1997

This is the expiration date for the product. It should be used before this date to assure full potency.

Manufacturer or distributor's name, address, and ZIP code

Provided for consumers by USP (U.S. Pharmacopeia); externalaffairs@usp.org. This information may be duplicated for educational purposes.

Over 40% of adults in the U.S. use nutritional supplementation on a regular basis.

The New Millennium brought with it buzzwords, such as antioxidants, phytochemcials, functional foods, and nutriceuticals. It is yet to be determined if these new compounds deserve the onslaught of press, print, and manufacture they so readily receive. When a new study has been completed that suggests a benefit from a nutrient, it is released immediately. Thousands of Americans rush to purchase the latest combination of vitamins, minerals, and nutritive supplements—spending billions of dollars on dietary supplements annually. Are they worth taking, and are the claims made by manufacturers true? Nutritional supplements may be helpful; but they may also be harmful. Taking supplements without knowledge of their actions and interactions could lead to imbalances of other nutrients, and potentially, toxicity. However, if taken properly and with forethought, supplements can increase general health and ward off some diseases.

When making the decision to take nutritional supplements, evaluation of the information available should be done in a carefully planned manner as part of a total nutrition program. If people hear of studies that seem to relate to their circumstances it is important for them to do some investigating on their own. Studies need to be assessed in the context they were performed, and their relationship to a person's particular situation. Health professionals can assist individuals in understanding what studies reveal. In any case, taking a supplement based on what has been read or heard in the news does not guarantee that a given person will have the same outcome.

The nutritional supplement industry is still in its infancy and grows exponentially each day. There continues to be an increasing variety of supplements readily available, which can be bought over the Internet, by mail order, at supermarkets, in drug stores, and other types of stores. Supplements are no longer the domain of natural food stores. The FDA regulates and oversees manufacturing, product information, and safety; and the Federal Trade Commission (FTC) regulates advertising of supplements. However, decisions regarding whether supplements should be taken, in what form, and how much, still remain a personal choice.

There is increasing interest among Americans to utilize nutritional supplements for optimum health. Some experts are also indicating a definite need for supplementation as part of a nutritional plan. Relying solely on diet to meet the body's needs for vitamins and minerals is fast becoming a thing of the past. We no longer eat food picked fresh from the local garden and cooked within hours. Additionally, many food preparation practices decrease the nutritive value of food.

Vitamins and minerals play an important role in optimum health and in reducing the risk of chronic diseases. But is the diet a person is consuming giving him or her enough nutrients and meeting individual needs? If so, then all that may be needed is a good quality multivitamin/mineral. However, if a person has poor nutritional habits; is under a great deal of stress; is pregnant or planning a pregnancy; or has a health problem, supplementation is a must. The supplements that are needed, how much of each, and for how long they need to be taken then becomes the issue. The research is promising, but for many nutrients, the results are still not definite.

KEY POINT

Supplements can never substitute for a healthy, sensible nutrition program where whole foods, containing hundreds of substances, working together synergistically, are consumed. Poor food choices and eating habits cannot be banished by supplementation.

Age, nutritional lifestyle, quality and quantity of food, gender, life stage, environment, family history, personal history, diet, exercise, and rest patterns should be considered in determining a person's need for nutritional supplementation.

As with all holistic approaches, knowledge, self-care, balance, and utilizing what nature provides are the keys. Individual nutritional needs can be determined by looking at the responses made on your Nutritional Lifestyle Survey (Chapter 1, Assessing Your Health Habits) and by considering several factors:

Age The need for nutrient supplementation increases with age. There are some nutrients that are not absorbed as well as a person ages, even if they are consumed in good quantity. Older adults may be affected by poor lifelong nutrition habits, social isolation, and chronic diseases that require special diets or affect food intake. Children need a balanced diet, along with a good quality multivitamin and limited sweets and fats to promote their growth and development.

Chronic health problems Some chronic conditions create special nutritional needs, while others produce symptoms that threaten a healthy nutritional status. If a person has a chronic health problem, is taking medication, and wants to take nutritional supplements, a thorough knowledge of drug–supplement interactions is necessary. Nurses and other health practitioners can help in this area.

Women Women who are pregnant, planning to become pregnant, breastfeeding, menopausal, or postmenopausal need added nutrients and/or supplementation. Different supplements are needed for different life cycles. Most recently the National Academy of Sciences has increased DRIs for folate and calcium for women (11, 12). These are of great import for women.

Lifestyle choices Cigarette and alcohol use reduce the levels of certain nutrients and predispose the body to diseases for which added protection is helpful. A stressful lifestyle can deplete nutrients. Deficiencies also can arise from the high consumption of caffeine and sugar.

If people presently take multivitamin/mineral supplements and believe they may benefit from taking additional supplements, they should first examine the labels of their food and supplements. They need to check the DVs (see discussion of DVs) of each vitamin and mineral listed. They should be receiving at least 100% for all nutrients from all food and supplements. If they are lower than 100%, they first need to determine if they can meet this need through a change in diet. If they cannot meet the requirements through diet, then supplements of specific nutrients may be necessary. If the DV is over 100% for some or all nutrients, they may want to cut back on that supplement. The guideline is to keep below 300% DV of any nutrient. A nutritional analysis can be used, also. A registered dietician (RD), nutritionist, or nutrition-knowledgeable healthcare professional can help with an analysis. Some Web sites offer free nutritional analysis (see Internet Resources at the end of this chapter).

KEY POINT

When using supplements, always read the labels. Know what you are taking, how easily it is absorbed, if it has United States Pharmacopeia (USP) initials, and when it expires. And, by all means, if you have any adverse affects—stop taking it.

Supplement Labels

Supplements come in many forms: tablets, capsules, softgels, powders, and liquids. The United States Pharmacopeia (USP) is the agency that oversees drug products and sets the standards for dietary supplements. All supplements now require labels, which are regulated by the USP. The USP has certain standards that must be met for single vitamins and those in combination, as well as dietary supplements, and botanical and herbal preparations. Figure 3–1 shows the information that is contained on a supplement label.

One facet of the dietary supplement label that is important to read is the Daily Value column. The DV is the percentage of the recommended daily amount of the nutrient that a serving gives. According to the USP, intake should be between 50% and 100% of the DV of each nutrient. One nutrient that would not provide 100% of the DV is calcium. If 100% of calcium were added to any supplement, it would be too big to swallow. Calcium should be taken in divided doses throughout the day.

The *bioavailability* of a particular nutrient is the amount of a nutrient that enters the blood stream and actually reaches the various organs, tissues, and cells of the body. Nutrients have greater bioavailability when they are taken with compounds that help their absorption.

Fruits and vegetables contain many compounds that, when eaten, allow for synergy to take place in the body, increasing bioavailability. Fruits and vegetables are especially affected by mode of storage and preparation. Those that have been exposed to heat, light, or air have lost some or all of their nutrients; their bioavailability is lowered.

Two important factors when considering the bioavailability of a supplement are ease of absorption and the benefit of taking it in combination with another supplement. *Disintegration* (how quickly a tablet/supplement breaks apart) and *dissolution* (how fast the supplement dissolves in the intestinal tract) (13) are two additional factors directly related to bioavailability. Vitamin C assists with the absorption of iron into the body. If taking iron as a supplement, people also should consider their vitamin C intake. Taking an iron supplement with a glass of orange juice would increase the bioavailability of the iron. On the other hand, calcium inhibits iron and magnesium absorption. This is important to remember when adding supplements to a nutritional plan, especially if iron, calcium, and vitamin C individually or in a multivitamin are being taken. More research is needed to determine and document supplement interactions. The NIH recently issued a call for research, mandated by Congress, "to explore the current state of our knowledge about the important issues related to bioavailability of nutrients and other bioactive components from dietary supplements" (14).

Birth Defects

One of the first vitamins addressed by the advisory committee on dietary supplements was folic acid. The original aim was said to reduce neural tube birth defects, *especially spina bifida*. The RDA for folic acid was doubled from 200 mcg/day to 400 mcg/day. The Centers for Disease Control, the USP, the FDA, and the March of Dimes have all recommended that women of childbearing age consume 400 mcg per day of folic acid, either through diet or supplements (15) (Figure 3–2). Women who are planning to become pregnant and who are of childbearing age should eat a varied diet and also take folic acid through supplementation. Sufficient folate is critical from conception through the first four-to-six weeks of pregnancy when the neural tube is formed. This means adequate diet and supplement use should begin well before pregnancy occurs.

Figure 3–2: Folic Acid

Folic acid is a B vitamin that everyone needs to help cells grow and divide. It is especially important for women who may become pregnant.

Why is Folic Acid So Important for Women?

Taken before and during early pregnancy, folic acid, also known as folate, reduces the chances of having a baby born with birth defects of the spine and brain (spina bifida and anencephaly). If you have already had a baby with spina bifida or anencephaly, see your doctor if you are considering another pregnancy.

For women of childbearing years USP (U.S. Pharmacopeia), the Centers for Disease Control and Prevention, the Food and Drug Administration, and the March of Dimes all recommend 400 mcg of folic acid daily.

You should not take more than 1,000 mcg daily unless your health care professional tells you to do so.

How Can I Get an Adequate Amount of Folic Acid?

It is possible to get folic acid by eating foods such as green leafy vegetables; cereal and cereal products; and citrus fruits and juices. Certain fully fortified breakfast cereals have 100% of the recommended daily amount of folic acid. Many women, however, prefer to take a multivitamin supplement.

What About a Dietary Supplement?

Folic acid may be taken as a tablet or as part of a multivitamin supplement. Make certain that the letters USP appear on the label to ensure that your vitamin/mineral product meets established standards for strength, quality, and purity.

Where Can I Find Additional Information About Pregnancy and Folic Acid?

Centers for Disease Control and Prevention
Mail Stop F 45
4770 Buford Highway N.E.
Atlanta, GA 30341-3724
770/488-7160
e-mail: pgm5@cdc.gov

Food and Drug Administration
HFE-88
5600 Fishers Lane
Rockville, MD 20857
800/332-4010
http://www.fda.gov

March of Dimes
1275 Mamaroneck Avenue
White Plains, NY 10605
888/663-4637
e-mail: resourcecenter@modimes.org

Spina Bifida Association of America
4590 MacArthur Blvd.
Suite 250
Washington, D.C. 20007
202/944-3285
e-mail: sbaa@sbaa.org

USP
12601 Twinbrook Parkway
Rockville, MD 20852
301/816-8223
e-mail: externalaffairs@usp.org

*Ask your health care professional
to help you determine your need for
folic acid supplements.*

Provided for consumers by USP (U.S. Pharmacopeia); externalaffairs@usp.org. This information may be duplicated for educational purposes.

The neural tube is a type of membrane that grows into the spinal cord and brain *in utero* (during pregnancy). Neural tube defects are problems in the development of the brain and spinal cord that arise during pregnancy. This is now believed to be a result of folate deficiency of the mother in the weeks before and in the early weeks of pregnancy. It is estimated that nearly 50% of all neural tube defects that occur can be arrested by adequate folate intake.

Antioxidants

Antioxidants play a crucial role in preventing or delaying the onset of cancer, heart disease, and premature aging. These are compounds that naturally protect the body from free radicals and help to depress the effects of metabolic by-products that cause degenerative changes related to aging. There is mounting evidence that antioxidants play a role in such diseases as cancer, stroke, arthritis, heart disease, immune problems, and neurological problems (16).

Free radicals have a helpful function in the body, but in higher levels they can damage cells and tissues. They are produced by the body's own metabolism, and generated from exposure to environmental factors and toxins. Antioxidant nutrients are said to neutralize the harmful free radicals that occur in the body constantly and arise from improper nutrition, eating fatty foods; smoking; drinking alcohol; taking drugs; exposure to environmental pollutants (such as herbicides and pesticides), toxins, carcinogens, iron, smog, and radiation.

The body has natural antioxidant enzymes that regulate the effects of free radicals. These enzymes are catalase, superoxide dismutase (SOD), and glutathione peroxidase. Vitamins A (as beta-carotene), C, and E and selenium assist the enzymes in the body to fight free radical damage.

Benefits vs. Risks of Antioxidant Supplementation

A diet low in fats, sweets, and animal protein that includes at least five fruits and vegetables per day, in variety, is a much safer way to obtain antioxidant protection than through supplementation. There is a greater chance of imbalances and toxicity when supplements are being used. (Please refer to the Tables 3–1 and 3–2 for guidelines for information on vitamins and minerals.) However, there continues to be increased evidence supporting antioxidant supplements as part of nutritional lifestyle.

Vitamin A

Vitamin A is necessary for good immune function, tissue repair, healthy skin and hair, bone formation, and vision. Fat-soluble vitamin A can cause toxicity and even

TABLE 3–1 VITAMINS

Vitamin	Lack of May Cause	How It Works	Excess May Cause	Best Foods to Eat
A	Night blindness; skin problems; dry, inflamed eyes	Bone & teeth growth; vision; keeps cells, skin, & tissues working properly	Birth defects; bone fragility, vision & liver problems	Eggs; dark green & deep orange fruits & vegetables; liver; whole milk
B1 Thiamin	Tiredness, weakness, loss of appetite, emotional upset, nerve damage to legs (late sign)	Helps release food nutrients and energy, appetite control, helps nervous system and digestive tract	Headache, rapid pulse, irritability, trembling, insomnia, interferes with B2, B6	Whole grains & enriched breads, cereals, dried beans, pork, most vegetables, nuts, peas
B2 Riboflavin	Cracks at corners of mouth, sensitivity to light, eye problems, inflamed mouth	Helps enzymes in releasing energy from cells, promotes growth, and cell oxidation	No known toxic effect. Some antibiotics can interfere with B2 absorption	Whole grains; enriched bread & cereals; leafy green vegetables; dairy; eggs; yogurt
Niacin	General fatigue, digestive disorders, irritability, loss of appetite, skin disorders	Fat, carbohydrate, & protein metabolism; good skin; tongue & digestive system; circulation	Flushing, stomach pain, nausea, eye damage; can lead to heart & liver damage	Whole wheat, poultry, milk, cheese, nuts, potatoes, tuna, eggs
B6 Pyridoxine	Dermatitis, weakness, convulsions in infants, insomnia, poor immune response, sore tongue, confusion, irritability	Necessary protein metabolism, nervous system functions, formation of red blood cells, immune system function	Reversible nerve injury, difficulty walking, numbness, impaired senses	Wheat & rice, bran, fish, lean meats, whole grains, sunflower seeds, corn, spinach, bananas
Biotin	Rarely seen because it can be made in body if not consumed. Flaky skin, loss of appetite, nausea.	Cofactor with enzymes for metabolism of macronutrients, formation of fatty acids, helps utilization of other B vitamins	Symptoms similar to vitamin B1 overdose	Egg yolks, organ meats, vegetables, fish, nuts, seeds; also made in intestine by normal bacteria there
Folic Acid	Anemia, diarrhea, digestive upset, bleeding gums	Red blood cell formation, healthy pregnancy, metabolism of proteins	Excessive intake can mask B12 deficiency and interfere with zinc absorption	Green, leafy vegetables, organ meats, dried beans
B12 Cobalamin	Elderly, vegetarians, or those with malabsorption disorder are at risk of deficiency-pernicious anemia, nerve damage	Necessary to form blood cells, promote proper nerve function, metabolism of carbohydrates and fats, builds genetic material	None known except those born with defect to absorb	Liver, salmon, fish, lean meats, milk, all animal products
Panto- thenic Acid	Not usually seen; vomiting, cramps, diarrhea, fatigue, tingling hands & feet, difficult coordination	Needed for many processes in body, converts nutrients into energy, formation of some fats, vitamin utilization, making hormones	Rare	Lean meats, whole grains, legumes
C Ascorbic Acid	Bleeding gums, slow healing, poor immune response, aching joints, nose bleeds, anemia	Helps heal wounds, collagen maintenance, resistance to infection, formation of brain chemicals	Diarrhea, kidney stones, blood problems, urinary problems	Most fruits, especially citrus fruits, melon, berries, & vegetables
D	Poor bone growth, rickets, osteoporosis, bone softening, muscle twitches	Calcium & phosphorus metabolism & absorption, bone & teeth formation	Headache, fragile bones, high blood pressure, increased cholesterol, calcium deposits	Egg yolks, organ meats, fortified milk, also made in skin when exposed to sun
E	Not usually seen, after prolonged impairment of fat absorption, neurological abnormalities	Maintains cell membranes, assists as antioxidant, red blood cell formation		Vegetable oils & margarine, wheat germ, nuts, dark green vegetables, whole grains
K	Tendency to hemorrhage, liver damage	Needed for prothrombin, blood clotting, works with vitamin D in bone growth	Jaundice (yellow skin) with synthetic form-flushing & sweating	Green vegetables, oats, rye, dairy; made in intestinal tract

TABLE 3–2 MINERALS

Minerals	Lack of May Cause	How It Works	Excess May Cause	Best Foods to Eat
Calcium	Rickets, soft bones, osteoporosis, cramps, numbness & tingling in arms & legs	Strong bones, teeth, muscle & nerve function, blood clotting	Confusion, lethargy, blocks iron absorption, deposits in body	Dairy, salmon and small bony fish, tofu
Phosphorus	Weakness & bone pain, otherwise rare	Works with calcium, helps with nerve, muscle, & heart function	Proper balance needed with calcium	Meat, poultry, fish, eggs, dairy, dried beans, whole grains
Magnesium	Muscle weakness, twitching, cardiac problems, tremors, confusion, formation of blood clots	Needed for other minerals & enzymes to work, helps bone growth, muscle contraction	Proper balance needed with calcium, phosphorus, & vitamin D	Nuts, soybeans, dried beans, green vegetables
Potassium	Lethargy, weakness, abnormal heart rhythm, nervous disorders	Fluid balance, controls heart, muscle, nerve, & digestive function	Vomiting, muscle weakness	Vegetables, fruits, dried beans, milk
Iron	Anemia, weakness, fatigue, pallor, poor immune response	Forms of hemoglobin & myoglobin, supplies oxygen to cell muscles	Increased need for antioxidants, heart disorders	Red meats, fish, poultry, dried beans, eggs, leafy vegetables
Iodine	Goiter, weight gain, increased risk of breast cancer	Helps metabolize fat, thyroid function	Thyroid-decreased activity, enlargement	Seafood, iodized salt, kelp, lima beans
Zinc	Poor growth, poor wound healing, loss of taste, poor sexual development	Works with many enzymes for metabolism & digestion, immune support, wound healing, reproductive development	Digestive problems, fever, dizziness, anemia, kidney problems	Lean meats, fish, poultry, yogurt
Manganese	Nerve damage, dizziness, hearing problems	Enzyme cofactor for metabolism, control blood sugar, nervous & immune functions	High doses affect iron absorption	Nuts, whole grains, avocados
Copper	Rare, but can cause anemia and growth problems in children	Enzyme activation, skin pigment, needed to form nerve & muscle fibers, red blood cells	Liver problems, diarrhea (most excess due to taking supplements, not dietary intake alone)	Nuts, organ meats, seafood
Chromium	Impaired glucose tolerance in low blood sugar and diabetes	Glucose metabolism	Most Americans have low intakes	Brewer's yeast, whole grains, peanuts, clams
Selenium	Heart muscle abnormalities, infections, digestive disturbances	Antioxidant with vitamin E, protects against cancer, helps maintain healthy heart	Nail, hair, & digestive problems, fatigue, garlic odor of breath	Meat & grains, dependent on soil in which they were raised
Molybdenium	Unknown	Element of enzymes needed for metabolism, helps body store iron	Gout, joint pains, copper deficiency	Beans, grains, peas, dark green vegetables

be fatal in amounts higher than 10,000 International Units (IU) per day. There may be greater risk of birth defects for babies whose mothers take preformed vitamin A during pregnancy—especially during the first trimester (17).

Beta-carotene, one of the family of carotenoids and a precursor to vitamin A, is a natural antioxidant, which enhances the immune system and may protect against certain cancers, cataracts, and heart disease. Beta-carotene is converted in the intestines and liver into preformed vitamin A; its sources are bright, orange-yellow fruits and vegetables.

Lycopene is another carotenoid and powerful antioxidant shown to reduce the risk of prostate and other cancers. The sources are fruits and vegetables of deep red to pink color. Some orange fruits and vegetables, some green leafy vegetables, and broccoli contain lutein, another carotenoid that has been found to arrest the development of macular degeneration and help protect the eyes from other diseases (18).

Vitamin C

Vitamin C is a popular supplement often consumed in large amounts. Recent research may be causing consumers of this supplement to rethink their intake. Between 100 mg and 200 mg of vitamin C is considered an optimum dose (19). High doses can easily upset bowel function, causing diarrhea. The dose for each person is highly individualized. Dr. Andrew Weil suggests a trial-and-error method for finding your optimum dose, which he recommends to be 3,000–6,000 mg per day (20). It is easy to have a 500 mg intake from eating at least six fruits and vegetables a day.

Vitamin E and Selenium

Vitamin E, discovered in the early 1920s, has antioxidant proprieties. It has been shown to decrease the risk of cardiovascular disease and some cancers, and may offer protection from Parkinson's disease and slow the progression of Alzheimer's disease.

Vitamin E together with selenium offers powerful antioxidant properties. Selenium has anticancer properties. Plants grown in selenium-rich soil are the best source. Vitamin E and selenium has been found to reduce some cancers by 37% and research has shown that the death rate from cancer was reduced by 50% in groups that took selenium supplements (21).

Vitamin E comes in two forms: natural and synthetic. The natural type is preferred and usually is listed on the label as d-alpha tocopherol (d-alpha tocopheryl) acetate. Synthetic vitamin E is listed on the label as dl-alpha tocopherol (tocopheryl) acetate.

There is little evidence of vitamin E toxicity, but at high levels it can increase the effect of anticoagulant (blood thinning) medications; and may also interfere with vitamin K's action in the body (blood clotting).

Vitamin E has been shown to help immune response, keep LDL cholesterol levels in check, and assist other antioxidants to be more available for use against free radicals. A diet including whole grains, wheat germ, nuts, sunflower oil, and corn oil will meet vitamin E RDAs. If you wish to consume 400–800 IUs per day, supplementation is necessary.

Phytochemicals

Phytochemicals (plant chemicals) are compounds that exist naturally in all plant foods and give them their color, flavor, and scent. They are the non-nutritive substances of plants and are not vitamins or minerals. Yet, phytochemicals have been associated with assisting the immune system, working as antioxidants, and fighting cancer (22). Foods that have been identified as having these health benefits are fruits, vegetables, legumes, grains, seeds, soy, licorice, and green tea. Researchers have discovered many classes of phytochemicals in food. Isoflavones (phytoestrogens) and lignins (soy), lycopene (tomato), anthocyanins and proanthocyanidins (grapes, blueberries, cherries, and other red crops), saponins (whole grains and legumes), flavonoids (cherries, tea, and parsley), isothiocyanates and indoles (broccoli, cauliflower, and cabbage), have antioxidant properties that may lower LDL (bad cholesterol levels) and curb growth of tumors (23).

One example of a vegetable that has gotten much press over the last several years is broccoli. Broccoli is in the cruciferous family, which includes cauliflower, cabbage, kale, brussels sprouts, bok choy, and Swiss chard. Cruciferous vegetables are excellent sources of fiber, beta-carotene, vitamin C, and other vitamins and minerals. Their cross-shaped flowers give them their name. The phytochemicals that have been found in these vegetables are indoles, isothiocyanates, and sulforaphane, which assist the body in triggering the formation of enzymes that block hormones and may protect cells against damage from certain carcinogens. Research is promising with regard to these and other phytochemicals and cancer; however more studies are needed.

Benefits and Risks of Phytonutrient Supplementation

The benefits of soy products have been clearly established in studies showing that soy fights cancer and lowers cholesterol levels. However, the use of soy products, especially in women who are vegetarians, has been linked to iron deficiency. One reason cited is that a vegetarian diet uses soy to replace the meat of conventional diets; therefore, supplementing the diet with vitamin C to enhance iron absorption is recommended (24).

Optimum levels for phytochemicals have not yet been determined. Individual foods contain different phytochemicals in varying amounts, and experts believe it is the combination of these compounds that may make the difference. Some scientists believe there are thousands of phytochemicals in a single food. Because researchers have advanced the most active phytonutrients found in fruits and vegetables over the last few years, it was inevitable that these components, in supplement form, would soon follow.

Though this provides an extremely convenient way of receiving the benefits of phytonutrients, supplements contain only isolated components and not the entire compound as it is found in the whole food state. At present, it would be best to consume phyto-chemicals by eating a variety of fruits, vegetables, grains, and legumes. Supplementation with isolated phytochemicals is discouraged until more information is obtained.

Cardiovascular Health

Heart disease is the number one killer of Americans, although it is largely preventable. The main issue leading to cardiovascular problems is arteriosclerosis (buildup of fatty deposits on the inner wall of arteries) more commonly known as hardening of the arteries. There has been a preponderance of literature explaining many factors affecting a person's risk of heart disease. Some factors include diet, stress, heredity, and lifestyle. Over the last several years, researchers have indicated the important role that some B vitamins—especially B6, B12, and folic acid—play in cardiovascular health by lowering blood levels of homocysteine.

Homocysteine, an amino acid, forms in the blood vessels and can accumulate there as a result of the breakdown of protein in foods (such as meats and dairy). High levels of homocysteine may be a leading cause of atherosclerosis. Secondly, research shows that people over the age of fifty have been found to have lower levels of vitamin B12. Although older adults may get sufficient vitamin B12 in their food, between 10% and 30% no longer have the ability to adequately absorb the naturally occurring form of B12, therefore, the National Academies of Science recommends those over age fifty should consume foods fortified with B12 and add supplements if necessary (25). B vitamins often work synergistically with each other as well as with other body processes, such as enzymes being activated; B vitamins in combination are the best way to supplement (see Exhibit 3–2).

EXHIBIT 3–2 RISKS WITH VITAMIN B GROUP SUPPLEMENTATION

There are risks associated with excess doses of certain vitamin B group vitamins, particularly niacin, B6, folate, and choline. Vitamin B6, when taken in amounts in excess of 100 mg per day can cause neuropathy (a disorder of the nerves), which could lead to weakness, pain, and numbness of the limbs. Niacin's upper level intake is 35 mg per day. Symptoms of overdose with niacin include flushing, itching, and warm sensation. The folate upper level limit is set at 1,000 mcg (1 mg); while choline is set at 3.5 grams per day. Excess choline may lead to low blood pressure.

Thiamine, riboflavin, B12, pantothenic acid, and biotin do not have upper limits set due to the lack of evidence suggesting adverse effects from high intakes of these B vitamins, however, excessive consumption of these B vitamins is not wise.

Vitamin A, as beta-carotene, vitamin C, calcium, magnesium, selenium, vitamin E, manganese, potassium, bioflavonoids, choline, and EFAs (essential fatty acids) are some nutrients that also have been linked to optimum cardiovascular health. These nutrients are needed to repair, protect, and prevent degeneration of the blood vessels.

Hypertension

High blood pressure responds very well to lifestyle changes. Increased fiber, low sodium intake, relaxation techniques, and exercise are helpful in lowering and maintaining blood pressure. The DASH diet, Figure 3–3, suggests foods that tend to be rich in potassium, magnesium, and calcium; these are the minerals experts believe to be important for controlling blood pressure. Food rich in potassium includes bananas, apricots, grapes, oranges, spinach, lentils, and almonds.

When diuretics (fluid pills) are used, the addition of magnesium as a supplement may be needed. Diuretics cause fluid loss and when fluid is lost from the body it takes potassium and magnesium with it. Magnesium assists potassium to keep blood pressure levels optimum.

Diabetes Mellitus

Diabetes is a chronic disease that is one of the major causes of blindness in the United States. It is caused from either a defect in or insufficiency of insulin that does not allow for the management of appropriate blood glucose levels.

Food is broken down and absorbed by the body when you eat. *Enzymes*—chemicals made by the body with the help of nutrients—turn protein into amino acids, and starches and sugars into their simple sugars. Fats are broken down into fatty acids. Once this happens there is usually a rise in blood sugar, leading to the hormone insulin being secreted by the pancreas (a gland located behind the stomach). Insulin assists in the movement of nutrients from the bloodstream into the muscles and fat tissues and also the liver. This allows the liver to stop producing glucose (blood sugar). If there is not enough insulin being excreted or if what is excreted is unable to be used then diabetes develops.

Chromium was first found to have a relationship with insulin control in the body in the mid-1950s, and in the late 1970s it was finally accepted as a nutrient (26). Chromium is a mineral, essential to the body, which acts cooperatively with other substances that control metabolism. It is a component of the glucose tolerance factor used to help with fat metabolism by transporting glucose to the cells (and being metabolized to produce

Figure 3–3: The DASH Diet

Following The DASH Diet

The DASH eating plan shown below is based on 2,000 calories a day. The number of daily servings in a food group may vary from those listed, depending on your caloric needs.

Use this chart to help plan your menus, or take it with you when you go to the store.

Food Group	Daily Servings (except as noted)	Serving Sizes	Examples and Notes	Significance of Each Food Group to the DASH Eating Plan
Grains & grain products	7–8	1 slice bread $1/2$ cup dry cereal* $1/2$ cup cooked rice, pasta, or cereal	whole-wheat bread, English muffin, pita bread, bagel, cereals, grits, oatmeal, crackers, unsalted pretzels, popcorn	major sources of energy and fiber
Vegetables	4–5	1 cup raw leafy vegetable $1/2$ cup cooked vegetable 6 oz vegetable juice	tomatoes, potatoes, carrots, green peas, squash, broccoli, turnip greens, collards, kale, spinach, artichokes, green beans, lima beans, sweet potatoes	rich sources of potassium, magnesium, and fiber
Fruits	4–5	6 oz fruit juice 1 medium fruit $1/4$ cup dried fruit $1/2$ cup fresh, frozen, or canned fruit	apricots, bananas, dates, grapes, oranges, orange juice, grapefruit, grapefruit juice, mangoes, melons, peaches, pineapples, prunes, raisins, strawberries, tangerines	important sources of potassium, magnesium, and fiber
Low-fat or fat-free dairy foods	2–3	8 oz milk 1 cup yogurt 1 $1/2$ oz cheese	fat-free (skim) or low-fat (1%) milk, fat-free or low-fat buttermilk, fat-free or low-fat regular or frozen yogurt, low-fat and fat-free cheese	major sources of calcium and protein
Meats, poultry, & fish	2 or less	3 oz cooked meats, poultry, or fish	select only lean; trim away visible fats; broil, roast, or boil, instead of frying; remove skin from poultry	rich sources of protein and magnesium
Nuts, seeds, & dry beans	4–5 per week	$1/3$ cup or 1 $1/2$ oz nuts 2 tbsps or $1/2$ oz seeds $1/2$ cup cooked dry beans	almonds, filberts, mixed nuts, peanuts, walnuts, sunflower seeds, kidney beans, lentils, and peas	rich sources of energy, magnesium, potassium, protein, and fiber

Figure 3–3: The DASH Diet *continued*

Food Group	Daily Servings (except as noted)	Serving Sizes	Examples and Notes	Significance of Each Food Group to the DASH Eating Plan
Fats & oils**	2–3	1 tsp soft margarine 1 tbsp low-fat mayonnaise 2 tbsps light salad dressing 1 tsp vegetable oil	soft margarine, low-fat mayonnaise, light salad dressing, vegetable oil (such as olive, corn, canola, or safflower)	besides watching fats added to foods, choose foods that contain less fat
Sweets	5 per week	1 tbsp sugar 1 tbsp jelly or jam 1/2 oz jelly beans 8 oz lemonade	maple syrup, sugar, jelly, jam, fruit-flavored gelatin, jelly beans, hard candy, fruit punch, sorbet, ices	sweets should be low in fat

* Serving sizes vary between 1/2 and 1 1/4 cups. Check the product's nutrition label.
** Fat content changes the serving sizes for fats and oils. For example, 1 tbsp of regular salad dressing equals 1 serving; 1 tbsp of a low-fat dressing equals 1/2 serving; 1 tbsp of a fat-free dressing equals 0 servings.

energy) and activates certain enzymes. The recommended daily allowance of chromium is 50–200 mcg. It is believed that only 10% of the population of the United States receives enough chromium in their diet. Deficiency or inadequacy of chromium effectively blocks insulin function, resulting in elevated glucose levels. Supplementation decreases fasting glucose levels and insulin levels, improves glucose tolerance, and suppresses cholesterol and triglyceride levels.

Essential Fatty Acids

The two essential fatty acids necessary for life and the proper function of the body are omega-3 (alpha-linolenic) and omega-6 (linoleic). EFAs enhance immune function, protect the lining of the gastrointestinal system, increase kidney blood flow, reduce inflammation, and inhibit platelet aggregation (cells of the blood sticking together). These fatty acids become converted with the help of enzymes eicosanoids. Prostaglandins are probably the most commonly known eicosanoids. One to two tablespoons of flaxseed ground fresh and sprinkled on food will provide and adequate amount of omega-3 oil for the average person. Cold-pressed and fresh canola, sunflower, and safflower oils are excellent sources of EFAs. These can be easily incorporated into your daily nutritional plan. Supplementation should be considered if a person has a health problem or does not include these nutrients in the diet.

KEY POINT

Omega-3 oils are found in fish oils and flaxseed; the omega-6 oil sources are borage (an herb), evening primrose, and black currant oils.

Osteoporosis

Calcium is an important mineral and may help prevent osteoporosis. When bones are calcium-rich they are less susceptible to fractures. The new Dietary Reference Intakes suggest Americans take between 1,000 and 1,300 mg of calcium per day. After menopause, some women may require up to 1,500 mg of calcium per day. The Upper Tolerable Limit (UTL) for calcium is set at 2,500 mg per day. Excess calcium can cause muscle cramps, kidney stones, high blood calcium, or poor absorption of iron, zinc, or magnesium (27).

When considering calcium intake, it is important to know that vitamin D is essential in metabolizing and absorbing the calcium you are ingesting (28); magnesium and phosphorus are minerals that work together with calcium. Meeting calcium requirements means consuming adequate supplies of calcium and vitamin D. If people depend on dietary sources for these nutrients they may have to eat a very large quantity of calcium-rich foods in addition to consuming foods that include vitamin D, phosphorus, and magnesium in the proper ratios. There are several forms of calcium available in supplements; the most bioavailable form is calcium citrate; the least absorbable is calcium carbonate.

Sorting It All Out

The concept that people must be constantly on guard and change course to follow the most recent scientific study, not really knowing if they are heading in the right direction, is ominous. Nutritional supplementation can seem like a daunting task and quickly becomes overwhelming, unless the basics are implemented. Rather than becoming overloaded with facts regarding optimum nutritional supplementation, people should focus on eating basic, well-balanced diets. When a balanced diet is eaten, many compounds are consumed that help with the protection, breakdown, absorption, and integration of all that is ingested. Nature provides what is needed with the proper ingredients in the right amounts for the body—if a nutritious and healthful food plan is followed. If people are confused or have any doubt regarding what or how much they should be taking, consulting a healthcare practitioner who is knowledgeable in nutrition and nutrition supplementation for guidance is beneficial.

Chapter Summary

Recommended Daily Allowances represent minimum standards of food intake to meet the needs of an average person while Dietary Reference Intakes go beyond RDAs to describe nutrient requirements for optimal health.

In 1994 the Dietary Supplement Health and Education Act required manufacturers to include the words *dietary supplement* on product labels and established an oversight office within the National Institutes of Health.

It is important to read supplement labels. Factors to consider when contemplating the use of supplements include age, the presence of chronic health problems, sex, and lifestyle habits. Supplements can never replace a healthy diet.

Antioxidants include vitamins A, C, E, and selenium. Phytochemicals are compounds that exist naturally in all plant foods.

Supplements can be beneficial in the treatment of many chronic conditions, however, they must be used wisely. People need to learn about the actions, interactions, and risks associated with the specific supplements they use.

References

1. Healthy People 2000. (2000). *National Health Promotion and Diagnosis Prevention Objective.* U.S. Department of Health and Human Services, Public Health Service, Centers for Disease Control, and the National Center for Health Statistics. Publication # PHS96-1256, p. 40.

2. U.S. Senate (the McGovern Report) Select Committee on Nutrition and Human Needs. (1977). *Dietary Goals for the U.S.,* 2nd ed. Washington, D.C.: U.S. Government Printing Office.

3. National Academies of Science (2002). New Eating and Physical Activity Targets to Reduce Chronic Disease Risk, *National Academies of Science Press Release,* September 5, 2002.

4. National Academies of Science (1997). Dietary Reference Intakes for Calcium, Phosphorus, Magnesium, Vitamin D, and Fluoride, *National Academies of Science News Release,* August 1997.

5. National Academies of Science (1998). Dietary Reference Intakes for Thiamin, Riboflavin, Niacin, Vitamin B6, Folate, Vitamin B12, Pantothenic Acid, Biotin, and Choline. *National Academy of Science Press Release,* April 7, 1998.

6. National Academies of Science (2001). Antioxidants' Role in Chronic Disease Prevention Still Uncertain; Huge Doses Considered Risky. *National Academy of Sciences Press Release,* April 10, 2000.

7. Russell, R. (2001). *Dietary Reference Intakes for Vitamin A, Vitamin K, Arsenic, Boron, Chromium, Copper, Iodine, Iron, Manganese, Molybdenum, Nickel, Silicon, Vanadium, and Zinc.* Opening Statement, Institute of Medicine, Public Briefing, Washington, D.C. January 9, 2001.

8. National Academies of Science (1997). New Report Recasts Dietary Requirements for Calcium and Related Nutrients. *The National Academy of Sciences Press Report.* August 13, 1997.

9. National Academies of Science (2001). *A Report of the Panel of Micronutrient, Subcommittee on Upper Reference Levels of Nutrients and of Interpretations and Uses of Dietary Reference Intakes, and the Standing Committee on Scientific Evaluation of Dietary Reference Intakes.* Washington, D.C.: Food and Nutrition Board, IOM, and National Academy of Sciences Press.

10. *What Are Dietary Supplements?* National Institutes of Health, Office of Dietary Supplements Web site, *www.ods.od.nih.gov* (accessed August 10, 2003).

11. National Academies of Science (1998). Dietary Reference Intakes for Thiamin, Riboflavin, Niacin, Vitamin B6, Folate, Vitamin B12, Pantothenic Acid, Biotin, and Choline, *National Academies of Science News Release*, April 1998.

12. National Academies of Science (1997). Dietary Reference Intakes for Calcium, Phosphorus, Magnesium, Vitamin D, and Fluoride, *National Academies of Science News Release*, August 1997.

13. United States Pharmacopeia (2003). *Dietary Supplements Lexicon* at *www.usp.org* (accessed August 10, 2003).

14. National Institutes of Health Office of Dietary Supplements (1999). *News and Events, Bioavailability of Nutrients and Other Bioactive Components from Dietary Supplements.* Washington, D.C.

15. National Academy of Sciences (1998). *Report on Dietary Intakes for Thiamin, Riboflavin, Niacin, Vitamin B6, Folate, Vitamin B12, Pantothenic Acid, Biotin, and Choline.* Washington, D.C.

16. Fann, Y. C. (1998). Free Radicals, Antioxidants and Your Health. *ITSS/NIEHS Connections*, Volume 6.

17. Rothman, K. J., Morre, L. L., Singer, M. R., et al. (1995). Teratogenicity of high vitamin A intake. *New England Journal of Medicine*, 333:1369–1373.

18. VERIS (2002). *Carotenoids and Eye Health.* LaGrange, IL: VERIS Research Information Services.

19. National Institutes of Health (1999). *Vitamin C News Release*, April 20, 1999.

20. Weil, A. (1997). *8 Weeks to Optimum Health: A Proven Program for Taking Full Advantage of Your Body's Natural Healing Power.* New York: Alfred A. Knopf Publishers, p. 57.

21. VERIS (1999). *Vitamin E Fact Book*. LaGrange, IL: VERIS Research Information Services, p. 13.
22. Pinto, J. (1999). *Phytochemicals Nutrient Information*. American Society for Nutrition Sciences Web page, *www.nutrition.org/nutinfo/* (accessed August 22, 2001).
23. American Dietetic Association (1995). Position of the American Dietetic Association: Phytochemicals and Functional Food. *Journal of the American Dietetic Association*, 95:493.
24. Carroll, K. (1991). Review of Clinical Studies on Cholesterol-Lowering Response to Soy Protein. *Journal of the American Dietetic Association*, 91:820–827.
25. National Academy of Sciences (1998). *Report on Dietary Intakes of Thiamine, Riboflavin, Niacin, Vitamin B6, Folate, Vitamin B12, Pantothenic Acid, Biotin, and Choline*. Washington, D.C.
26. *Chromium and Diabetes Workshop Summary*. Washington, D.C.: Office of Dietary Supplements, November 14, 1999.
27. National Academies of Science (1998). Report on Dietary Reference Intakes for Calcium, Phosphorus, Magnesium, Vitamin D, and Fluoride. *National Academies of Science News Release*, August 13, 1998.

Suggested Reading

Igloe, R. S. and Hui, Y. H. (2001). *Dictionary of Food Ingredients*, 4th ed. New York: Chapman and Hall.

MacWilliam, L. (2003). *Comparative Guide to Nutritional Supplements*, 3rd ed. Oswego, NY: Northern Dimensions Publishing.

Mindell, E. (1999). *Earl Mindell's Vitamin Bible for the 21st Century*. New York: Warner Books.

Murray, M. (1998). *Encyclopedia of Nutritional Supplements*, 2nd ed. Rocklin, CA: Prima Publishing.

Ulene, Art. *Complete Guide to Vitamins, Minerals, and Herbs*. New York, N.Y.: Avery Books.

Weil, Andrew. (1997) *8 Weeks to Optimum Health: A Proven Program of Taking Full Advantage of Your Body's Natural Healing Power*. New York: Alfred A. Knopf Publishers.

Internet Resources

American Council on Science and Health
1995 Broadway
New York, NY 10023
212-362-7044
www.acsh.org
Covers many issues regarding nutrition and health with links to other sites.

Ask Dr. Weil Bulletin
www.drweil.com
Online information featuring Dr. Andrew Weil, founder of the Integrative Medicine Program, University of Arizona Health Sciences Center, Tuscon, AZ. Offers many topics on integrative medicine and health.

National Heart, Lung, and Blood Institute
P.O. Box 30105
Bethesda, MD 20824-0105
301-592-8573
Facts About the DASH Eating Plan
www.nhlbi.nih.gov
This site offers the DASH diet plan with recipe suggestions for downloading or to order by mail.

Healthfinder Web Page
www.healthfinder.gov
Online consumer health information service provided by U.S. Department of Health and Human Services. Links to medical journals and databases with special resources on health.

National Institutes of Health
Office of Dietary Supplements
9000 Rockville Pike
Bethesda, Maryland 20892
www.ods.od.nih.gov
IBIDS (International Bibliographic Information on Dietary Supplements) database provides access to bibliographic citations and abstracts from published international, scientific literature on dietary supplements. This database was set up to help consumers, healthcare providers, educators, and researchers.

National Library of Medicine
8600 Rockville Pike
Bethesda, MD 20894
www.nlm.nih.gov

Nutrient Data Laboratory USDA Agricultural Research Service, Beltsville Human
Nutrition Research Center
4700 River Rd., Unit 89
Riverdale, MD 20737
301-734-8491
www.nal.usda.gov/fnic/foodcomp/
This database gives facts about the composition of food, a glossary of terms, and
links to other agencies.

PlaneTree Health Library
Mission Oaks
15891 Los Gatos-Almaden Rd.
Los Gatos, CA 95032
408-358-5667
www.planetreesanjose.org
A consumer health and medical library which is free and open to the public with
the aim of providing access to information to make informed decisions about health.
There is a range of information from professional/technical to easy-to-understand
materials for all areas of medical treatment. They also offer some materials in
Spanish and Vietnamese.

CHAPTER 4

EXERCISE: MINDFULNESS IN MOVEMENT

Objectives

This chapter should enable you to:

- List at least ten benefits of regular physical activity
- Describe rib cage breathing
- Define aerobic exercise
- Calculate target heart rate
- List at least six activities that provide an aerobic workout
- State an example of a muscle-strengthening exercise
- Describe the benefits of Hatha Yoga and T'ai Chi Chuan

The body is made to move. As you read this page, your heart is pumping, blood is coursing through hundreds of miles of the cardiovascular network, your lungs are expanding and contracting, your eyes are moving, your eardrums are vibrating, and neurons are firing. Thousands of processes are transpiring to promote the essence of your being…and you have not even lifted a finger to turn a page.

The body is not intended to be stagnant. Every movement, each effort of the muscles to pump blood brings the life force to every cell and flushes or removes from the body all that is no longer needed.

What does it mean to exercise? How does it change us? Why does the body require exercise? What does it look and feel like? These are questions to explore when using a model for holistic movement that is life sustaining and promotes wellness.

Reflection   What attitude do you have toward exercise? What about your family background, experiences, and education contributed to that attitude?

What Does It Mean to Exercise?

For the last several decades the public has been bombarded with the importance of exercise. In the 1960s President John F. Kennedy implemented the President's Council on Physical Fitness, which launched the fitness craze. Children were tested and rewarded for their ability to climb a rope, do sit-ups and push-ups, throw a softball, and speedily run the 100-yard dash. This was the country's attempt to address the health hazards of a sedentary lifestyle for children. Today, physical fitness of youth remains an unmet goal. The U.S. has an increasingly overweight population with evidence of hypertension and atherosclerosis beginning in the childhood years. Lifestyle-related diseases are beginning earlier as people become increasingly physically inactive and technologically dependent. *Labor-saving* devices are not *life saving*, and there is significant physical and spiritual deterioration evident among all ages.

Improved physical fitness also has been a priority for those interested in positively impacting the aging process. Congress, in 1975, broadened the definition of the Older Americans Act to include "… services designed to enable older persons to attain and maintain physical and mental well being through programs of regular physical activity and exercise." With the launch of the new millennium it is now more evident than ever that the country must reconsider its commitment to a healthy population for all citizens: young, old, rich, poor, and all ethnic populations that make up the diverse tapestry of the U.S.

KEY POINT

Research shows benefits of regular physical activity include improved cardiopulmonary function, reduced risk of coronary artery disease, lowered risk of colon cancer, heightened immune function, decreased susceptibility to depression, increased self-esteem, and improved quality of life.

Fitness is not limited to youth; growing old does not mean a loss of good physical condition and function. Further, it is a misconception that persons with physical limitations cannot engage in a health-promoting movement activity. Aging or disease does not mean weakening or sacrificing the abundance life has to offer. Hypertension control, bone and muscle strength, recovery from illness and injury, weight management, functional ability, and a general sense of well being are all enhanced with regular physical activity.

Gentle movement programs can produce an enhanced immune response that is vital for resilience and physical/emotional integrity. Muscles respond to movement—the demand to contract and relax. Muscles are made to work and just as the human spirit thrives when given a task or job to do, so does the body when put into motion.

KEY POINT

It is a myth that an aging person or someone with a health condition must experience *physical decline, dysfunction, disability,* and *dependency.* These outcomes are related to inactivity and a sedentary lifestyle—not the person's chronological age.

Commonly held, although limited, definitions of exercise bring images of calisthenics, sweaty workouts to loud music, strenuous weight lifting, and sessions of breathlessness to near exhaustion. It is time to evolve into a new view of exercise that is gentler and deeper, and lasts a lifetime. This revised view emphasizes the significance of movement that engages the muscles and enhances the flow of body fluids and energy. Insufficient movement can show its effects in all areas of the self. Immobility causes muscles to shorten and weaken, and joints to become stiff and less able to move or rotate smoothly. Sluggish digestion, slower elimination, and removal of toxins and waste products are outgrowths of inactivity. Inadequate physical movement affects the mind as well—evidenced by mild depression or a lack of enthusiasm and zest for living.

KEY POINT

To keep the body in good health is a duty...
otherwise we shall not be able to keep our minds strong and clear

—Buddha

Benefits of Exercise

There are many benefits to exercise. Regular physical activity improves muscle strength and tone. Regular deliberate movement tones muscles, which has a positive impact on appearance, posture, body image, and the ability to engage in self-care activities. It also improves the efficiency of the body's metabolism. It helps use fat for fuel, and when you eat nutritious meals, it uses the energy for activity.

Regular aerobic exercise helps to regulate blood sugar or glucose levels. The increased demand for oxygen during exercise (which is what makes movement *aerobic*) improves the regulation and utilization of insulin, necessities for bringing glucose into the cells for metabolism or energy production. Exercise helps stabilize and keep the body's blood sugar levels balanced. Developing a regular movement program is a major preventative measure for adult-onset diabetes, heart disease, and atherosclerosis, as well as disorders of mood and thinking.

Endurance is enhanced by regular aerobic exercise. Exercise helps increase the efficiency of the heart and lungs, aiding in creating a greater capacity for coping with life challenges.

KEY POINT

When regularly challenged through aerobic activity (jumping, walking, jogging, biking, swimming, etc.) the heart and lungs learn to accommodate the body's increased demand for oxygen.

Oxygen is the essence of the life force, every cell of the body requires it for proper functioning. The gentle exertion of exercise challenges the organs to work more efficiently to draw the oxygen in more rapidly. Heart rate, breathing rate, and circulation increase allowing each cell to receive nourishment and eliminate wastes.

There also is a dilatation or widening effect to the blood vessels because the heightened demand for oxygen causes the vessels to open wider to accommodate the increased fluid flow. Openness promotes flow. Again, let metaphor bring wisdom and empowerment to a holistic lifestyle. When the mind/body is open it can receive new information and new possibilities, more of what is necessary and good. Strength and endurance become characteristics for the whole person not just of the physical being, but also of emotional and spiritual facets.

Blood and lymphatic fluids carry the oxygen and nutrients necessary for the feeding of every cell. These fluids are the vehicles for removal of all unnecessary and unwanted waste products from the body. The increased demand for blood flow stimulates the bone marrow to produce more blood cells to carry the oxygen. In a very short period of time, usually less than one month, improvements in cardiorespiratory function can be experienced. This challenge to the heart and lungs makes them stronger and more efficient. At rest their rate goes down, meaning that they need to work less to get the same amount of work done. For this reason, resting blood pressure decreases. Weight bearing/resistance activities, such as walking, swimming, weight training, jumping, running, yoga, and T'ai Chi enhance the ability of the bones to keep calcium in the skeleton. A regular movement program is a major factor in the prevention of osteoporosis.

Exercise stimulates the circulation of endorphins—the neurohormonal transmitters responsible for feelings of well being and psychospiritual hardiness, which can relieve stress. (For more information on stress see Chapter 6, Flowing with the Reality of Stress.)

Regular exercise helps reduce chronic physical pain. Premenstrual cramping, headache, and joint stiffness can be relieved by movement. It can also help to prevent falls or injuries, and shorten recovery time. The fit body is more resilient to the effects of gravity. Having the strength and balance to recover from falls is an important advantage to being in good physical condition.

Exercise has social, psychological, and emotional benefits. The release of hormones and various neuropeptides from regular activity help decrease pain, alleviate anxiety, promote feelings of well being, and suppress fatigue. Exercise improves circulation to the brain, which enhances alertness, clarity of thought, and memory; it sharpens the mind. It increases "regularity" and "flow" of the gastrointestinal tract, which assists with digestion and bowel elimination.

Exercise promotes the flow of lymph fluid. Lymph fluid is not driven by a pump like the heart, rather it *undulates*, or moves in wave-like fashion, in response to muscle contraction. The lymph pathways are laced within the body much like a fishnet stocking from the top of the head to the bottom of the toes. Lymph fluid flows from deep within towards the superficial layers of the skin and returns back to the thoracic duct in the neck. From the thoracic duct it joins with the general circulation. Circulation of fluid lubricates the joints, moistens the body—keeps us flowing within.

Exercise normalizes hormonal balance of the body. Not only is insulin better utilized for blood sugar stability, but cortisol, from the adrenal glands, is better modulated through aerobic activity. The modulation of cortisol is extremely important for reduction of the detrimental effects of stress. (Modulating cortisol is one of the important ways of keeping calcium in the bones and out of the blood stream where it tends to make the vascular system hard (atherosclerosis)).

What Does Exercise Look and Feel Like?

You do not need to sweat, pant, or hurt to benefit from action that is taken deliberately and in a context of wellness promotion. You simply need to develop a movement program that circulates fluid, contracts muscles, resists gravity, and symbolizes fun and value for you. This idea transcends the notion that exercise is done to give us the outside appearance of a "perfect body." The commercial world promotes an ideal body that is an unrealistic image for most people.

Movement is one of the non-negotiable laws of life. The body, like all life-forms, thrives on movement. It is a metaphor of life itself. There is an automatic rhythm within and outside us that doesn't cease until death—the cyclic motion of breathing, the expanding and contracting of lungs. It is only through the breath that we have life and the more breath we have the more vital and alive we feel.

Reflection   Take a moment right now, put down the book, let yourself get comfortable in your seat, and take a long deliberate inhalation in through your nose down to your lungs. Let your lungs be so full that you feel the entire rib cage rise and fill to capacity. Slowly let the air leave you, let your body sink in the exhalation. What do you observe about the effects?

The Mechanics of Breathing

The mechanics of breathing primarily involve the diaphragm—a large, dome-shaped muscle that separates the abdominal and chest cavities—and the intercostals, which are the muscles between the rib bones. The process of inspiring and exhaling depends on the surface tension between the alveoli—or air sacs of the lungs, the elasticity of the lungs within the chest wall, and the integrity of the large airways or bronchial tree to support the transport of air into the body.

When the diaphragm contracts or shortens, it flattens downward, increasing the chest cavity and creating a negative pressure that draws air into the lungs and produces the inspiration phase of the breathing cycle. Every breath inhaled can be considered an opportunity to "inspire the life force," to "bring in spirit" (inspiration) for the soul to be fed or nurtured through the energizing of the body. (See Exhibit 4–1).

EXHIBIT 4–1 RIB CAGE BREATHING

Inhale deeply while raising your extended arms from your side to straight above your head. Exhale as your arms are returned to your side. Enjoy the sensation of a fully expanded rib cage. Keep the movement of the arms smooth and slow. Count 1 and 2 inhaling and moving the arms up; count 3 and 4 exhaling and moving the arms down. This is an excellent exercise for pulmonary hygiene—to fully expand the lungs, bringing oxygen to the very deepest aspects of the lungs. It is a wonderful way to cleanse lung tissue, bringing in life-giving oxygen and flushing out waste products that no longer serve the body. Do rib cage breathing four-to-six times to a session. It is a powerful way to renew and refresh as well as to put the lungs and ribs through their "full range of function."

A conscious effort to deep breathe can be incorporated into activities, such as walking, yoga, T'ai Chi, dancing, swimming, jogging, or cycling. Diaphragmatic breathing is a potent health-promoting exercise and has benefits beyond helping to bring greater amounts of oxygen into the body.

There is a large collection of lymph nodes in the belly region. Each "full-bellied breath" massages this lymphatic center. The movement of the diaphragm "milks" the lymph fluid back up to the heart. (Please see Chapter 5 on Immune Enhancement for a discussion of the lymphatic system and the role of exercise in promoting healthy immune integrity.)

Aerobic Exercise

Aerobic exercise is one of the most important and efficient methods of attaining muscular and cardiovascular fitness. Aerobic exercise is accomplished when enough demand is put on the muscles to increase their need for oxygen, causing the heart to beat faster and the lungs to work harder. This not only increases cardiovascular endurance, but also helps to prevent heart attacks by strengthening the heart and increasing the flow of blood through the vascular system, thereby keeping the arteries open and elastic. Fresh oxygen in the blood improves the functioning of all cells in the body. It helps to burn away fat from the muscles and build new, lean muscle tissue. This increases the metabolic rate of the whole body even during sleep and is valuable for losing weight and keeping it off.

In order to gain aerobic benefits, the heart rate must be elevated and maintained for the duration of the workout within the *target heart rate*. The target heart rate range is the range between the maximum and minimum calculated heart rate based on age. When an aerobic exercise is started, a person should keep the heart rate down toward the lower end of the range, gradually moving toward the higher.

KEY POINT

To find your *target heart rate*, subtract your age from 220. This gives you your *maximum heart rate*. Multiply your maximum heart rate by .50 and .75 to get your *target heart rate range*.

To get aerobic it is easiest to use the legs; remember, the quadriceps are the largest muscles of the body and so they require the most oxygen and, thus, will burn the greatest amount of energy in the shortest amount of time. Examples of moderate activities that use the legs and provide an aerobic workout are listed in Exhibit 4–2.

EXHIBIT 4–2 ACTIVITIES FOR AEROBIC EXERCISE

- Fast dancing for 30 minutes
- Swimming laps for 20 minutes; water aerobics for 30 minutes
- Walking—this includes on a treadmill—for 2 miles in 30 minutes
- Bicycling—either outside or on a stationary bike—for 5 miles in 30 minutes
- Stair walking for 15 minutes
- Jumping rope or jumping on a trampoline for 15 minutes
- Ball sports, such as tennis, handball, racquetball, soccer, or basketball for 15 minutes
- Jogging or running 1.5 miles in 15 minutes

Rebounding or jumping on a trampoline is a particularly beneficial form of exercise. Most forms of aerobic exercise demand the body move forward, or horizontally, along the earth. Running, cycling, swimming, or walking allows the body to move in a measurable distance. Jumping on a rebounder or trampoline, on the other hand, gives the body the unique experience of moving vertically allowing gravity to act upon the cells, tissues, organs, and muscles in a way that literally squeezes out toxins and waste products. This activity also challenges every cell in the body (approximately 60 trillion) to improve integrity, strength, and function. The action of jumping up and down causes the body to adapt to and resist the force of gravity. This act of resistance promotes stronger bones, firmer muscles, and improvement in the circulation of all body fluids. Jumping or rebounding puts exceptional challenge on the venous and lymphatic systems to return the blood and lymph back to the heart. The main restriction to someone developing a rebounding program is lower back pain or injury. Lumbar back injury or strain would prohibit safe and enjoyable jumping.

By engaging in a moderate aerobic activity for at least 20–30 minutes a day, 3–5 days a week, improvements in all areas of mind/body/spirit will be noticed. Changes can usually be seen after 3–5 weeks of starting the exercise program.

KEY POINT

Any aerobic activity you choose will serve you well if you *enjoy* doing it. There is no "right or wrong" movement, if you pay attention to your body. Pain, injury, and discontent are the symptoms of an inappropriate activity. Joy, enthusiasm, and commitment to the habit are indications that an aerobic activity is a well-suited one.

Muscle Strengthening Exercises

Strength is an essential, functional component of much of what we do. The lack of strength is responsible for many injuries. Weight training is useful in developing muscle strength. Lifting weights is good for increasing the size and strength of specific muscles. This kind of training can be useful for people who wish to develop particular muscles or muscle groups for a specific sport in which they are involved. It also is used for bodybuilding.

KEY POINT

- Muscle bulk is attained by using weights, doing 12–20 repetitions.
- Muscle strength is developed by using the heaviest weights manageable by the person, doing 2–6 repetitions.
- Muscle endurance and definition is increased by lighter weights, while doing 40–50 repetitions.

When working out, the principle of overload must be employed. That is, the number of repetitions, the amount of weight, and the speed and intensity of the effort put out, must continually increase if there is to be any real benefit from the practice.

Energy-Building Exercises

Exercise systems such as *Hatha yoga* and *T'ai Chi chuan* are aimed at the development of energy that flows through the external body structure. The process of *Qi* (or *Chi*) development produces an effect in the physical body often seen as increased strength, attention, endurance, and vitality. As you work on your energy you will enhance your physical body.

Hatha yoga develops poise, balance, strength, and amazing agility and limberness. The postures (*asanas*) massage and revitalize the internal organs and harmonize the Qi of the body, imparting internal strength and youthfulness. There is no strain as one assumes the postures and lets the muscles relax and stretch into place. Special attention is paid to alignment of the spine and development of spinal flexibility, because the spine is the center of the energetic and nervous systems and energy blocked here affects the entire system.

Through T'ai Chi Chuan, some of the world's most advanced techniques for the training of the mind and body in harmony are available. In Taoist philosophy the *T'ai Chi*, or the source and terminus of the universe manifest as a unity, is composed of two interacting and complementary forces called *yin* and *yang*. In T'ai Chi Chuan this idea is expressed through a beautiful, coordinated series of postures that through regular practice, develop and coordinate the body, under the control of Qi, to a level of perfection not otherwise attainable. Proper alignment of the spine is maintained and the mind is stilled through the slowness of movement with the focus of attention placed on the lower abdomen.

Any Activity Can Benefit Your Health

Regular structured activity, such as walking, yoga, swimming, trampoline jumping, T'ai Chi, or any number of other movement programs enhances health by causing:

- Muscles to grow
- Metabolism to increase, causing more efficient utilization of the energy of food
- Fat stores to be reduced
- Blood vessels to multiply
- Bones to stay harder
- Thinking processes to be more clear
- Mood to be positive and elevated

An exercise program also promotes vitality and enthusiasm in your relationships. Just as movement of fluids flushes toxins out and allows energy to flow more freely into you, it also opens your social experiences by increasing your confidence and sense of competence.

KEY POINT

The yin/yang concept of balance is promoted in many Eastern philosophies. Applying some of these concepts to movement is helpful when developing a lifestyle fitness program.

Yang energy is assertive, thrusts outward, masculine in nature, and supportive. It is strength and protection; the ability to "stand up for oneself." Developing an aerobic exercise program that uses the largest muscles of the body (thighs or quadriceps) most efficiently circulates blood, strengthens the cardiovasculature, releases toxins through sweat, and in general promotes strength, endurance, and resilience. It is yang activity.

Yin activity, the softer type, is just as necessary for a balanced life. Examples include T'ai Chi and other forms of "moving meditation" and yoga. Yin activity brings oneself inward and quiet. It develops focus, balance, and a sense of "center."

Lifetime fitness means to be active throughout the life span. All that is needed for a lifetime fitness program is finding the activity that resonates with the heart's desire to move. It is best to do the chosen activity at least 3–4 times a week, month to month, season to season. It doesn't take long for the activity to become a habit. Maintaining a regular, realistic, and pleasurable movement program is a key to radiant health. Each individual is the best care-provider and custodian of his or her own heart and soul.

Chapter Summary

Physical fitness is important for people of all ages. Exercise strengthens and tones muscles, improves efficiency of body, enhances cardiovascular function, prevents bone loss, relieves stress, helps reduce chronic pain, speeds healing, elevates mood, sharpens the mind, increases regularity and flow of the gastrointestinal system, promotes lymphatic fluid flow, and normalizes the body's hormonal balance.

Aerobic exercise involves putting ample demand on the muscles to increase their oxygen requirement, thereby causing the heart and lungs to work harder. To gain benefit from aerobic exercise, the heart rate should be maintained within the target heart rate range during exercise. Target heart rate range is the range between maximum and minimum heart rate, calculated by using the individual's age. Other forms of exercise include weight training, which is useful in developing muscle strength, and Hatha yoga and T'ai Chi Chuan, to enhance energy flow. Exercise plans that are sustainable and most effective are those that are regular, realistic, pleasurable, and individualized.

Suggested Readings

Anderson, B., Anderson, J., and Turlington, C. (2003). *Stretching*. Bolinas, CA: Shelter Publications.

Brooks, L. (1999). *Rebounding to Better Health*. Albuquerque, NM: Ke Publishers.

Clark, C. C. (1996). *Wellness Practitioner: Concepts, Research, and Strategies*. New York: Springer.

Douillard, J. (1994). *Body, Mind, and Sport*. New York: 3 Rivers Press.

Hahn, F., Eades, M. R., and Eades, M. D. (2002). *The Slow Burn Fitness Revolution: The Slow Motion Exercise That Will Change Your Body in 30 Minutes a Week*. New York: Broadway Books.

Jahnke, R. (2002). *The Healing Promise of Qi. Creating Extraordinary Wellness Through Tai Chi and Qigong*. New York: McGraw-Hill Contemporary Books.

Khalsa, S. K. (2000). *Kundalini Yoga*. Darya Ganj, New Delhi: DK Publishers.

Kirsh, D. (2002). *Sound Mind, Sound Body. David Kirsh's Ultimate 6-Week Fitness Transformation for Men and Women.* New York: Rodale Press.

Siler, B. (2000). *The Pilates Body. The Ultimate At-Home Guide to Strengthening, Lengthening, and Toning Your Body without Machines.* New York: Doubleday.

CHAPTER 5

IMMUNE ENHANCEMENT: MIND/BODY CONSIDERATIONS

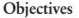

Objectives

This chapter should enable you to:

- Describe the peripheral lymphatic system
- Describe diaphragmatic breathing
- List at least three signs of an imbalanced immune system

The germ is nothing … the terrain is everything.
—Louis Pasteur

It is your immune system's resilience that protects you from overwhelming infection, from getting knocked out cold in the ring of life's daily matches. Your susceptibility to infections and diseases, from the simple cold to catastrophic cancers, is deeply influenced by the health and integrity of the immune system. Likewise, chronic illnesses and imbalances can threaten the immune system.

The reflective saying, "as within—so without" represents a way of understanding immune function. Immune integrity can be viewed as a metaphor of your ability to "stand up for yourself." Just as you need to have a good communication network in your personal and professional lives, you also need exquisite communication pathways between each cell and system within the body.

The immune system represents an understanding of "boundaries" and harmonious living in community with others. Your integrity, resilience, and support lie within the immune system's ability to mobilize, defend, communicate, and hold peace and balance within. A primary role of the immune system is to "serve and protect." The capacity and success of this system to function optimally and be ever vigilant are important aspects of radiant health.

Components of the Immune System

The immune system consists of a lacy network of pathways capable of transporting immune cells throughout the body. It also has a collection of organs, tissues, and cells dispersed strategically throughout the body (Table 5–1). This system is intricately connected to the nervous system (brain) and the endocrine system (hormonal).

The lymph fluid of the body is constantly "oozing" toward the heart from the farthest reaches of the body and is then reintroduced into the general lymphatic circulation. There are two layers of lacy lymph networks just under the skin that return the lymph fluid to the heart. The purpose of these redundant lymphatic pathways is to provide a passage for the return of lymph fluid to the heart.

Keep in mind that lymph fluid is the consistency of an egg white—it is quite thick and moves very slowly. Lymphatic fluid does not have a pump to force it through the body like the heart forces blood with every beat. Lymph fluid movement is dependent on the muscles that provide movement.

Function of the Lymphatic System

All lymph fluid passes through lymph nodes. The lymph nodes are depots where special white blood cells, called T-cells, wait on alert for foreign material, such as bacteria or viruses to be brought into the nodes for identification and security check.

Lymph nodes are located strategically throughout the body. Seventy percent of the body's immune system surrounds the abdominal area. The reason there is a large number of lymph nodes and vessels in the gut is to make sure that all the foreign, non-self material that is ingested becomes user-friendly and beneficial. Imagine the amount of infection and disease you could suffer if you did not have strong, vigilant immunity to counter all of the bacteria and other foreign material that is carried on food or produced by the process of digestion.

The rest of the body's lymph nodes are located where major bones articulate, or meet, and where the body has openings to the outside world. There are lymph nodes at the ankles, knees, around the groin area, elbows, armpits, and chest and chains of lymph nodes along the neck and collarbone.

TABLE 5–1 THE IMMUNE SYSTEM

Component	Function
Spleen	Bloody organ in the upper left quadrant of the abdomen that produces antibodies, maintains cellular immunity, recirculates white blood cells, and receives B cells, T cells, antigens, macrophages, and antigen-reactive cells from the blood.
Bone marrow	Located in the hollow interior of long bones, produces red blood cells and macrophages; B and T cells undergo development here.
Lymph nodes	Pea-shaped organs throughout the body that are connected by a network of vessels that receive drainage and filter antigens from this lymphatic fluid.
Thymus gland	Located beneath the breastbone, this gland reaches its full size in early childhood and then progressively shrinks. It produces and stores T cells.
Other organs	Tonsils are groups of lymphoid tissues located in the throat that contain B and T cells. The appendix, Peyer's patches (accumulations of lymphoid cells under mucous membranes that produce nodules), and intestinal nodes are sites of B-cell maturation and antibody production for the intestinal region.
Cells:	
Macrophages	Large white blood cells produced in bone marrow, responsible for phagocytosis.
B cells	Bone marrow–derived cells that produce antibodies that neutralize or destroy antigens.
T cells	Thymus-derived cells consist of T-helper cells that induce B cells to respond to an antigen and T-suppressor cells that halt specific activity of immunologic response. T-helper and T-suppressor cells are in a delicate balance that must be maintained for adequate immune response.
NK (natural killer) cells	NK cells kill foreign invaders on direct contact without B-cell involvement by producing cytotoxin, a cell poison.

There are two reasons lymph must pass through nodes on its return trip to the heart. One reason is to carry protein molecules to the general circulation because proteins are too big to be circulated back through the venous circulation. This helps keep the fluid levels of the body balanced. The second reason all lymph fluid passes through lymph nodes is to identify *pathogens* (bacteria, fungi, viruses) that are foreign to the body.

The purpose of immune cells is to recognize what is self and what is not self. Just as the eyes sense or recognize what is outside of self and retain a memory of that image for life, so, too, the immune cells recognize and remember for a lifetime an encounter with a particular organism—be it a bacteria, virus, fungi, food, or an environmental allergen. Your immunity provides you with the surveillance mechanism to defend and protect from the day you are born until your last breath.

The immune system is intimately connected to the nervous and endocrine systems. Not only does it respond to physical factors, such as invading pathogens or germs, but also it is very sensitive to your thoughts and emotions. How you think and decide to interpret the world around you influences the kind of activity that either enhances immune resilience or promotes immune disorders.

The immune cells are on patrol and in action every day of your life. They do not die off like skin cells, organ cells, and most other cells of the body that have a particular life span ranging from a day to a few months. Immune cells always perceive and remember the biochemical interactions between self and substances foreign to the body. The cells are mobile and, when optimal conditions exist, able to transport unwanted materials from the body, keeping the host victorious against infection or compromise.

KEY POINT

It is the job of the immune system to maintain balance.

Enhancing Lymphatic Flow

The most important muscle for the movement of your immune system is the diaphragm—the thin, dome-shaped muscle separating the lungs from the abdominal cavity like a parachute. Every deep breath and every step you take has the effect of massaging or oozing lymph fluid along its way. Vigorous deep breathing, as occurs during brisk walking or any aerobic activity, or *conscious breathing*, such as that done in yoga and other meditative practices, enhances the flow of lymph fluid through a type of breathing called *diaphragmatic* or *belly breathing*. Babies come into the world belly breathing and it is something that needs to be re-learned to promote optimal immune function. Deep breathing with the diaphragm is an activity that is extremely useful in improving immune integrity.

KEY POINT

Diaphragmatic breathing is the process of contracting the diaphragm, the thin, dome-shaped muscle covering the stomach and liver, to create a deep inhalation. During the in breath, an effort is made to push the stomach out as the diaphragm flattens down onto the abdomen. This enables the lungs to more fully expand. The rhythm produced by this breathing enhances lymphatic fluid movement and helps milk the removal of toxins and waste products from lymph fluid.

Making a habit of practicing belly breathing is a powerful yet subtle means of stress management. Deep breathing helps the heart beat more regularly and perform more competently. Carbon dioxide is more efficiently removed with diaphragmatic breathing. One will be more alert and fit when the breath is attuned with other rhythms of the body. Changing the breathing style to belly breathing rather than chest breathing will bring more oxygen into the cells, increase the energy available for activity and performance, and enhance the innate harmony between breath, heart rate, sense of well-being, and enthusiasm for life. Belly breathing promotes relaxation and maintains calmness in situations of perceived stress through the action of the diaphragm synchronizing its rhythm with the heart's rhythm and other processes of the body. A state of peace and harmony helps to conserve the immune system.

Physical exercise has the ability to increase the vessels that carry blood and lymph throughout the body. The more vessels available to carry blood and lymph, the more efficiently the heart functions and fluids flow. Just as the Dan Ryan Expressway in Chicago opens its collaterals or extra lanes to accommodate the increased number of vehicles, the body also has the ability to develop collateral circulation to relieve congestion and keep the flow moving easily and effortlessly.

> **KEY POINT**
>
> The job of the peripheral lymphatic system is to clear germs and cancer cells from the body. This lacy network accomplishes this through the massaging movement of the muscles of motion and breathing. Regular physical activity and deep breathing help the efforts of the immune system.

Signs of Imbalanced Immune Function

You may be beginning to notice a relationship between immune integrity, exercise, nutrition, positive attitude, and the other aspects of healthful living. The body and mind are an interconnecting network of systems affecting each another and making up the total being. It is the immune system's lacy network covering the body from the top of the head to the tips of the toes that links the nervous and endocrine systems with thoughts and perceptions. This is why consideration of how well people are in rhythm with themselves and life around them is of equal importance as the quality of the air they breathe or the amount of exercise they get. Social alienation is compromising to the immune system. For example, it has been shown that spouses have a much greater chance of becoming gravely ill during the first year after the loss of their mate than other persons in the same age group. Loneliness and the lack of feeling that you belong to others is as depleting of the immune system as any other essential nutrient deficiency.

Reflection   Immune integrity has as much to do with the quality of your relationships as it does with the quality of your air and water. Are you as concerned about your psychosocial environment as you are with your physical environment?

In addition to physical signs of disease, there are symptoms affecting the mind and spirit that can help people to realize that they are not in balance; these can be categorized under the headings of *disorientation*, *disorganization*, *disidentification*, and *disintegration*. Some questions that can aid in exploring the presence of imbalance are described in Exhibit 5–1.

EXHIBIT 5–1 QUESTIONS TO REVEAL IMBALANCES OF MIND AND SPIRIT

Disorientation. Are you feeling disconnected to your life's calling, your life's purpose? Do you love the work you do or do you grudgingly face the world each day with a dark feeling of being out of sync? Is energy flowing abundantly through you or steadily being drained without replenishment?

Disorganization. Look around you. Does your house and office reflect how you feel about your home or your work? Are your living and work spaces organized and manageable or are you overwhelmed and taken over by stuff that no longer serves you? Do your possessions create a sense of peace and sacredness or bring you stress and frustration?

Disidentification. Are you working on becoming the person you truly want to be? Are you honoring your life's calling? Are you tending to all the others in your life and ignoring your own needs? Do you nourish your spirit and soul?

Disintegration. Are you feeling more torn down than renewed? Do you have regular infections? Are you chronically tired or fatigued? Is there an air of zest and enthusiasm in your daily life?

Boosting Immunologic Health

Diet

In addition to a good basic diet, there are some foods that can positively affect immunity. These include milk, yogurt, nonfat cottage cheese, eggs, fresh fruits and vegetables, nuts, garlic, onions, sprouts, pure honey, and unsulfured molasses. A daily multivitamin and mineral supplement is also helpful; specific nutrients that have immune-boosting effects are listed in Exhibit 5–2. Due to their negative effect on the immune system, intake of refined carbohydrates, saturated and polyunsaturated fats, caffeine, and alcohol should be limited.

Fasting

Fasting, the abstinence of solid foods for 1 to 2 days, is becoming increasingly popular as a means to promote health and healing. The effects of fasting on the immune system include (Chaitow, 1998; Muller, 2001):

- Increased macrophage activity and neutrophil antibacterial activity
- Raised immunoglobulin levels
- Improvement of cell-mediated immunity, ability of monocytes to kill bacteria, and natural killer cell activity
- Reductions in free radicals and antioxidant damage

EXHIBIT 5–2 IMMUNE-ENHANCING NUTRIENTS

Protein

Vitamins A, E, B_1, B_2, B_6, B_{12}, C

Folic acid

Pantothenic acid

Iron

Magnesium

Manganese

Selenium

Zinc

For most persons, a day or two without food is safe; however, an assessment of health status is essential before beginning a fast because some health conditions and medication needs can be altered. Also, it is essential that good fluid intake be maintained during a fast.

Exercise

Any form of exercise, done regularly, can be of benefit to the immune system. Exercise needn't be strenuous; low-impact exercise, such as yoga and T'ai Chi, has a positive effect on immunity. (See Chapter 4 for more information on exercise.)

Stress Management

The thymus, spleen, and lymph nodes are involved in the stress response; therefore, stress can affect the function of the immune system. Some stress-related diseases, including arthritis, depression, hypertension, and diabetes mellitus, cause a rise in serum cortisol, a powerful immunosuppressant. Elevated cortisol levels can lead to a breakdown in lymphoid tissue, inhibition of the production of natural killer cells, increases in T-suppressor cells, and reductions in the levels of T-helper cells and virus-fighting interferon.

Individuals need to identify stress reduction measures with which they are comfortable so that they will practice them on a regular basis. It makes no sense for a person to attempt to engage in meditation if he or she is uncomfortable with that activity, because it will be more stress-producing than stress-reducing. Some stress reduction measures that could be used are progressive relaxation, meditation, prayer, yoga, imagery, exercise, diversional activity, and substitution of caffeine and junk foods with juices and nutritious snacks.

> KEY POINT
>
> The ability of our psychological state to affect physical health is recognized; in fact, the specialty of *psychoneuroimmunology* has emerged in recognition of the fact that thoughts and emotions affect the immune system.

Psychological Traits and Predispositions

Studies have identified traits consistent with strong immune systems to include the following (Cohen, 2002; Cohen and Miller, 2001):

- Assertiveness
- Faith in God or a higher power
- Ability to trust and offer unconditional love
- Willingness to be open and confide in others
- Purposeful activity
- Control over one's life
- Acceptance of stress as a challenge rather than a threat
- Altruism
- Development and exercise of multiple facets of personality

Individuals could improve their immune health by developing and nurturing some of these characteristics.

Reflection How many traits consistent with a strong immune system do you possess? What can you do to nurture those traits and to develop additional ones?

Caring for the Immune System by Caring for Self

As people support and nurture themselves, their immune systems will respond by helping them to feel:

Reorientated   A renewed sense of belonging and purpose. Perceptions of *belonging* and *connectiveness* help people feel grounded and secure. This is in contrast to having perceptions of *alienation* and *aloneness*, which cause the immune system to stay vigilant and on the defense, which can be an exhausting stance over time.

Reorganized   Being able to discern what is and isn't truly needed for one's highest good. This can include letting go of what no longer serves one whether it is old clothes, appliances, or relationships that tear down instead of building up, and making revisions on priorities in life. These are ways that people can empower themselves without the stress of trying to take charge over those things that cannot be controlled.

Reidentified   A renewed definition of one's identity and purpose. This can be achieved through developing ways of nourishing your body, mind, and spirit. Meditation, solitude, and prayer are among the practices that can assist with this.

Reintegrated   A renewed belief and confidence in self. As the mind/body is supplied with what it needs for optimal function there is renewal of hope and zest for life. Reducing the fear and anxiety that people feel about daily life eases the burden on the immune system by reducing its need to protect and defend.

It is the ability to *adapt* and *endure* that gives people healing powers to recover from disease and move from darkness into light. Beliefs can lay the foundation for the body to restructure or reform its physical self. How people think and feel connected has an enormous influence on the strength and vitality of immune function. The health and well-being of the mind and spirit can be just as important to the immune response as nutrition or immune-boosting herbs like echinacea.

There are a variety of additional measures that can assist in enhancing the function of the immune system. Some of these are discussed in the chapters on Healthful Nutrition, Exercise, Flowing with the Reality of Stress, Herbal Remedies, and Environmental Effects on the Immune System.

Chapter Summary

The immune system is a lacy network consisting of organs, tissues, and cells. It monitors the body for disease-producing organisms and initiates defenses to eliminate them.

It is helpful for people to be concerned about the health of their immune systems and to engage in practices to promote immune health. Physical exercise and diaphragmatic breathing promote the movement of lymphatic fluid throughout the body.

Individuals can take action to enhance their immune function, such as eating specific foods, fasting, exercising, managing stress, and developing psychological traits consistent with strong immunity.

An imbalanced immune system can create a variety of physical signs, such as increased ease and frequency of infection. In addition to physical signs, an imbalanced immune system can cause disorientation, disorganization, disidentification, and disintegration.

References

Chaitow, L. (1998). *Antibiotic Crisis: Antibiotic Alternatives*. London: Thorsons.

Cohen, S. (2002). Psychosocial stress, social networks, and susceptibility to infection. In H. G. Koenig and H. J. Cohen eds. *The Link Between Religion and Health: Psychoneuroimmunology and the Faith Factor*. NY: Oxford University Press.

Cohen, S. and Miller, G. E. (2001). Stress, immunity, and susceptibility to upper respiratory infections. In R. Ader, D. Felten, and N. Cohen (eds.), *Psychoneuroimmunology, Third Edition*. NY: Academic Press.

Muller, H. (2001). Fasting followed by vegetarian diet in patients with rheumatoid arthritis: A systematic review. *Scandanavian Journal of Rheumatology, 30*(1):1–10.

Suggested Readings

Ader, R., Felten, D., and Cohen, N. eds. (2001). *Psychoneuroimmunology, Third Edition*. New York: Academic Press.

Cheraskin, E. (1999). Are antibiotics our best choice? *International Journal of Integrative Medicine, 1*(3)36–38.

Fazzari, T. V. (1997). Stability of individual differences in cellular immune responses to acute psychological stress. *Advances: The Journal of Mind-Body Health, 13*(3):36–37.

Gallucci, B. B. (1997). Neuroendocrine and immunological responses of women to stress. *Advances: The Journal of Mind-Body Health, 13*(3):36.

Golczewski, J. A. (1998). *Aging: Strategies for Maintaining Good Health and Extending Life*. Jefferson, NC: McFarland.

Goldsby, R. A., Marcus, D. A., Kindt, T. J., and Kuby, J. (2003). *Immunology*. New York: W.H. Freeman and Company.

Jason, E. and Ketcham, K. (1999). *Chinese Medicine for Maximum Immunity*. Three Rivers, MI: Three Rivers Press.

Moldawer, N. and Carr, E. (2000). The promise of recombinant interleukin-2. *American Journal of Nursing, 100*(5):35–40.

Stern, E. (1997). Two cases of hepatitis C treated with herbs and supplements. *Journal of Alternative and Complementary Medicine: Research on Paradigm, Practice, and Policy, 3*(1):77–82.

CHAPTER 6

FLOWING WITH THE REALITY OF STRESS

Objectives

This chapter should enable you to:

- List the three stages of response to stress that Selye identified
- Define *psychoneuroimmunology*
- Describe different types of stress
- Outline the response of the sympathetic nervous system to stress
- Describe factors to consider in the self-assessment of stress
- List four common elements of stress-reduction measures
- Describe a progressive muscular relaxation exercise
- List at least three measures that can aid in stress reduction

You are unable to escape stress. On a daily basis, people are exposed to numerous events, issues, and circumstances that challenge them. When faced with stress, some people rise to the occasion, thriving and prospering, while others experience a myriad of negative physical and psychological effects. Why is this so? The answer, despite much research on the subject, is not clearly understood, but is strongly connected to how an individual *manages* stress.

95

The Concept of Stress

In the 1950s, Dr. Hans Selye, recognized as the father of stress research, laid the foundation for much of the work that has since unfolded in the field of stress (1). His premise was that all organisms have a similar response when confronted with a challenge to their well-being, regardless of whether that challenge was seen as positive or negative. He called that response the *general adaptation syndrome* (GAS), which he defined as "the manifestations of stress in the whole body, as they develop in time." He identified three stages of the general adaptation syndrome.

KEY POINT

The three stages of response to stress that Selye identified are the *alarm reaction*, the *stage of resistance*, and the *stage of exhaustion*.

The first stage is the *alarm reaction*, more commonly known as the fight-or-flight response, a physiologic process first described by a psychologist, Dr. Walter Cannon, in the early 1900s. In this stage the body gears up physically and mentally for battle or energizes to escape the threat. Often referred to as an *adrenaline rush*, it can be recognized as the pounding heart, dry mouth, cold hands, and knot in the stomach felt when you perceive yourself to be threatened. In the *stage of resistance* the body maintains a state of readiness, but not to the extent of the initial alarm reaction. If the threat is not eliminated and this heightened state of readiness persists, Selye believed that the *stage of exhaustion* would be reached. At this point the body, having spent its existing energy reserves, is no longer able to sustain the workload of constant readiness. It is here that it may begin to fail, resulting in the onset of illness and possibly death.

Decades of continuing research into the mechanisms and effects of stress have yielded much information. However, interpretations of that information vary greatly and are sometimes considered controversial. A major development in the area is the field of *psychoneuroimmunology*. This has brought new definitions of stress that address the mind-body connection, such as the one offered by Seward that stress is "the inability to cope with a perceived or real (or imagined to be real) threat to one's mental, physical, emotional, or spiritual well-being, which results in a series of physiologic responses and adaptations" (2).

KEY POINT

Psychoneuroimmunology is the in-depth study of the interaction of the mind, the central nervous system, and the immune system, and their impact on our health and well-being.

Most authors and researchers now agree that there is a difference in the body's response to good stress and bad stress. Good stress (termed *eustress* by Selye) motivates and has pleasant or enjoyable effects, such as that resulting from a job promotion or a surprise birthday party. Although it causes an alarm response, the strength and duration of that response is usually short lived. Conversely, bad stress (termed *distress* by Selye), like that experienced when involved in a confrontation with a spouse or being involved in a car accident, most often fully initiates the fight-or-flight response and may also have a prolonged impact on your well-being. This distress is what people usually are speaking of when they use the word *stress* (3).

Stress can also be viewed as *acute*, which has a sudden onset and is usually very intense, but ends relatively quickly. The body quickly recovers and the symptoms of acute stress subside. *Chronic stress* is stress that lasts over a prolonged period of time, but may not be as severe or intense as the acute type. Chronic stress is believed to be a major culprit in the development of stress-related diseases (4).

> **KEY POINT**
>
> An example of acute stress could be losing your wallet containing your paycheck. Initially, when you discover you have lost your wallet, your stress level is very high. Once you find your missing wallet under the front seat of your car, the crisis is over.
>
> A prolonged illness of a loved one or lengthy unemployment can cause chronic stress, exhausting all of your coping resources over time.

The Body's Physical Response to Stress

When your brain perceives a threat to your well-being, a series of events made up of chemical reactions and physical responses occurs rapidly. The first of these is the activation of your sympathetic nervous system (SNS), which stimulates the release of *epinephrine* from the outer layer of the adrenal gland (medulla) located on top of the kidney and *norepinephrine*, also from the adrenal glands and from the ends of nerves located throughout our bodies. When these hormones are released, the fight-or-flight response is triggered. Your heart, blood vessels, and lungs are strongly impacted by these hormones. The force and rate of the heart's contractions increase, and the rate and depth of our breathing increases. The *arteries*, vessels carrying oxygen and nutrient-rich blood to your vital organs, widen or dilate to ensure extra blood flow to the heart, lungs, and major muscles. At the same time, the arteries to areas that are not essential (the skin and digestive tract) narrow or constrict. This provides extra blood for the vital organs. One of the other major outcomes of sympathetic nervous system stimulation is a large increase in the production of glucose, your body's primary energy source. The overall net result is an increase in the available amount of glucose and oxygen for the organs and tissues that need it.

Additionally, the pituitary gland, located in the brain, is actively involved in the stress response. The anterior pituitary gland releases a hormone called *adrenocorticotrophic hormone (ACTH)*. This hormone stimulates the outer layer of the adrenal gland (cortex) to release *aldosterone* and *cortisol*. Aldosterone, along with a hormone produced by the posterior pituitary gland *vasopressin* or *antidiuretic hormone*, works to preserve blood volume by limiting the amount of salt and water the kidney is allowed to excrete. Cortisol increases the production of glucose and assists in the breakdown of fat and proteins to provide the additional energy needed to protect the body from the perceived threat. The hormones released during the stress response have many effects on the body (Exhibit 6–1).

Sources of Stress

The sources of stress in daily life are different for each individual. One person may find a 20-mile drive home through a mountain pass after work tedious and frustrating while another may view it as a source of pleasure and relaxation. Other sources of stress can be associated with the physical environment, job, interpersonal relationships,

EXHIBIT 6–1 EFFECTS OF STRESS	
Physiologic	
Increased heart rate	Grinding of teeth
Rise in blood pressure	Insomnia
Dryness of mouth and throat	Anorexia
Sweating	Fatigue
Tightness of chest	Slumped posture
Headache	Pain, tightness in neck and back
Nausea, vomiting	Urinary frequency
Indigestion	Missed menstrual cycle
Diarrhea	Reduced interest in sex
Trembling, twitching	Accident proneness

EXHIBIT 6–1 EFFECTS OF STRESS *(continued)*

Emotional

Irritability	Tendency to cry easily
Depression	Nightmares
Angry outbursts	Suspiciousness
Emotional instability	Jealousy
Poor concentration	Decreased social involvement
Disinterest in activities	Bickering
Withdrawal	Complaining, criticizing
Restlessness	Tendency to be easily startled
Anxiety	Increased smoking
Increased use of sarcasm	Use of drugs or alcohol

Intellectual

Forgetfulness	Errors in arithmetic and grammar
Poor judgment	Preoccupation
Poor concentration	Inattention to detail
Reduced creativity	Blocking
Less fantasizing	Reduced productivity

Work Habits

Increased lateness, absenteeism	Low morale
Depersonalization	Avoidance of contact with coworkers
Excess breaks	Resistance to change
Impatience	Negative attitude
Reluctance to assist others	Carelessness
Verbal or physical abuse	Poor quality and quantity of work
Threats to resign	Resignation

Source: Eliopoulos, C. *Nursing Administration Manual for Long-Term Care Facilities*, 6th ed., Health Education Network, 2001. Reprinted with permission.

past experiences, or psychological makeup. Identifying what stresses them and how they react to that stress is the first step for people to take in developing effective personal stress-management strategies. There are a variety of tools that can help people to identify the stresses in their lives, one of which is offered in Exhibit 6–2.

Reflection   Take a few minutes to complete the self-assessment in Exhibit 6–2. What are the three major stresses in your life that you have identified?

EXHIBIT 6–2 HOLISTIC SELF-ASSESSMENT OF STRESS

There are hundreds of surveys and questionnaires designed to assess one's level of stress. Most, if not all of these, are based on a mechanistic approach to health, not a holistic one (where the whole is considered greater than the sum of parts). The purpose of this self-assessment is to begin to have you look at your problems, issues, and concerns holistically.

1. **First, make a list of your current stressors and explain each one:**

    1. _____

    2. _____

    3. _____

    4. _____

    5. _____

    6. _____

    7. _____

    8. _____

    9. _____

    10. _____

EXHIBIT 6–2 HOLISTIC SELF-ASSESSMENT OF STRESS *(continued)*

2. Next, from the list you have just made, reorganize it into acute (short-term) stressors and chronic (prolonged) stressors.

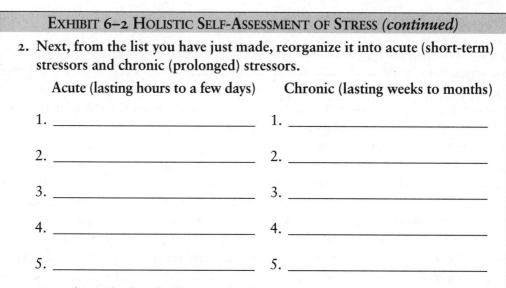

Acute (lasting hours to a few days)	Chronic (lasting weeks to months)
1. _____	1. _____
2. _____	2. _____
3. _____	3. _____
4. _____	4. _____
5. _____	5. _____

3. Now, from the first list you made, determine whether each stressor is mental, physical, emotional, or spiritual.

Mental	Physical	Emotional	Spiritual
			Relationships/
Overwhelmed/ bored	*Injuries/ sickness*	*Anger or fear based*	*Values/Purpose of Life*
1. _____	1. _____	1. _____	1. _____
2. _____	2. _____	2. _____	2. _____
3. _____	3. _____	3. _____	3. _____
4. _____	4. _____	4. _____	4. _____
5. _____	5. _____	5. _____	5. _____

Source: Brian Luke Seward, Ph.D. *Managing Stress: Principles and Strategies for Health and Wellbeing.* 1999, Sudbury, MA: Jones and Bartlett Publishers. Reprinted with permission.

Stress and Disease

As mentioned, the recognition of the link between the mind and the body is not new. However, the specific mechanism to explain the link between stress and disease is still unclear despite years of scientific research. It is widely believed that the impact of stress—especially chronic stress—on the human body greatly increases the risk of developing a variety of diseases such as asthma, arthritis, cancer, hypertension, heart disease, migraine headaches, strokes, and ulcers just to mention a few. Statistics from a variety of sources state that 50 to 90 percent of health-related problems are linked to or aggravated by stress (5,6). Nearly every consumer-oriented publication from hospitals, public health departments, health maintenance organizations, and physician's offices recommends or offers some type of stress-management program.

Most people probably are able to recognize the major physical symptoms of stress in their lives. They also need to be aware of other important behavioral, emotional, or mental symptoms that may be stress related, such as compulsive eating, drinking or smoking, restlessness, irritability or aggressiveness, boredom, inability to focus on the task at hand, trouble thinking clearly, memory loss, or inability to make decisions (7). The self-assessment tool shown in Exhibit 6–3 contains common physical symptoms often related to stress to help people assess how they are affected by stress in their lives. It is helpful for healthcare professionals to encourage people to engage in a self-assessment as a means to gain insight into the impact of stress in their lives. This is not only important to maintaining a state of wellness, but also as part of living with chronic conditions.

Stress-Reduction Measures

Once people recognize the symptoms of stress in their lives they can minimize the impact of stress on their physical, mental, emotional, and spiritual well-being by using one or a combination of measures designed for stress reduction. The ultimate goal of stress reduction or stress management is the *relaxation response*, "a state of profound rest ... of cultivating an attitude of greater equanimity ... of letting go of troubling or worrisome thought... " (8). The term *relaxation response* was first used by Dr. Herbert Benson in his book of the same name. He cites four elements that are essential to and found in most stress-reduction measures (8):

1. A quiet environment
2. A mental device, such as a word or a phrase that should be repeated over and over again

EXHIBIT 6–3 STRESS AND DISEASE: PHYSICAL SYMPTOMS QUESTIONNAIRE

Look over this list of stress-related symptoms and circle how often they have occurred in the past week, how severe they seemed to you, and how long they lasted. Then reflect on the past week's workload and see if you notice any connection.

	How Often? (number of days)	How Severe? (1 = mild, 5 = severe)	How Long? (1 = 1 hour, 5 = all day)
1. Tension headache	0 1 2 3 4 5 6 7	1 2 3 4 5	1 2 3 4 5
2. Migraine headache	0 1 2 3 4 5 6 7	1 2 3 4 5	1 2 3 4 5
3. Muscle tension (neck and/or shoulders)	0 1 2 3 4 5 6 7	1 2 3 4 5	1 2 3 4 5
4. Muscle tension (lower back)	0 1 2 3 4 5 6 7	1 2 3 4 5	1 2 3 4 5
5. Joint pain	0 1 2 3 4 5 6 7	1 2 3 4 5	1 2 3 4 5
6. Cold	0 1 2 3 4 5 6 7	1 2 3 4 5	1 2 3 4 5
7. Flu	0 1 2 3 4 5 6 7	1 2 3 4 5	1 2 3 4 5
8. Stomachache	0 1 2 3 4 5 6 7	1 2 3 4 5	1 2 3 4 5
9. Stomach/ abdominal bloating/ distention/gas	0 1 2 3 4 5 6 7	1 2 3 4 5	1 2 3 4 5
10. Diarrhea	0 1 2 3 4 5 6 7	1 2 3 4 5	1 2 3 4 5
11. Constipation	0 1 2 3 4 5 6 7	1 2 3 4 5	1 2 3 4 5
12. Ulcer flare-up	0 1 2 3 4 5 6 7	1 2 3 4 5	1 2 3 4 5
13. Asthma attack	0 1 2 3 4 5 6 7	1 2 3 4 5	1 2 3 4 5
14. Allergies	0 1 2 3 4 5 6 7	1 2 3 4 5	1 2 3 4 5
15. Canker/cold sores	0 1 2 3 4 5 6 7	1 2 3 4 5	1 2 3 4 5
16. Dizzy spells	0 1 2 3 4 5 6 7	1 2 3 4 5	1 2 3 4 5
17. Heart palpitations (racing heart)	0 1 2 3 4 5 6 7	1 2 3 4 5	1 2 3 4 5
18. TMJ	0 1 2 3 4 5 6 7	1 2 3 4 5	1 2 3 4 5
19. Insomnia	0 1 2 3 4 5 6 7	1 2 3 4 5	1 2 3 4 5
20. Nightmares	0 1 2 3 4 5 6 7	1 2 3 4 5	1 2 3 4 5

	How Often? (number of days)	How Severe? (1 = mild, 5 = severe)	How Long? (1 = 1 hour, 5 = all day)
EXHIBIT 6–3 *(continued)*			
21. Fatigue	0 1 2 3 4 5 6 7	1 2 3 4 5	1 2 3 4 5
22. Hemorrhoids	0 1 2 3 4 5 6 7	1 2 3 4 5	1 2 3 4 5
23. Pimples/acne	0 1 2 3 4 5 6 7	1 2 3 4 5	1 2 3 4 5
24. Cramps	0 1 2 3 4 5 6 7	1 2 3 4 5	1 2 3 4 5
25. Frequent accidents	0 1 2 3 4 5 6 7	1 2 3 4 5	1 2 3 4 5
26. Other (please specify)	0 1 2 3 4 5 6 7	1 2 3 4 5	1 2 3 4 5

Score: Look over the entire list. Do you observe any patterns or relationships between your stress levels and your physical health? A value over 30 points may indicate a stress-related health problem. If it seems to you that these symptoms are related to undue stress, they probably are. While medical treatment is advocated when necessary, the regular use of relaxation techniques may lessen the intensity, frequency, and duration of these episodes.

Source: Brian Luke Seward, Ph.D. *Managing Stress: Principles and Strategies for Health and Wellbeing*, 1999, Sudbury, MA: Jones and Bartlett Publishers. Reprinted with permission.

3. The adoption of a passive attitude (which is perhaps the most important of the elements)

4. A comfortable position

For purposes of clarification, a *passive attitude* is one in which a person is open to a free flow of thoughts without analysis or judgment.

KEY POINT

Numerous studies of the results of stress reduction have demonstrated positive findings to include the reduction of blood pressure in individuals with hypertension, improved sleeping patterns in individuals suffering from insomnia, decreased nausea and vomiting in chemotherapy patients, and reduction in the multiple symptoms of women diagnosed with premenstrual syndrome or who are experiencing menopausal symptoms (9).

Individual preferences and circumstances will influence the selection of stress-reduction measures. Some stress-management techniques are simple, while others require some initial instruction. Regardless of the choice of method or combination of methods, *all* require practice and need to be used on a regular basis to be effective. Nurses and other healthcare professionals provide a valuable service by instructing, assisting, and coaching people in the use of stress-reduction techniques. Some of the specific measures that can be employed are described in the remainder of this chapter.

Exercise

In the early days of human existence most threats were physical and demanded an immediate, intense physical response to ensure survival. The response was literally "fight" or "flight." All the stress hormones released were quickly consumed and their physical effects were diminished in that burst of activity. In today's environment, the majority of the sources of stress are much less physical and more complex. They usually result from cumulative factors, such as multiple, often simultaneous demands at home and at work.

Physical, emotional, and mental well-being depends on finding a way to dissipate the negative effects of those stressors. " ... a single bout of aerobic exercise burns off existing catecholamines and stress hormones by directing them towards their intended metabolic functions, rather than allowing them to linger in the body to undermine the integrity of vital organs and the immune system" (10). A consistent exercise program has also been demonstrated to help decrease the level of reaction to future stressors (11). The key to utilizing exercise for stress reduction is to develop an individualized program that is tailored to one's physical abilities, time constraints, and finances. Additionally, selecting an activity that does not increase stress by emphasizing competitiveness rather than relaxation and enjoyment benefits stress reduction.

Progressive Muscular Relaxation (PMR)

When you are stressed, anxious, angry, or frightened your body automatically responds by increasing muscle tension. You may have experienced the effects of that response resulting in muscular aches and pains in various parts of your body after an unpleasant encounter or a hectic day. Progressive muscular relaxation (PMR) was developed in the 1930s by Dr. Edmund Jacobson, a physician–researcher at the University of Chicago, as a method to reverse this tension and elicit the relaxation response. Moving sequentially from one major muscle group or area of the body to another, for example, from head to toes or vice versa, muscles will be consciously tensed and then relaxed. This conscious muscular activity interrupts the stress response by interfering with the transmission of stress-related tension via the sympathetic nervous system to the muscle fibers.

The physiologic effects of PMR reported by Dr. Jacobson included decreases in the body's oxygen usage, metabolic rate, respiratory rate, and blood pressure. These early findings have been demonstrated in clinical studies with patients diagnosed with hypertension and chronic obstructive lung disease (12). Additionally, PMR has been shown to be a useful pain management tool in some patients with cancer and chronic pain (13).

PMR is relatively easy to learn. The method cited Exhibit 6-4 is only one of the variations on the original technique designed by Dr. Jacobson (14).

Meditation

Meditation is one of the oldest known techniques for relaxation, dating back to the 6th century B.C. There are as many definitions of *meditation* as there are types of

---

EXHIBIT 6–4 PROGRESSIVE MUSCULAR RELAXATION EXERCISE

Progressive muscular relaxation (PMR) can be done from a sitting or lying position and usually takes 20–30 minutes to complete. As you take in a deep breath, tighten or tense individual groups of muscles to the count of five. A common sequence to follow is:

- Forehead
- Eyes
- Jaw
- Neck
- Back
- Shoulders
- Upper arm
- Lower arm
- Hands
- Chest
- Abdomen
- Pelvis/buttocks
- Upper legs
- Lower legs
- Feet

After the completion of the five count, exhale slowly and allow the muscles to relax. This process is repeated twice for each major muscle group or body area.

meditation, but basically it can be understood to be a practice that quiets and relaxes the mind. During a meditative state the individual strives to let go of all connections to physical senses and conscious thoughts. All focus and awareness is turned inward with the ultimate goal of peace and harmony in mind and body (15). As a stress-reduction measure, daily or twice-daily meditation sessions increase resistance to negativity and former stressors, significantly dampening the stress response (16). Studies have shown that anxiety, a major symptom of acute stress, was significantly reduced with the regular use of meditation (17). As stated earlier, there are many techniques for meditation, some with rituals or rules for that specific technique. In *Minding the Body, Mending the Mind*, Joan Borysenko, PhD presents a simple, eight-step process for meditation that is easily understood (18):

1. Choose a quiet spot where you will not be disturbed by other people or by the telephone.
2. Sit in a comfortable position.
3. Close your eyes.
4. Relax your muscles sequentially from head to feet.
5. Become aware of your breathing, noticing how the breath goes in and out, without trying to control it in any way.
6. Repeat your focus word silently in time to your breathing.
7. Don't worry about how you are doing.
8. Practice at least once a day for between 10 and 20 minutes.

Reflection Have you built a time for meditation into your daily routine? If not, why? Consider developing a plan to incorporate this practice into your days for the next week. Designate a quiet space, schedule the time period, and leave yourself a written affirmation (I honor my body, mind, and spirit by taking time to meditate daily). Evaluate your efforts and responses after one week.

Imagery

"Imagery is a mental representation of an object, place, event, or situation" (19). People use images regularly when they describe feelings or concepts in their conversations. For example, when stressed they might say they feel tied up in knots or if they receive recognition from an employer for closing a major deal they may say they feel like they are on top of the world. Those images can convey powerful messages and can be utilized as a stress-reduction method. In her book, *Creative Imagery in Nursing*, Karilee Halo Shames defines two types of imagery: *therapeutic imagery* and *guided imagery*. Therapeutic imagery is a process that "allows us to use the senses and the mind to create whatever it is that we desire, as well as to solve problems and conflicts; in guided imagery the subject is led with specific words, symbols, and ideas to elicit a positive response" (20).

Other

There are other measures that can be used to help reduce stress, such as music therapy, biofeedback, and diversional activities. Other chapters in this book (Herbal Remedies, Aromatherapy, and Humor), offer additional insights into measures that assist with stress management. It is beneficial for the nurse or other healthcare professional to help people understand the dynamics of stress, identify individual sources and responses to stress, develop effective stress-management strategies, and reinforce the significance of efforts to manage stress.

Chapter Summary

Hans Selye identified the three stages of stress as the *alarm reaction*, the *stage of resistance*, and the *stage of exhaustion*. Some stress is positive (*eustress*) in that it motivates or has pleasant effects. *Distress* is the bad stress and has negative effects.

The sympathetic nervous system is activated when a person is stressed, which produces many effects in the body. *Psychoneuroimmunology* is the study of the interaction of the mind, the central nervous system, and the immune system, and their impact on health.

Identifying and understanding stressors is essential in changing the way stress is managed. Elements of most stress-reduction exercises include a quiet environment, a mental word that can be repeated, adoption of a passive attitude, and a comfortable position. Exercise, meditation, and imagery are among the measures beneficial in stress reduction.

References

1. Selye, H. (1984). *The Stress of Life*. New York: McGraw-Hill, pp. 29–40.
2. Seward, B. L. (1999). *Managing Stress: Principles and Strategies for Health and Wellbeing*. Sudbury, MA: Jones and Bartlett, p. 5.
3. Ibid., p. 8.
4. Girdano, D., Everly, G. S., and Dusek, D. E. (1997). *Controlling Stress and Tension*, 5th ed. Boston: Allyn and Bacon, p. 4.
5. Seward, B. L. (1999). *Managing Stress: Principles and Strategies for Health and Wellbeing*. Sudbury, MA: Jones and Bartlett, pp. 38–39.

6. Pelletier, K. R. (1977). *Mind as Healer, Mind as Slayer.* New York: Dell Publishing, p. 7.

7. Stuart, E. M., Webster, A., and Wells-Federman, C. L. (1992). Managing stress. In Benson, H. and Stuart, E. M. eds. *The Wellness Book.* New York: Simon & Schuster, pp. 180–182.

8. Benson, H. (2000). *The Relaxation Response.* New York: HarperTorch, p. 110–111.

9. Domar, A. D. and Dreher, H. (1997). *Healing Mind, Healthy Woman.* New York: Henry Holt and Company, pp. 20–21.

10. Girdano, D., Everly, G. S., and Dusek, D. E. (2000). *Controlling Stress and Tension,* 6th ed. Menlo Park, CA: Addison Wesley, p. 262.

11. DeGeus, E. J. C., Lorenz, J. P., Van Doormen, L. J. P., and Orlebeke, J. F. (1993). Regular Exercise and Aerobic Fitness in Relation to Psychological Make-up and Physiologic Stress Reactivity. *Psychosomatic Medicine,* 55:347–363.

12. Gift, A. G., Moore, T., and Soeken, K. (1992). Relaxation to Reduce Dyspnea and Anxiety in COPD Patients. *Nursing Research,* 41:242–246.

13. Sloman, R. (1995). Relaxation and the Relief of Cancer Pain. *Nursing Clinics of North America,* 30:697–709.

14. Domar, A. D. and Dreher, H. (1997). *Healing Mind, Healthy Woman.* New York: Henry Holt and Company, pp. 52–54.

15. Girdano, D., Everly, G. S., and Dusek, D. E. (2000). *Controlling Stress and Tension,* 6th ed. Menlo Park, CA: Addison Wesley, p. 241.

16. Kabat-Zinn J., Massion A. O., Kristeller, J., Peterson L. G., Fletcher, K. E., Pbert, L, Lenderking, W. R., and Santorelli, S. F. (1992). Effectiveness of a Meditation-Based Stress Reduction Program in the Treatment of Anxiety Disorders. *American Journal of Psychiatry, 149*(7):936–943.

17. Miller, J. J., Fletcher, K., and Kabat-Zinn, J. (1995). Three-Year Follow-up and Clinical Implications of a Mindfulness Meditation-Based Stress Reduction Intervention in the Treatment of Anxiety Disorders. *General Hospital Psychiatry, 17*(3):192–200.

18. Borysenko, J. (1993). *Minding the Body, Mending the Mind.* New York: Bantam Books, pp. 42–44.

19. Post-White, J. (2002). Imagery. In Snyder, M., and Lindquist, R. *Complementary/Alternative Therapies in Nursing.* New York: Springer Publishing Company, p. 103.

20. Halo-Shames, K. (1996). *Creative Imagery in Nursing.* Albany, NY: Delmar Publishers, p. 33.

Suggested Readings

Appel, L. J. (2003). Lifestyle Modification as a Means to Prevent and Treat High Blood Pressure. *Journal of the American Society of Nephrology, 14*(7), (Supplement 2): S99–S102.

Banga, K. (2000). Stress Management: A Step-By-Step Process. *Nurse Educator, 25*(3): 130, 135.

Bartol, G. M. and Courts, N. F. (2000). The Psychophysiology of Bodymind Healing. In Dossey, B. M., Keegan, L., and Guzetta, C. *Holistic Nursing: A Handbook for Practice*, 3rd ed. Gaithersburg, MD: Aspen, pp. 69–88.

Benson, H. and Stuart, E. M. (1992). *The Wellness Book: The Comprehensive Guide to Maintaining Health and Treating Stress-Related Illness*. New York: Simon & Schuster.

Chrousos, G. P. (1998). Stressors, Stress, and Neuroendocrine Integration of the Adaptive Response: The 1997 Hans Selye Memorial Lecture. *Annals of the New York Academy of Sciences*, 851:311–335.

Clark, A. M. (2003). 'It's Like an Explosion in Your Life': Lay Perspectives on Stress and Myocardial Infarction. *Journal of Clinical Nursing, 12*(4):544–553.

Davidson, R. J., Kabat-Zinn, J., Schumacher, J., Rosenkranz. M. N., et al. (2003). Alterations in Brain and Immune Function Produced by Mindfulness Meditation. *Psychosomatic Medicine, 65*(4):564–570.

Eriksson, J., Burell, G., Andersson, H., et al. (2003). A Stress Management Program that Improves Metabolic Control and Blood Pressure in Type 2 Diabetes Patients. *Diabetes*, 52 (supplement): A412.

Forester, A. (2003). Healing Broken Hearts. *Journal of Psychosocial Nursing & Mental Health Services, 41*(6):44–49.

Haight, B. K., Barba, B. E., Tesh, A. S., and Courts, N. F. (2002). Thriving: A Life Span Theory. *Journal of Gerontological Nursing, 28*(3):14–22.

Jones, M. C. and Johnson, D. W. (2000). Reducing Stress in First Level and Student Nurses: A Review of the Applied Stress Management Literature. *Journal of Advanced Nursing, 32*(1):66–74.

Jones, M. C and Johnson, D. W. (1997). Distress, Stress, and Coping in First Year Nursing Students. *Journal of Advanced Nursing, 26*(3):475–482.

Kenney, J. W. (2000). A Women's 'Inner Balance': A Comparison of Stressors, Personality Traits and Health Problems by Age Groups. *Journal of Advanced Nursing, 31*(3):639–650.

Lambert V. A., Lambert, C. E., and Yamase, H. (2003). Psychological Hardiness, Workplace Stress and Related Stress Reduction Strategies. *Nursing and Health Sciences, 5*(2):181–184.

Mimura, C. and Griffiths, P. (2003). The Effectiveness of Current Approaches to Workplace Stress Management in the Nursing Profession: An Evidence-Based Literature Review. *Occupational & Environmental Medicine*, 60(1):10–15.

Richardson, S. (2003). Effects of Relaxation and Imagery on the Sleep of the Critically Ill Adults. *Dimensions of Critical Care Nursing*, 22(4):182–190.

Sapolsky, R. M. (1999). *Why Zebras Don't Get Ulcers*. New York: W. H. Freeman & Company.

Seaward, B. L. (2000). *Managing Stress: Principles and Strategies for Health and Wellbeing*, 2nd ed. Sudbury, MA: Jones & Bartlett.

Seaward, B. L. (1999). *Stressed Is Desserts Spelled Backwards*. New York: Barnes & Noble Books.

Shealy, C. N. (1999). *90 Days to Stress-Free Living*. Boston: Element Books.

Sloman, R. (2002). Relaxation and Imagery for Anxiety and Depression Control in Community Patients with Advanced Cancer. *Cancer Nursing*, 25(6):432–435.

Thorpe, K. and Barsky, J. (2001). Healing Through Self-Reflection. *Journal of Advanced Nursing*, 35(5):760–768.

Yonge, O., Myrick, F., and Hanse, M. (2002). Student Nurses' Stress in the Preceptorship Experience. *Nurse Educator*, 27(2):84–88.

PART II

Developing Healthy Lifestyle Practices

CHAPTER 7

GROWING HEALTHY RELATIONSHIPS

Objectives

This chapter should enable you to:

- Identify the characteristics of a healthy relationship
- Discuss the difference between one's little ego and higher ego
- List four defense mechanisms that people use to protect themselves
- Describe what is meant by a *body memory*
- List at least five personal characteristics that aid in developing healthy relationships

Throughout life we encounter and form innumerable relationships. Each relationship, no matter how loving or distasteful, how short- or long-term it may be, contains within it a storehouse of information about our own and others' unique personalities. Each relationship, should we choose to view it with a new openness of mind, offers a rich opportunity to re-examine our innermost selves and to re-form, if necessary, the ways in which we perceive and behave in our relationships with other people and in given situations.

But how do we determine healthy versus unhealthy relationships; constructive versus destructive ones? How do relationships become so out of control and out of balance, perhaps to the point of ultimately becoming toxic and disease producing to a person's core being? And precisely what can be done to change these uncomfortable or intolerable relationships in which people tend to repeatedly find themselves?

Identifying Healthy versus Unhealthy Relationships

To begin to answer these questions, we first need to know how to identify a healthy relationship.

KEY POINT

A healthy (human) relationship is one in which there is ongoing mutual trust, respect, caring, honesty, and sharing that is given and received in an environment of nonjudgment and unconditional love; an environment that provides a safe place for physical, mental, emotional, and spiritual growth for all persons involved.

A *healthy relationship* can be defined as, "A healthy sense of connection in which two or more persons agree to share hurts, failures, learning, (and) successes in a nonjudgmental fashion (in order) to enhance each other's life potentials" (1). A healthy relationship requires a balance of both healthy dependence and healthy independence (2). (See Table 7–1).

TABLE 7–1 TASKS IN HUMAN DEVELOPMENT AND FORMATION OF HEALTHY AND UNHEALTHY BOUNDARIES

Development of Healthy Boundaries and Relationships	Tasks*	Approximate Age in First Cycle	Realm of Being	Development of Unhealthy Boundaries and Relationships	Stage in Recovery
• Continued search for self and God • Recycles many of the items listed below	Be Co-create Extend love Transcend ego Self-realize	Later in life, usually second half, when a sense of self that can let go is developed	Spiritual	• Continued search for self and God • Possibility for adult-child healing including working through healthy developmental tasks and boundaries • Recycle most of below	3
• Explores intimate relationships	Recycle	19		• Dysfunctional attempts at intimate relationships	
• Struggle for further self-identity			Emotional	• Continued distorted boundaries and sense of self	
• Begins to separate from parents and family	Evolve and grow	13		• Unhealthy separation from parents and family	
• Continues developing healthy social roles	Regenerate (heal)			• Social roles a detriment to self	
• Continues exploring, with a growing sense of self	Evaluate Develop morals, skills, and values Create (make)	6		• Parents, parent figures, and others continue to stifle the child's healthy exploring and self-esteem	

TABLE 7–1 TASKS IN HUMAN DEVELOPMENT AND FORMATION OF HEALTHY AND UNHEALTHY BOUNDARIES

Development of Healthy Boundaries and Relationships	Tasks*	Approximate Age in First Cycle	Realm of Being	Development of Unhealthy Boundaries and Relationships	Stage in Recovery
• Continues learning how he is the same and different from others	Master	4		• Distortion of sameness into codependence and differentness into low self-esteem	2
• Models behavior and thinking after parents and close others	Cooperate	3			
• Parents begin to let go of (A) below, allowing child to individuate	Think		Mental	• Unhealthy boundaries are solidified by parent's modeling and demanding boundaries are too rigid and/or too loose	
• Begins to test limits	Separate	2			
• Begins to realize is separate from parents and begins to explore the world in more depth	Initiate Explore			• Wounded themselves, parents disallow child to separate and explore for itself	1
• Mother-infant symbiosis helps infant organize perceptions and feelings in a healthy giving and receiving, similar to a sort of "healthy projective identification" (A)	Trust Feel Love	1	Physical	• Narcissistic or otherwise distracted parents mistreat and mold infant to be an extension of their wants and needs. Parents may also neglect children causing an insecure, fragile environment	0
• Older infant believes he is an extension of his parents	Connect			• Same as healthy	
• Infant believes he is a part of and is fused with parents. Parents begin to "mirror" (See A above)	Be	0		• Same as healthy	

* We recycle through these tasks regularly throughout our life. Healthy adolescents repeat the first 14 to 16 tasks. Parents usually cycle in parallel with their children.

In order to form healthier relationships it is necessary for people to learn about:

- Their own unique personalities and idiosyncrasies
- The defensive coping mechanisms they use to react or respond to unconscious or conscious emotions, such as anxiety, anger, fear, conflict, loneliness, envy, and jealousy

This learning *may* best take place in the context of a professional yet trusting relationship with a mental health professional and involve the gradual conscious experiencing of previously unconscious (or unrecognized) feelings (3). This process or journey, though at times painful and difficult, can lead to new insights and ways of feeling and being that, perceived through a positive lens, can fill one's life with an expanded consciousness creating richer meaning and healthier patterns or ways of living and relating to others.

KEY POINT

> To take relationships beyond the human sphere, you must also include those you have with yourself, the universe, the planet, animals, your work, your hobbies, material objects, such as money; behaviors, such as eating, smoking, and alcohol consumption; and even the relationships you form with your own bodily illnesses and pain, to mention only a few.

Your Relationship to Self

The most important relationship you will ever form is the one you create with your true self. This is also the only relationship over which you will ever have any actual or ultimate control. Because the way you relate to your own self significantly impacts how you choose to relate to others, it is imperative, before delving into external or *other* relationships, that you take a look at the meaning of *self* and the inner relationships you have formed with aspects of your many *selves* rooted in your earliest experiences, learning, perceptions, and understanding.

You might think of yourself as consisting of two major selves: your *lower, false self* or *little ego*, and your *authentic, divine self* or *higher ego*. The little ego is the part of you that is dominated and controlled by the emotion of fear. It is the part that creates such feelings as *not good enough, not deserving enough, not smart enough;* all of those *not enoughs* prevent you from moving forth to pursue and manifest your dreams. In contrast, your higher ego is defined and directed by the emotion of unconditional love (4). With your higher ego as your guiding force, you find that you genuinely love yourself and others. This kind of love allows you to believe in yourself and have the confidence that whatever you seek to do or be in life can be envisioned and created in abundance.

Reflection Are there any not enoughs *that limit you? How do they affect your life?*

Love and fear are the two basic emotions from which all other emotions evolve and it is difficult for these two emotions to co-exist within one simultaneously. Unfortunately, most people operate from the perspective of their little ego. They choose to see possibilities as *im*possibilites. Relationships often have an underlying theme of, "Sure, they like me now, but when they find out who I *really* am, they won't want anything to do with me." Their little ego is deathly afraid of being found out, and so they may go about presenting a false face and, consequently, a false self to the world. This classically represents the wisdom of the words, "As within, so without." In the fear of confronting and coming to know the true self, they hide it both in their relationship to their inner self and in their outer relationships with others.

Carl Jung, one of the most renowned and respected psychiatrists of our time, contended that each of our personalities is structurally made up of four archetypes or models, and that these archetypes significantly influence our interpersonal behaviors and (therefore) our relationships. His four models include our *persona*, the social mask or face that we reveal to the public, our *shadow*, the parts of ourselves that we disown or deny, our *anima-animus*, the part of us that contains both our male and female characteristics, and our *self*, the part of the personality Jung considered the most significant because it embodies each person's longing for unity and wholeness. Jung also believed that the goal of personality development is self-realization, or, as I would interpret this, a remembering, realizing, and reclaiming of our true, authentic self. In our process of seeking and finding our selfhood, Jung proclaimed that we as human beings are transformed from biological creatures into spiritual individuals (5).

The Search for the Authentic Self

We begin to develop our relationships as infants and young children as we watch and interact with significant people in our lives—parents, siblings, grandparents, extended family and friends, and other authority figures—and to our environment in general. As we grow, we listen, observe, and absorb what is being said and acted out around us. We see how the authority figures in our lives respond and react to different situations and people. And with them as our role models, we tend to embrace the same or similar kinds of patterns in our own lives. If there is a lot of fear and anxiety within the family unit, we may tend to react with that same kind of fear. If there is trust and contentment, our responses, rather than spontaneous defensive reactions, tend to be on a more trusting, calm, and balanced plane. In most families, there will be a mixture of these types of feelings, behaviors, reactions, and responses. Depending on their individual makeups, people perceive, think, and feel about situations and relationships in their own unique ways.

Children from the same households with the same parents and circumstances, and with very little, if any, notable differences in upbringing, are often extremely different personality-wise.

There are numerous theories as to why individual differences exist. One, of course, has to do with genetic makeup. One child may "take more" after one side of a family or individual in that family. Another contributing factor is the manner in which one chooses to perceive given events, situations, or people. What one person chooses to take personally and get extremely upset or fearful about, another may take in stride with an attitude of calmness and trust and a certain *knowing* that all will work out as it needs to. If the stimuli in a given situation is overwhelmingly negative, people may develop misperceptions about the world as a whole. They may decide that *all* people, good or bad, are not to be trusted, and that *all* situations are either black or white with no gray in between (6). When young, people are essentially powerless over the circumstances of where and with whom they live. If people are abused or perceive themselves as being wounded in some way, it is natural to look for ways to deny, escape, manipulate, react, or do whatever it takes to ultimately survive in settings that may otherwise be intolerable or literally destructive to their very bodies, minds, souls, and spirits.

Through ages seven or eight, people are much like sponges soaking up whatever is taking place within the world. They have not yet formed any type of protective psychological barrier or screen through which they can filter or sort out the tremendous amount of information and stimuli that is being received. They are left to deal with overwhelmingly negative people, circumstances, and stimuli, with both the good and the bad in life, in the best ways they can manage.

KEY POINT

When so-called childhood nurturers fail to heal from the wounds of their childhood, there is a strong probability that their wounds will impact their children.

Few people enter adulthood with a totally positive self-esteem. Within most people, there dwells a significant amount of unhealed toxic shame. This shame is the result of low self-esteem born out of painful childhood situations in which people had no ability or permission to choose, and during which times their innermost selves felt vulnerable and inappropriately exposed (7). The psyche was stripped naked. Over and over they may have been told negative things about themselves and even called names that were demeaning. This type of relating from role models cultivated fear and distrust, not only of and for them, but, because of the childhood inability to see themselves apart from their role models, it also created fear and distrust within themselves. People can grow to literally hate aspects of themselves that were identified as the bad, negative, or ugly child. And throughout their lives, until they begin to recognize and heal those self *mis*perceptions, they are doomed to repeat the same words, feel the same feelings, and, in essence, play the same tapes over in their minds that prove to them again and again that they are not good or competent human beings, and that no matter what they do, it is never enough.

Even if people didn't grow up in the worst of circumstances, they face problems and difficulties that require the development of some type of coping strategies. What must be emphasized here is the fact that in given circumstances, whether what has happened in the past or what is happening in the present is perceived rightly or wrongly, people develop their own unique coping mechanisms that actually work or at least work well at certain times and in given situations.

In the physical realm, people *appear* to be totally separate from others, and given that perception, they naturally form certain defense and coping patterns that serve to act as barriers to anyone or anything that may seem a threat to their well-being. However, from the holistic perspective, there is no such thing as true separation. The body is an energy field that interconnects energetically to others by the vast oceanic universe in which we live (8).

> **KEY POINT**
>
> Some of the more common defense mechanisms used by people in efforts to protect themselves include *denial, displacement, rationalization,* and *regression.*
>
> *Denial* allows people to refuse to see anything that may cause pain or that they don't want or know how to deal with.
>
> *Displacement* causes people to place blame on other people or situations rather than taking on personal responsibility for whatever is happening in their lives.
>
> *Rationalizations* are simply mental justifications for the inappropriate actions, feelings, and thoughts people have.
>
> *Regression* is a reverting back to more primitive or childish behaviors, such as whining, pouting, yelling, cursing, and even physical hitting or beatings. It occurs when feeling out-of-control and is connected to feelings of loss of control or power.
>
> These unhealthy coping mechanisms, along with a large score of others, are fear-based and create barriers between people that block the ability to form loving, intimate relationships.

Intimacy versus Isolation, Love versus Fear

The coping mechanisms that people develop, as noted previously, may have helped them to survive the otherwise intolerable times in their lives. It is only later, when they are older and free from a toxic family and/or environment that they may undergo an "ah-ha" experience. At this time they realize that these particular ways of relating, these old patterns of behavior, are simply not working for them any longer. They may feel a desperate need to change, to relate differently, but they simply don't know how.

Old patterns of thinking and behaving can become so entrenched, so much a part of who a person is, that even the *suggestion* of change can feel too overwhelming, frightening, and threatening.

The process of change can feel as though some sort of death is occurring. And, in a very real sense, this is true. Even though people are not *really* dying—they actually are healing and transforming old parts of themselves—but the very act of moving through that incredible process can feel extremely scary. Anytime people go from what is familiar and "fits like an old shoe," and metaphorically step into a new pair of shoes representing a new, unknown, and unfamiliar world, their natural human instinct is to resist. Intellectually, they may realize that the changes they are choosing to make are all in their own best interest. Still, their emotional tendency is to hold tight to what has felt right for such a long time.

It is at times such as these that the soul is searching to find what has been missing from life all along. People begin to develop an awareness that there are others who appear to have something missing from them. That something, though it may not be easily identified or defined right away, is the ability to love and form intimate relationships without the anxiety and fear of rejection or abandonment.

Reflection Intimacy *is the ability to form close or intense (as in marriage) relationships in which you share your life easily and openly with others who have also developed this capacity. With whom do you share intimate relationships? Are they satisfying? Nurturing?*

Intimate relationships do not have to be limited to other humans. People can form them with pets, certain causes that they support, or their creative efforts. When we think about marriage or any relationship akin to a lifelong partnership between two people, intimacy grows out of the capacity these two people have for mutual love and their ability to pledge a total commitment to each other. This intimacy goes far beyond any sexual relationship they may have. Rather than a person, this type of commitment could be formed with a particular career, cause, or endeavor that one chooses to devote his or her life. No matter with whom or what one decides to become intimately involved, personal sacrifices will be made in the giving of self. The ability for this kind of intimacy is learned when, as children, people have been the recipients of unconditional love and of giving within their family unit (9).

The inability to form intimate relationships results in withdrawal, social isolation, and loneliness. People may seek what they think is intimacy through numerous superficial friendships or sexual contacts. No career is established; instead they may have a history of job changes. Or, they may so fear change that they remain most or all of their adult lives in undesirable job situations (9).

Body Memories as Blocked Manifestations of Relating

In the holistic framework, your body does not end with your skin. Surrounding you are mental, emotional, and spiritual subtle bodies that are invisible to the average human eye. These bodies are sometimes referred to as *auras* and are reported to be seen by certain people who are sensitive to that particular energy. When all of these bodies are in harmony, both with your internal and external worlds, there is a constant circulating free flow of energy. However, when that balance is disturbed and the energy is blocked on one or more levels, you experience imbalance and disharmony. Left unattended and untreated, the imbalance eventually leads to discomfort and/or disease on all levels. These energetic "holding patterns," or *body memories*, can be and often are, literally *stuck* emotions within your physical, mental, emotional, and/or spiritual bodies.

By definition, body memories are events stored within the physical body at the cellular level. These memories may be of a pleasant or unpleasant quality. Body memories may be of a conscious or unconscious nature. It appears that some type of stimulus is necessary for recall, especially of traumatic memories. Body memories of an unconscious nature tend to be more traumatic in origin; they contain strong emotions related to the event, and are thought to manifest as frozen or blocked energy inside the body making them more resistant to recall (10).

Jung noted that illness of any kind—including mental, physical, emotional, and spiritual—originates, for the most part, from disharmony between different aspects of one's perceived self (11). An individual only heals completely by addressing every facet of the whole; each person is responsible for his or her own healing. How much you choose to heal is a decision that you, as a responsible individual, must make.

Every relationship encountered, be it with a friend or perceived foe, brings back a part of self that was missing. And when that part resonates within, it is transformative, drawing a person closer to wholeness. Healing seldom, if ever, occurs in a vacuum. Healing doesn't involve or affect just one person. Rather, people are continually, whether knowingly or unknowingly, consciously or unconsciously, participating together as copartners in healing—in their relationships with others, and their relationship with the planet and a higher power.

The Role of Forgiveness in Relationships

He drew a circle that shut me out—
Heretic, rebel, a thing to flout.
But love and I had a way to win:
We drew a circle that took him in

Unknown

More than any other quality in your life, the ability to forgive is the key to inner peace. Mentally, spiritually, and emotionally, it transforms fear into love. Many times the perceptions of other people and situations become a battleground between the ego, or the lesser self's desire to judge and find fault, while the higher authentic self desires to accept people as they are. The lesser ego is a relentless fault finder in both self and others. However, the places in which a person estranges from love are not faults, but wounds. The authentic self seeks out its innocence and never seeks to punish, but rather to heal self and others.

KEY POINT

Forgiveness is selective remembering—a conscious decision to focus on love and let the rest go (12). It is easy to forgive those who have never done anything to make you seriously upset or angry. However, it is the people who trigger you, who push your buttons, who create fear and self-doubt, who are your best teachers. They measure your capacity to love unconditionally. And it is this very love that brings healing to all the lives involved, including your own.

Why, a person might ask, would I *not* judge or find fault with something I know to be wrong? The emphasis here needs to be placed on the behavior or the action as opposed to the person. When one perceives the action and the person as the same, it is impossible to see the person as innocent and his or her actions as unhealed wounds.

Personal Characteristics in the Development of Healthy Relationships

Dorothea Hover-Kramer (1) has identified eight major personal characteristics that can be tremendously helpful in developing healthy relationships. The following is a modification of her list:

1. Being willing to take a genuine look at one's own faulty personal defenses and blind spots and begin the process of identifying and letting go of these defense patterns

2. Creating a correct sense of self-worth, confidence, and self-esteem; having no grandiosity, yet not putting oneself down

3. Developing flexibility; looking at people and situations from different perspectives; a willingness to "walk in another's shoes"

4. Developing a willingness to take personal responsibility for all of one's feelings or actions

5. Setting conscious awareness of one's spiritual essence and wholeness experienced as a sacred space of inner calm, and setting boundaries that allow for a clear sense of purpose, goal orientation, and direction

6. Making the effort to be understood, persevering to find common ground; seeking and integrating (genuinely taking in) feedback

7. Developing sincere empathy and mutual respect for others without appeasing, complying, or attempting to be overly pleasing

8. Committing oneself to a willingness to revisit, rethink, and redefine previous decisions; accepting the possibility of being wrong and allowing others the space to acknowledge their mistakes

These are characteristics that can be easily identified in effective communicators and negotiators. They bring integrity and balance to the art and skill of successful communication, which is necessary to the building, maintenance, and enhancement of healthy relationships.

In his book, *The Seven Spiritual Laws of Success*, Deepak Chopra (13) also outlines principles for success in life that correlate and correspond with what it takes to have, maintain, and grow healthy relationships. His seven principles, as described here, summarize all that has been talked about in this chapter toward growing healthy relationships. Chopra strongly emphasizes that success is a journey, not a destination and you should never expect to "arrive"; that you will continue throughout your life to learn and hopefully grow from your experiences.

The first need on Chopra's list of seven laws is that of daily *stillness*; meditation or prayer time during which people can go within and listen to the silence from which comes the wisdom of their spiritual and innermost beings. It is through this silence that they ultimately get in touch with their ability to heal old faulty ways of thinking and behaving, to manifest and create their bliss; and it is also through this practice that, over time, they come to realize that low self-esteem (relationship to self) combined with a large dose of fear and negative thinking are the only barriers between themselves and what they desire most in life.

Giving is another crucial ingredient for successful relationships. What is given doesn't have to be extraordinary, but it does have to be genuine. It may take time, energy, and monies that could be spent elsewhere, and experiencing life as more pleasant and less demanding in that moment. This type of giving does not demand nor expect anything in return and is given in the spirit of unconditional love.

Receiving, the third component, can be the hardest for many people. If people grew up never feeling worthy or deserving, then accepting anything given freely to them by others can be most difficult. In order to grow they need to have the ability to receive. Chopra notes that it is helpful to affirm oneself with such thoughts as, "Today I will gratefully receive all the gifts that life has to offer me, including the gifts of sunlight, birds singing, spring showers, or the first snow of winter. I will be open to receiving from others and will make a commitment to keep (positive relationships) circulating in my life by giving and receiving life's most precious gifts: the gifts of caring, affection, appreciation, and love"(14).

Next comes acute awareness of the choices made in each moment and how, in the mere witnessing of these choices, they are brought into conscious realization. One begins to understand that the best way to prepare for any future moment is to be fully conscious in the present.

Acceptance of people, situations, circumstances, and events as they occur is another key part of fully entering into a state of peace with self, others, and the world. One can know that the moment is as it should be and consciously choose not to struggle against what cannot be changed.

KEY POINT

When people accept, they take *responsibility* for problems, choosing not to blame anyone or anything (including themselves) for what is happening. Rather, they recognize all events and situations as opportunities in disguise … opportunities that they can take and transform into a greater benefit for all involved.

It is necessary, says Chopra, that awareness remain established in defenselessness. People must let go of the need to defend their point of view. The need to persuade or convince others to accept a point of view is a use of energy that could be much better spent elsewhere. Remaining open to all points of view and not rigidly attaching to any one of them, allows for a plethora of choices and opportunities that people may have been blind to within their defensiveness.

Chopra's seventh and last principle is that of *detachment*. Detachment, he says, allows an individual and others the freedom to be who they are and travel their life paths as they must, while remaining unattached to the outcome. This detachment does not mean that people don't care. On the contrary, they deeply care and are concerned about those with whom they relate. And they are there for others in loving, caring ways. But once again, they must not interfere or try to do others' processes for them. People must learn in their own way and at their own pace what feels right for them. They may have later come to the conclusion that a person who gave them advice was right all along, but what is significant is that they chose to act on it in their own time and at their own pace.

Reflection Do you tend to force your opinions and advice on others when you are confident that you know what is in their best interest? If you think for just a moment about how resentful and angry you felt when others have attempted to take over or force your choices in a particular direction, it doesn't take long to see how your attempts to do the same with others can so easily backfire.

As people begin to understand and absorb the principles Chopra outlines, they can gradually unblock painful and disease-producing energy that has been kept in, and in doing so, allow that energy to become more balanced and free flowing. This action frees them to discover their unique talents and to create and manifest long held dreams. At the same time they also are freed up to serve and respond to others with an unconditional and unbounded love.

In this global, multicultural world, people are continually encountering a wide variety of people from different cultures, beliefs, backgrounds, skills, and education. Access to advanced technology through the Internet and other avenues has given people the means to bring different parts of the world right into their own homes. In doing so, they are forced to a greater extent than ever before, to deal with other people, cultures, ideas, information, and beliefs that may be profoundly different from their own. However, if individuals are willing to crack the door to the possibility of experiencing a new consciousness, they can begin the step forward toward the creation of richer, healthier relationships and lives filled with an abundance of experiences, learning, and growth that previously would have been unimaginable.

Chapter Summary

A healthy relationship is one in which there is ongoing mutual trust, respect, caring, honesty, and sharing that is exchanged in an environment of nonjudgment and unconditional love. Learning about oneself fosters the building of healthy relationships.

Healthy relationships are not built on neediness, but on love and caring. Major personal characteristics are helpful in developing healthy relationships, such as a willingness to look at oneself honestly, creating a realistic sense of self-worth, flexibility, being aware of spiritual essence, making an effort to be understood, having empathy and respect for others, and acknowledging one's own mistakes.

Deepak Chopra describes seven laws of success that include the need for stillness, giving, receiving, awareness of choices, acceptance of people and circumstances, defenselessness, and detachment. With an understanding of these principles, people can gradually unblock painful and disease-producing energy that has been long held within, and be freed to serve and respond to others with an unconditional and unbounded love.

References

1. Hover-Kramer, D. (2000). In Dossey, B. M., Keegan, L., and Guzzetta, C. E. eds. *Holistic Nursing: A Handbook for Practice*, 3rd ed. Gaithersburg, MD: Aspen, p. 642.
2. Whitfield, C. L. (1991). *Co-Dependence: Healing the Human Relationship*. Deerfield Beach, FL: Health Communications, Inc.
3. Lego, S. (1985). Psychoanalytically oriented individual and group therapy with adults. In Critchley, D. L. and Maurin, J. T. eds. *The Clinical Specialist in Psychiatric Mental Health Nursing: Theory, Research and Practice*. New York: John Wiley & Sons Publications, Inc., p. 196.
4. Bradshaw, J. (1988). *Healing the Shame That Binds You*. Deerfield Beach, FL: Health Communications, Inc.
5. Carson, V. B . and Arnold, E. N. eds. (2000). *Mental Health Nursing: The Nurse-Patient Journey*, 2nd ed. Philadelphia: W. B. Saunders & Co.
6. Burns, D. D. (1990). *The Feeling Good Handbook*. New York: Penguin Group.
7. Bradshaw, op cite.
8. Manhart-Barrett, E. A. ed. (1990). *Visions of Rogers' Science-Based Nursing*. New York: National League for Nursing, p. 119.
9. Townsend, M. C. (2003). *Psychiatric Mental Health Nursing: Concepts of Care*. Philadelphia: F. A. Davis Co., pp. 44–45.
10. Belcher, I. W. *Body Memory: In Search of a Definition*. (Unpublished Masters Thesis, Georgia State University, 1995).
11. Jacobi, J. and Hull, R. F. C. ed. (1973). *C.G. Jung: Psychological Reflections: A New Anthology of His Writings 1905–1961*, Princeton, NJ: Princeton University Press.
12. Williamson, M. (1996). *A Return to Love: Reflections on the Principles of a Course in Miracles*, New York: HarperCollins.

13. Chopra, D. (1995). *The Seven Spiritual Laws of Success: A Practical Guide to the Fulfillment of Your Dreams*, San Rafael, CA: co-published by Amber-Allen Publishing and New World Library, p. 2.
14. Ibid., p. 36.

Suggested Readings

Autry, J. A. (2002). *The Spirit of Retirement. Creating a Life of Meaning and Personal Growth.* New York: Prima Press.

Barnum, B. S. (2003). *Spirituality in Nursing.* 2nd ed. New York: Springer Publishing Company.

Bender, M., Bauchham, P., and Norris, A. (1999). *The Therapeutic Purpose of Reminiscence.* Thousand Oaks, CA: Sage.

Borysenko, J. (1998). *A Woman's Book of Life: The Biology, Psychology, and Spirituality of the Feminine Life Cycle.* New York: Riverhead Books.

Carson, V. B. and Arnold, E. N. eds. (2000). *Mental Health Nursing: The Nurse-Patient Journey*, 2nd ed. Philadelphia: W. B. Saunders & Co.

Carter-Scott, C. (1998). *If Life Is a Game, These Are the Rules.* New York: Broadway Books.

Cary, C. (1998). *A Foxy Old Woman's Guide to Living with Friends.* Freedom, CA: Crossing Press.

Conway, J. (1997). *Men in Midlife Crisis.* Colorado Springs, CO: Chariot Victor Publishers.

Cox, A. M. and Albert, D. H. (2003). *The Healing Heart: Communities.* Gabriola Island, Canada: New Society Publishers.

Felton, B. S. and Hall, J. M. (2001). Conceptualizing Resilience in Women Older than 85: Overcoming Adversity from Illness or Loss. *Journal of Gerontological Nursing, 27*(11):46–53.

Hertz, J. E. and Anschutz, C. A. (2002). Relationships Among Perceived Enactment of Autonomy, Self-Care, and Holistic Health in Community Dwelling Older Adults. *Journal of Holistic Nursing, 20*(2):166–186.

Hillman, J. (1999). *The Force of Character and the Lasting Life.* New York: Random House.

Kaiger-Walker, K. (1997). *Positive Aging: Every Woman's Quest for Wisdom and Beauty.* Berkeley, CA: Conari Press.

Lemme, B. H. (1999). *Development in Adulthood*, 2nd ed. Boston: Allyn & Bacon.

Levey, J. and Levey, M. (1998). *Living in Balance. A Dynamic Approach for Creating Harmony and Wholeness in a Chaotic World.* New York: MJF Books.

McGinnis, A. L. (1997). *The Balanced Life. Achieving Success in Work and Love.* Minneapolis, MN: Augsburg Press.

Moore, S. L., Metcalf, B., and Schow, E. (2000). Aging and Meaning in Life: Examining the Concept. *Geriatric Nursing, 21*(1):27–29.

Puentes, W. J. (2000). Using Social Reminiscence to Teach Therapeutic Communication Skills. *Geriatric Nursing, 21*(3):318–320.

Quadagno, J. S. (1999). *Aging and the Life Course: An Introduction to Social Gerontology.* Boston: McGraw-Hill College.

Semmelroth, C. (2002). *The Anger Habit Workbook. Proven Principles to Calm the Stormy Mind.* Calrsbad, CA: Writers Club Press.

Snowden, D. (2001). *Aging with Grace: What the Nun Study Teaches us about Leading Longer, Healthier, and More Meaningful Lives.* New York: Random House.

Thomas, E. L. and Eisenhandler, S. A. (1999). *Religion, Belief, and Spirituality in Late Life.* New York: Springer.

Thomas, K. (1999). *Simplicity. Finding Peace by Uncluttering Your Life.* Nashville: Broadman and Holman Publishers.

Wallace, S. (2000). Rx RN: A Spiritual Approach to Aging. *Alternative and Complementary Therapies, 6*(1):47–48.

Wilt, D. L. and Smucker, C. J. (2001). *Nursing the Spirit.* Washington, D.C.: American Nurses Publishing.

Wolf, T. P. (2003). Building a Caring Client Relationship and Creating a Quilt. A Parallel and Metaphorical Process. *Journal of Holistic Nursing, 21*(1):81–87.

CHAPTER 8

SURVIVAL SKILLS
FOR FAMILIES

Objectives

This chapter should enable you to:

- List at least five types of families
- Describe at least three assumptions about families
- Discuss the body, mind, and spirit of a family
- Outline at least six questions that can be used to explore the balance of work and family needs
- Describe seven major components of a Healthy Options Assessment
- List the six steps of goal setting
- Describe what is meant by holistic parenting

Family is a word that represents something very personal, yet common, to each of us. Families can be youthful, seasoned, single-parented, childless, multigenerational, married or partnered, divorced, or blended.

Reflection What meaning does family *hold for you? Examining your personal beliefs about the meaning of family and the cultural and social influences that surround* family *is one step towards developing successful survival skills as a family.*

The last three decades have seen a major shift in the composition of the American family. During the 1960s and 1970s much attention was given to the nuclear family.

According to Michael Gordon this term refers to a unit consisting of husband, wife, and dependent offspring (1). In *The Ties That Stress* Dr. David Elkind points out (2):

> In the 1960s the demands for recognition and legitimization of human diversity ... by minorities, women, and gays, among others ... challenged the idea that only one kind of kinship structure was suited to the function of meeting the emotional needs of family members. The postmodern permeable family includes not one but many different relationship patterns.

This type of family structure—the *permeable family*—evolved because of influences such as the civil rights movement, the women's movement, and the acceptability of premarital sex. This shift created a structure where the rules and boundaries became less clear and continually in flux (3).

KEY POINT

Anyone who is a member of any of the following groups may be acutely aware that our culture still has a long way to go in learning about and respecting all types of families:

- Blended families
- Single-parent families
- Families with one child
- Families with many children
- Same gender partner families
- Grandparents raising grandchildren
- Young parent families
- Older parent families
- Couples without children

Just as there is a cultural evolution redefining the description of family, there is a personal one as well. Each family changes with time. Even with the same people and the same composition individual family members age, develop new interests, gain new friends, move to other communities, or change jobs. Each change that happens to one person within a family has an affect on the whole. Accepting and acting on this principle of holism is a step toward developing successful survival skills for families.

> ### KEY POINT
>
> Assumptions about families:
>
> - Each family is unique in its beliefs, identity, composition, gifts, and challenges
> - Each family influences, and is influenced by, its community and its culture
> - Each family shares many things in common with other families
> - Each family deserves respect and opportunities to be successful
> - Each family has the responsibility to respect and care for each of its members while accepting each person as an individual and encouraging their personal health and growth

Family Identity

> What's in a name? That which we call a rose,
> By any other name would smell as sweet.
>
> — *William Shakespeare* (4)

When was the last time you looked at your birth certificate? Among the spaces that include the date, time, and place of your birth are the spaces for your mother's maiden name and your father's name. This record of birth, completed or not, forms part of your identity. You are far more than a piece of paper, yet this document follows you through life and represents your heritage.

What meaning do those names hold for you? Were you named after someone, living or deceased? Do you have a middle name? Are you called by the name inscribed there, or over the years have you gained and lost nicknames? Did any of those nicknames stick and become the name to which you now respond?

The names on a birth certificate may give a clear picture of the origins of a family going back to the "old country." Perhaps names have been altered to fit the late-nineteenth-century view of what it meant to be an American. Somewhere in the dusty stacks of a family's history are the storytellers who know. They carry the tales and the details of where a family originated and how long a family has been in this country. There are the tales of courage, of those who traveled, learned a new language, received an education, and raised a large, successful family. When one stops to think about it, the challenges faced by ancestors are amazing.

Even when the stories are shadows or memories created from a need to know more about family background, people gain an appreciation for the courage and life of their ancestors that brought them here and gave them life. Those names and stories, whether clear or hazy, contribute to their identity and that of their family.

Reflection Sunday Dinner: A Guided Reflection

How far back in your childhood can you remember? Were you two, three, or four years old? If someone asked you to talk about Sunday dinner when you were 10, how would you respond? You may have clear memories of special foods, aromas, the time of day, your place at the table, who was present, and who was not. In your family who prepared the meal, set the table, cleared the dishes, cleaned up? Compare that with your Sunday dinner last week. Answer the same questions. Are there similarities between Sunday dinner then and now? What were the differences? Ask each adult in your family to reflect on those similarities, and the differences, then and now.

What does identity have to do with balancing family, work, and leisure? Balance, be it on ice skates, a bicycle, or juggling the many needs and desires of a family, happens when people know where they are in space; they have focus, and they understand their purpose. They know who they are, where they've come from, and where they're headed.

KEY POINT

One interesting dynamic about families is that each represents a merging of the identity, needs, and desires of two or more people. People may be different as individuals, but when joined together as a family, their success depends in part on their ability to develop a unique definition of family that all members can accept and value. Finding and maintaining a balance between the needs of the family and those of each individual member contribute to a family's survival skills.

Family identity is based on many things and may change over time, as individuals mature, children leave the nest, and life presents new opportunities, challenges, and surprises. This identity is reflected in where families live, what foods they prefer, religious or spiritual beliefs, political values, lifestyle preferences, educational interests, and vocational choices. It can include their rest/activity patterns, favored forms of entertainment and recreation, and the nature of their personal relationships.

Articulating family identity requires people to sit in peace and equality, each as individuals contributing to the family unit. Each person brings together what he or she desires personally and what each is able to contribute to the whole.

Exhibit 8–1 offers a Family Identity Exercise. It could be beneficial for you to complete this yourself prior to using it with others. As you complete this exercise, focus on your family and what is needed for its health and success while acknowledging each person's need for respect and opportunities for growth. Maintaining such a focus contributes to the holistic awareness of your family's unique composition. As you proceed with this exercise think in terms of *body, mind,* and *spirit.*

The *body* of the family describes the physical connection—how they are joined genetically, legally, and emotionally. Body acknowledges how things get done within the system: the responsibilities of child care, transportation, home maintenance, meal preparation, financial management, and the myriad daily things a family has to do.

Mind includes the common belief systems, and how the family thinks, reviews the past, plans for the future, and adjusts to life through learning. Mind touches on the many realms of human life; it influences communication and relationships and the ability to adapt to change.

Spirit acknowledges the awareness that there is something beyond the here and now. Some families manifest their spirituality by adopting a specific lifestyle, others do so through their religions, or by contributing to their communities. Still, others define themselves as perpetual seekers, desiring an intense "something":

They want their children to embrace the vitality and wonder of the natural world. They hope to see their children become strong, ethical, responsible people. They yearn for their family to feel part of a soulful community and of the eternal continuum of life (5).

As families explore their unique connections with and contributions to the whole, words and practices may become apparent that help to clarify a family's unique expression of their spirituality. Defining that which is meaningful from the heart and uplifting in daily life supports a family's sense of spirit.

As you go through this exercise think of key words and phrases to describe your family in selected categories. Under *Food Choices* a family that has some vegetarian members while others eat meat may describe themselves as being *mixed* or *varied.* This description acknowledges that variety and choice are welcome. Their food choice statement might mention that "variety is the spice of life" and then go on to list favorite menus.

A family that limits use of technology by using television or radio only for special broadcasts could include the word *selective* in their media use description. Those who read newspapers, magazines, and journals can find words or phrases that reflect their reading style. Their identity may be varied, reflective of popular culture, or aligned with their recreational interests.

You will notice that some areas overlap. This is holism at work; those topics that thread between *body, mind,* and *spirit* are supporting wholeness within your family's

EXHIBIT 8–1 FAMILY IDENTITY EXERCISE

The following categories of body, mind, and spirit include topics to think about and discuss in relation to your family's identity. These lists can be lengthened or shortened. The purpose is to stimulate conversation about who you are and who you want to be as a family. Try reviewing them as a family unit.

Body

Type of area where you live (country, city, suburbs; region of the nation):

_____

Your dwelling place is a(n) (apartment, condominium, house, ranch):

_____

Your food preferences are: _____

_____

Your physical recreation is: _____

Your overall health is: _____

You receive your health care from: _____

You describe your financial situation as being: _____

Mind

Your educational achievements include: _____

Your educational interests and goals for your children (if applicable) include: _____

Your reading interests, individually, and as a family are: _____

_____

The forms of arts and entertainment you enjoy are: _____

You use these types of media and technology: _____

_____

Your political preference is: _____

Voting habits of adults in the family are: _____

Your favorite topics of conversation are: _____

_____

Favorite activities that nurture your creativity include: _____

You participate in the following groups and community activities: _____

_____

EXHIBIT 8–1 FAMILY IDENTITY EXERCISE

Spirit

Traditions, rituals, and spiritual practices that are honored by your family include: _____

You realize meaning and purpose in your life through: _____

_____

Your religious preference, if any, is: _____

You intentionally engage with nature in these ways: _____

_____

You consider the following volunteer activities to be part of your spiritual experience: _____

People who are very dear to you include: _____

---

life. A family who lives in the country, reads magazines focused on country living and spends leisure time outdoors, feels very much a part of the natural world. Their identity with nature is strong and influences the choices they make throughout their lives.

As you complete and reflect upon the Family Identity Exercise, think about your current situation and what you want for the future. The family in the country may be longing for a move to the city. They want more social diversity and a greater variety of arts and entertainment right at their doorstep. Those who live in the city may wish for the peace and open space of the country. Such interests have the potential to determine choices they will make in their work, dwelling place, and community activities.

The descriptions chosen in the Family Identity Exercise will offer guidance in determining how to achieve balance between family, work, and leisure.

Family and Work

Work for most families is a necessity. Livelihood is literally our bread and butter, the means for the roofs over our heads. For some, work or career becomes an expression of who they are. A person's job can affect the family and, in turn, family needs may affect the job.

Creating balance between work and family occurs in an atmosphere of mutual respect. There are workplaces that are family friendly, offering flexible hours, health insurance, vacation hours, child-care benefits, and employee-assistance programs. The best employers are understanding of families while having reasonable work expectations.

When the family is respectful of the work of its members, people are able to be punctual, have good attendance, and maintain focus while at work. Consistency in these areas should mean that an employee is treated courteously when they are then called away for family needs.

Salary or hourly wages are important, but may not account for the most desirable aspects of a job. Questions that explore how work life aligns with your family life are offered in Exhibit 8–2.

Creating a balance between work and family responsibilities can be achieved, even partially, by having a clear understanding of the needs and limitations of each. Once these are established it is important to convey your limits to both family and work. Sample statements are:

- "I'll be able to go on your field trip if I get approval from my supervisor."

EXHIBIT 8–2 EXPLORING WORK AND FAMILY NEEDS

1. Do the hours of business create a reasonable match for family responsibilities and desires?
2. What benefits, written and unwritten, are provided to employees at various pay levels?
3. Is there flexibility in where I do my work? Am I able to work at home when my child has a day off from school?
4. Is the employer one that meets or exceeds the conditions of the federal government's Family and Medical Leave Act?
5. Is my workplace a reasonable commute from home?
6. Is my workplace free of hazards, and does it actively promote staff health and safety?
7. Is there support for continuing education with both allocation of time and financial reimbursement?
8. Is there a wage and benefit package that allows me to provide for my family as I wish?
9. Is this a workplace and job that supports my personal and family values and beliefs?
10. Does this workplace embrace employee suggestions and involvement?
11. Are customers of this business viewed holistically and with respect and dignity?

- "I'm available to attend one evening meeting three weeks a month. I'll need to check with my family if I'm requested to work extra evenings."
- "I prefer flexing my hours to working overtime."
- "I'll be working a little late on Thursday and would like to have supper ready when I get home at 7:30."

While following guidelines such as these, it is advisable for people to know and understand their employee rights and obligations. An employer's attitude toward family and flexibility can vary over time or with a change in supervisors. Ultimately it is the responsibility of the individual employee to know the employer's limitations and to advocate for change if warranted.

Another point to consider in balancing family and work is that each family/work scenario is unique. What works for one family may not work for another. Part-time employment may not have exciting financial benefits, but may provide the time to become more involved in a child's activities and education. The family as a whole can determine the best mix for their current situation. When circumstances change, family/work balance can be re-evaluated and new combinations developed as desired. Exhibit 8–3 lists questions that can guide families in exploring these issues.

EXHIBIT 8–3 QUESTIONS TO REFLECT ON REGARDING YOURSELF, YOUR FAMILY, AND FAMILY ROLES IN RELATION TO WORK

- What days and hours do I want or need to be home with my family? Are there certain times of day that I want to be available for them?
- Does my family understand my profession/career/job and its responsibilities?
- What messages do I convey to my family about my workplace, my career, and my work-related goals?
- Do I/we have backup plans for child care, transportation, and illness?
- Who assumes the responsibilities for chores, meal preparation, and family coordination? Are household and family tasks shared cooperatively?
- Do I foresee that I will need to plan for family changes over the coming years? These may include the needs of dependent adults or a change in the number and ages of children.
- Are there established ground rules related to my work? Examples include accepting phone calls or leaving during business hours for family appointments and activities.

Families and Leisure

According to the *Random House Dictionary*, leisure is defined as freedom from the demands of work or duty, free or unoccupied time, and unhurried ease (6).

Families today are very much on the go, continually on the move, around town and across the country. Everyone has much to do—responsibilities to home and family, a job or career, and health and fitness. When and how can anyone plan for fun? With all that needs to be accomplished, how can leisure happen?

Creating leisure, whether personal or for the family, often requires planning. People have busy lives. Spontaneity would be wonderful fun, but it often doesn't fit in with the structure of the average life.

Reflection Say these words unhurried ease *aloud three times; say them slowly. What sort of images arise for you? Time to smell the roses, ladies twirling parasols in a green grassed Monet, the sweet schuss of powder snow beneath skis. As your imagination creates more pictures of what you'd do with free time, what you'd do with unhurried ease, shift to your body. Has your breathing relaxed? Have your muscles softened? Hopefully the answer to these questions is yes. If so, you are experiencing the importance of leisure. Day dreaming, spacing out, doing nothing, taking a nap, and taking your time are simple yet important acts that are a forgotten art for many. Wildlife and animals are excellent models for how to enjoy each moment, time to live with unhurried ease. Observe the bird as it perches to preen its feathers, a cat lounging in the afternoon sun, a moose and her young browsing on rich swamp delicacies.*

Making a commitment to leisure is making a commitment to oneself. Relaxation is a practice, as are playing the piano, meditating, and woodworking. Daily practice encourages people to become skilled and proficient in the art of leisure and relaxation. By pausing, even for a brief moment, during the busiest days to focus on breath, an individual takes the time to renew.

In their book *Everyday Blessings*, Myla and Jon Kabat Zinn (7) remind us that mindfulness means moment-to-moment, nonjudgmental awareness. It is cultivated by refining our capacity to pay attention, intentionally, in the present moment, and then sustaining that attention over time as best we can. In the process, we become more in touch with our lives as they are unfolding.

A family commitment to leisure acknowledges that free-time needs vary from one person to another. Quiet contemplation is meaningful to one while creating garden space is the height of joy for another. Rock music and rock climbing may symbolize unhurried ease to some, not to others.

Ideally, a plan to create balance through leisure includes individual as well as family relaxation periods. Scheduling unstructured family time works because it affirms commitment to self and the family unit. When a block of time is set aside for family, individual members can go with the flow or plan an activity that has group meaning. They may go somewhere for hours or days, or stay at home and plan something out of the ordinary. The key is to remain focused on their together time and to avoid old patterns of distraction.

Some families set aside a Family Day, a time to be together, exceptions occurring only for special reasons or occasions. This form of structure opens the way for group leisure and time together that can lead to spontaneous moments such as a cookout, a walk in the park, or a drive to the shore. Families can be encouraged to make a wish list of activities to do with unhurried ease and tailor it to the moment.

Reflection As you think about leisure and how to use it to create balance in your life, go back to your family identity descriptions. Who are you now as a family? Are there ways in which you want to change? Do you see where leisure will enhance your overall well-being, uplifting your spirit while moving your body and quieting your mind?

As people take steps toward creating balance between family, work, and leisure, they'll begin to note shifts in their behaviors or those of others around them. It becomes easier to say no to extra duties … anywhere. Sunsets last longer. They *do* learn to focus on their breath. They *do* share a kiss and hug when leaving for work. The roses somehow *do* smell sweeter than they did in the past.

Healthy Habits for Families

Habits are patterns of behavior. They are established or discarded over time and with practice. Once habits are firmly in place they can be hard to change because people act almost without thinking. Recall the time when seat belts first came into use. Many would forget to wear them, buckling up only after a friendly reminder from the car itself or from a fellow passenger. Fastening a seat belt is now as automatic as starting the car.

Decision making and choices enter into this topic area as well. How do people decide when it is time to adopt one behavior over another? Is it an area in which they feel free to choose or does it tend to result from the suggestion of another person? Are they choosing this habit because they were told it would be good for them or because it is something they believe in and embrace with a full heart? Is it something they are trying for someone else's benefit in hopes that it will improve their relationship? Is the habit they are adopting healthy for their entire family, and have they been respectful of others' needs while seeking to meet their own?

The discussion of healthy habits for families will align with and build on the Family Identity Exercise. Comments and thoughts summarized in this activity will help to assess if current habits or those being sought, contribute to the family's individuality, thereby promoting overall health.

Body includes where people live, their type of dwelling, food choices, physical activity, and finances. These are the most basic needs, to have food and shelter and the ability to pay for them. People need to be able to physically move from one place to another and may depend on others or physical means to do so.

The city or town in which they live and the dwelling in which they reside can help to promote family identity and the life people choose to lead. They may find that their neighborhood has some limitations or influences that are unhealthy for what they want in their lives. Exhibit 8–4 depicts the numerous elements of country, city, or village life to consider when assessing the current or future situation. As each item is reviewed, evaluate how the community contributes to or detracts from the family's identity, goals, and well-being.

If a family is considering a move in the future, it should consider its dream town. The qualities that are most important for the family's health and well-being need to be prioritized and used as a guide for their search.

EXHIBIT 8–4 HOW DOES YOUR COMMUNITY'S PROFILE CONTRIBUTE OR DETRACT FROM YOUR FAMILY'S IDENTITY, GOALS, AND WELL-BEING?

- Environment/climate/geography
- Population density
- Overall safety
- Infrastructure: Roads, government, utilities, transportation, and fire/police/rescue
- Service base: Education, health care, and social services
- Spiritual life/civic organizations
- Recreation/arts/cultural events
- Employment options/economic base/sustainability
- Tax base
- Overall quality of life/acceptance of diversity

The sense of place is then moved from a community focus to a family focus. This includes household members and home. Families need to think about the living space, both common areas and private areas. Does the home provide designated places for people to gather for meals and conversation? Does it assure that people have rooms or corners to call their own? Even in crowded situations, the surroundings can be adapted by consciously choosing behaviors that contribute to privacy. To do so is respectful because expectations are clarified about space, times for bathing, quiet hours, and meals.

Healthy Options

Attending to their relationships while planning for privacy contributes to the manner in which family members nurture or nourish each other. The topic of nourishment includes providing for the mind and spirit as well as feeding the body. Each statement in the Healthy Options Assessment (Exhibit 8–5) represents the behaviors and practices of families who exhibit balanced living. When surveying the Healthy Options list you will notice that following these guidelines requires commitment, communication,

---

EXHIBIT 8–5 HEALTHY OPTIONS ASSESSMENT

Consider the following nourishment statements and note your level of agreement (*most of the time, sometimes,* or *rarely*) with each. This activity is not intended to be scored or to rate you on your abilities; the purpose is to determine your family's individual patterns and establish if there are changes you would like to make.

	Most of the Time	Sometimes	Rarely
A. Food			
• We are satisfied with our diet and believe it is healthy.	____	____	____
• We eat together as a family every day.	____	____	____
• We eat our meals at the table.	____	____	____
• We eat without distractions such as TV.	____	____	____
• We honor each other's food choices.	____	____	____
• We limit our use of stimulating or depressing substances.	____	____	____

	Most of the Time	Sometimes	Rarely
EXHIBIT 8–5 HEALTHY OPTIONS ASSESSMENT *(continued)*			

B. Communication and Displays of Affection

- We communicate about our schedules (work, games, meetings, etc.). ____ ____ ____
- We routinely check in with each other by phone, notes, or e-mail. ____ ____ ____
- We support each other with positive statements. ____ ____ ____
- We each have opportunities to express our opinions. ____ ____ ____
- We use hugs, kisses, and healthy touch to communicate with each other. ____ ____ ____
- We use and practice effective listening skills. ____ ____ ____
- We practice the arts of apology and forgiveness. ____ ____ ____

C. Physical Activity

- We exercise three to five times a week for at least 20 minutes a session. ____ ____ ____
- We incorporate activity in our family and work lives as much as possible. ____ ____ ____
- Our fitness plan includes stretching and rest periods. ____ ____ ____
- We choose exercise that is enjoyable. ____ ____ ____
- Our exercise plan includes activities that can be done individually or as a family. ____ ____ ____
- We use safety equipment, such as helmets and pads, when exercising. ____ ____ ____

	Most of the Time	Sometimes	Rarely
• We limit use of TV and other sedentary activities.	____	____	____

D. Rest and Relaxation

	Most of the Time	Sometimes	Rarely
• We honor each individual's sleep, rest, and relaxation patterns.	____	____	____
• Our children have regular bedtimes with calming bedtime rituals.	____	____	____
• Adults get seven-to-nine hours of sleep; children sleep nine-to-twelve hours depending on their age.	____	____	____
• We set aside time every week to relax and have fun as a family.	____	____	____
• Nap or quiet time is planned for those who choose or need it.	____	____	____
• We practice daily relaxation, such as breath work and meditation.	____	____	____

E. Financial Security/ Household Responsibilities

	Most of the Time	Sometimes	Rarely
• Household chores and responsibilities are shared.	____	____	____
• Our income allows us to pay our bills on time.	____	____	____
• We have a long-range financial plan.	____	____	____
• Children have chores in addition to care of their possessions.	____	____	____
• We continually upgrade our work-related skills.	____	____	____
• The work we do honors us as individuals and as a family.	____	____	____

EXHIBIT 8–5 HEALTHY OPTIONS ASSESSMENT *(continued)*

	Most of the Time	Sometimes	Rarely
F. Family/Friends/Community			
• We have a nearby network of family and/or friends.	___	___	___
• We feel connected to our community.	___	___	___
• We participate in community groups and/or activities.	___	___	___
• Our community offers a positive quality of life for our family.	___	___	___
• We have regular get-togethers with family and/or friends.	___	___	___
• We are spiritually fulfilled through our religion and/or other spiritual activities.	___	___	___
G. Creative Expression			
• Family members are encouraged to use their individual talents.	___	___	___
• Family artwork is honored and displayed.	___	___	___
• Financial resources are allocated for lessons, equipment, or materials used in creative expression.	___	___	___
• All forms of creativity are valued, including culinary, financial, and athletic skills.	___	___	___
• We have rituals and celebrations that are unique to our family.	___	___	___

---

and coordination. Each family must decide for itself which guidelines have meaning and which to disregard. Feel free to add any that will create an individualized profile of nourishing habits.

Patterns/Repatterning

Once this exercise has been completed, it should be reviewed and put away for a few days. Resist the temptation to judge or analyze behaviors when you return to it. Survey the responses, looking for patterns that emerge. Exhibit 8–6 offers issues that can be reviewed to help identify patterns within the family.

It is useful for people to identify those Healthy Options areas that reflect their family's optimal functioning. This can be followed by noting those areas in which they would like to create change over the coming weeks or months. They should be guided in staying focused on keeping their goals reasonable and in alignment with their family identities. They may want to begin their change process with small goals that can be readily accomplished. Once they have celebrated success and developed an atmosphere that fosters growth, they can select more challenging goals.

Goal Setting

There are steps families can follow to make concrete action plans that will help them to create what they want for the future (Exhibit 8–7). This process is enriched by establishing equality: Each person has a chance to be heard, to state opinions, to offer suggestions, and to describe their role in family goal setting and goal attainment.

Changing habits and adopting new life patterns can often be accomplished through small shifts in behavior. For example, if people want to become more physically active,

---

EXHIBIT 8–6 ISSUES FOR DISCUSSION TO AID IN IDENTIFYING PATTERNS WITHIN THE FAMILY

- Identify those choices that promote balance and simplicity.
- Do you have a healthy amount of time together as a family? Do these occasions contribute to your well-being?
- Note how your choices support individual and family wellness.
- Determine if your responses align with your family identity. Observe where they vary and explore the meaning of that variation.
- Ask yourself if your choices contribute to the health of your community.
- Which areas elicit an intuitive response of satisfaction, consternation, or anything in between? An intuitive response arises when you have observed something that has significance for you. Such an observation can indicate a pattern to continue because of its benefits. Conversely, your response may be rooted in a pattern that does not support health and warrants change.

EXHIBIT 8–7 GOAL-SETTING STEPS

1. *Plan a time for the family to meet about a specific purpose,* such as planning meals, choosing a pet, or selecting a vacation destination.

2. *Set the goal.* What is it you want to do? Does it fit within the picture of your family identity? Is it a reasonable goal given your resources of time, skills, and finances? Do you have a clear picture of what your goal will look and feel like once it has been reached?

3. *Plan the process for reaching your objective.* Design a long-term plan with steps that can be accomplished in two-to-four weeks. This will make your efforts seem more reasonable because your gains will be readily visible. Working on short-term steps allows room for course corrections as your project unfolds.

4. *Set aside time to review and celebrate your successes.* It makes it easier to focus on your next steps when you can look back and pat yourself on the back for a job well done. Reflection serves to remind the whole family that everyone's in this together, no matter what the individual roles and responsibilities are.

5. *Review and revise goals as needed.* Sometimes in the course of a project, the goal changes. It may be altered enough to look like a whole new goal. It may no longer be relevant, being dropped entirely or reframed into a new goal. For instance, a family was in the process of planning to purchase a larger home. They explored their options and decided that, given low interest rates and love of their current home, it was better to build an addition than to purchase a new home.

6. *Recognize goal attainment.* This is an opportunity to review your change process and to identify alterations you will make in it when you establish goals for future projects. It also is a time to celebrate success in reaching desired outcomes.

---

they can increase activity at work by going for a ten-minute walk rather than taking the usual coffee break.

KEY POINT

Adopting small actions that can be readily woven into a daily routine increases the likelihood of staying with a plan. For example, remembering to spend a few moments focusing on breathing and doing gentle stretches can awaken the senses and enhance the body's flexibility (8).

These ideas aren't new. Most people have heard them before, time and again. If behavior changes have been attempted in the past without success, perhaps there has been an intent to alter too much at once. Change takes time and a modest approach. Look for small, healthy changes that can be easily accomplished. Remember that habits are developed over time. Weeks or months of practice may be needed before positive effects of actions are noted (9).

Reflection   One action-oriented example of a healthy change involves your daily routine travel. Whether you travel by car, train, or bus, take three breaths when you arrive at your destination. The 15 or 20 seconds you invest in this routine will clear your mind and cleanse your body. Do you think you are worthy of this modest investment?

Holistic Parenting

In human relations, ends depend on means, and outcome depends on process. Personality and character flourish only when methods of child rearing are imbued with respect and sympathy.

— *Dr. Haim Ginnott (10)*

Holistic parenting is based on mindfulness, kindness, respect, and reflection. Through the parent/child relationship people learn more about themselves while learning about their child. They come to honor their individuality as much as you cherish their common traits. They learn to listen to their hearts, the wisdom centers that will guide them to parent in a way that is respectful and prepares their children and themselves for the future. They learn that discipline is another way of caring.

Parenting, once started in a holistic and loving way, lasts a lifetime. Parents become the family elders. As people age and grow in their parenting experiences, they will reflect more on their own lessons; they will see that their children also have lessons to learn through their own experiences. They will stand as guides and supporters, pointing the way and offering a heart and hand when the going is rough.

KEY POINT

The challenge of being a parent is to live our moments as fully as possible, charting our own courses as best we can, above all, nourishing our children, and in the process, growing ourselves. Our children and the journey itself provide us with endless opportunities in this regard.

Myla and Jon Kabat Zinn (11)

Topics that are discussed in this section will build on or reflect back to the exercises completed in the section Balancing Family, Work, and Leisure. Through holistic awareness people will develop a realization that there are many paths to follow when parenting a child. Although there are those who will suggest, prod, coerce, even mandate that people parent in a specific manner, ultimately all parents are responsible to their own children and to themselves for the form their parenting will assume.

Holistic parenting is based on strength-oriented practice. It maintains a focus on personal competence while promoting positive traits and behaviors. The child is honored for whom he or she is and the attributes radiated as a unique person while being guided with clear, reasonable, and healthy expectations. This practice does not disregard less-desired behaviors, actions, and words; rather, it educates on how to keep them in perspective. It is centered on the art of offering love and respect to a child while discussing challenging, frustrating, or painful situations.

KEY POINT

Mindful parenting does not mean being overindulgent, neglectful, or weak; nor does it mean being rigid, domineering, and controlling (12).

Holistic parenting can begin at any time; it is never too late. Humans are resilient and respond well to those who focus on their gifts and treat them with respect. When people parent from a heart center, they learn to apologize and to forgive with integrity and without the burden of guilt for either themselves or their children. This is a discipline; practice is necessary. Mindfully, they will do the best they can for today, and tomorrow they will arise and engage in their heart-centered practice again. At times, parents may feel that their parenting skills are developing more slowly than desired. Parents need to be encouraged to hold on to their intentions and to focus on their desires to have open, balanced relationships with their children.

Parent Education from a Holistic Perspective

Parenting education, until recent years, has been primarily experiential. We learned about parenting as children from our parents. We took those lessons and applied them to our children, making adjustments as each child grew or another came along. Anticipatory guidance, or what to expect in a child's development and how to prepare for and manage it, came primarily from well-meaning family and friends and information gathered during pediatrician visits. To add to our overall inexperience and confusion, points of view often varied, sometimes being contradictory.

Today there are parenting classes and support groups, books and videotapes, and community resources that provide specialized support and guidance for families. Many of these will ask parents to do the same thing: *begin at the beginning*. How do parents begin at the beginning when their child is six years old and they feel bogged down by patterns that are already established? Part of the beginning is going back to their own childhoods, to those earliest memories of their families. Parents can be guided to recall the faces and relationships, the good times and the bad. Questions can be asked: When were you happy? What made you run and hide? What do you do or say now that seems like a flashback from those long ago years?

Remembering those times and family patterns that brought them joy—or pain— can offer parents hints for what to do and avoid with their own children. Thinking back to those years can help people to become mindful parents. Moment by moment they will become aware of verbal habits, facial expressions, and mannerisms that have become embedded in their behavior patterns. The manner with which their children respond to their words and actions will give parents clues about which behaviors to continue and which to change. When parents release an unhealthy behavior from their past, they may be ending a family cycle that has been in place for generations. The legacy of their actions has the potential to extend past the lives of their children.

Another way to begin at the beginning is to study child development. This commitment, to learn about development from the earliest moments of life *in utero* (in the uterus/womb), can help parents to understand children's behaviors. They will be less confused by the once friendly seven-month-old who now melts into tears as a reserved ten-month-old. They will understand why their practical four-year-old has suddenly developed an intriguing relationship with an imaginary friend.

KEY POINT

Parents really need to know what a two-year-old is like, what a three-year-old is like, what a six- or seven-year-old is like. There are characteristic patterns and predictable rhythms of growth and development for those age groups (13).

Learning about development helps parents appreciate their children in relation to others of the same stage while gaining a sense of each child's temperament and talents. They learn to respect and have compassion for those parents whose child is intense, very shy, or has special needs. Sharing their joys and frustrations with other parents can help them to learn new techniques while guiding others by the example of their lessons. They come to realize they are not alone and that being with someone who listens fully while acknowledging their feelings is a precious gift.

When parents gain an understanding of child development they are better able to:

- Understand their children's words and actions.
- Adjust their expectations to match their children's current level of ability and understanding.
- Use behavioral guidance and discipline that is appropriate for a child's developmental level.
- Anticipate what stages will come next and how to prepare for coming changes.
- Provide a safe environment for a child.
- Plan family activities that match a child's interests and abilities.
- Offer foods that are interesting, safe, and nutritionally sound.
- Help others to understand their children's individual talents, preferences, and challenges.
- Understand the variations in development from one child to another and typical milestones. (A *milestone* is the average age at which most children will develop a skill such as sitting up, talking, and walking.)
- Know when they, their children, or their family need professional guidance and support regarding health, development, behaviors, or relationships.
- Accept their children and others for the people they are and the individuals they are becoming.
- Identify, acknowledge, and balance their personal needs with those of their children.

Reflection (for parents)

As you reflect on your own childhood experiences and what you have learned about "typical" (usual, average, expected) child development, pause to reflect on the thoughts that arise as you complete these statements:

- *I became a parent because* _____
- *I knew I wanted to be a parent when I* _____
- *I hoped for a child who* _____

Sit with your responses, breathing gently into your heart. As you continue to breathe, release emotions that have manifested with your statements. Release any fear, sadness, and anger and allow yourself to be filled with peace, suspended in this eternal moment.

Hold that sense of peacefulness and proceed by completing these statements:

- *As a parent I wish I could* _____
- *The greatest gift I have given my child is* _____

- *The greatest gift my child has given me is* _____
- *The best advice I could give a new parent is* _____
- *The person who is most supportive of me as a parent is* _____
- *This person shows their support by* _____

Put your responses aside and breathe quietly for a few minutes. Review your statements without judgment. As you reflect on your statements, consider the following:

- *Those that are strength based, containing words that are positive, offering affirmation and a feeling of hope.*
- *Those statements that surprise you.*
- *Those that bring up emotions: your joy, sadness, and anger.*
- *Note where there are patterns of similarity or contradiction.*

Write a page on what you have learned about how your original desires and expectations of parenting differ from your present reality. Define steps you can take to become a more effective parent over the coming year. Use your affirmative statements as the building blocks for what you want to accomplish. For instance, you could say, "I will use supportive listening and open dialogue to guide my child in seeking new solutions for problems at school."

Seeking Guidance

Disruption may signify that professional guidance is needed to help resolve a situation. That support could be available from a healthcare provider, a rabbi or minister, or a counselor. Today, there are numerous support groups and therapies, both traditional and complementary, for families who are seeking wisdom and solace.

Mutual trust and respect are two of the cornerstones on which a therapeutic relationship is based. People need to give themselves permission to search for the right match for their family. They should talk with the professional person about their beliefs and values, and the hopes they have for their parent/child relationship. They can then invite that person to partner with them as their parenting develops and as their children grow in life awareness.

Parents need to take time to center and find renewal in personally satisfying ways. When they feel whole and refreshed they have greater resources to bring to their relationships with their children. The children, in turn, will learn from their parents' example that personal time is important for maintaining health and balance. Parents need to encourage their children to find their own methods for relaxing and attaining personal fulfillment.

Family Comes Full Cycle

Our days go from dawn to dusk; our years flow from spring through winter. So it is with our lives and those of our family members.

We have touched on survival, balance, and each family's unique qualities. A person's individuality is embraced in the family's inherent rhythms and cycles. By pausing to recall past and plan for the future, a person becomes more keenly aware of those patterns.

Chapter Summary

Families come in a variety of forms, including blended, single parent, one child, multiple children, same-gender partner, grandparents raising grandchildren, younger parents, older parents, and couples without children. There are some basic assumptions when working with families that can guide a professional's actions. Each family is unique, influences and is influenced by its community and culture, shares many things in common with other families, deserves respect and opportunities for success, and has responsibility to respect and care for its members while accepting the individuality of its members. Each family has a unique body, mind, and spirit.

The Healthy Options Assessment offered in this chapter can be useful in guiding families in the discussion of their patterns in regard to food, communication, display of affection, physical activity, rest and relaxation, financial security, household responsibility, family, friends, community, and creative expression. From this, plans can be made for repatterning.

Parenting should be viewed as a holistic process. It is based on mindfulness, kindness, and reflection. It is a strength-oriented practice. With reflection, knowledge, and practice, parenting patterns can improve.

References

1. Gordon, M. (1972). *The Nuclear Family in Crisis: The Search for an Alternative.* New York: Harper & Row, Publishers, p. 1.
2. Elkind, D. (1994). *The Ties That Stress.* Cambridge, MA: Harvard University Press, 1994, p. 31.
3. Elkind, D. (1997). Dr. David Elkind on Raising Kids Today. *Scholastic Parent & Child,* 4(5):50.
4. Shakespeare, W. (1936). Romeo and Juliet. In Clarke, Mary, ed.: *Best Loved Plays of William Shakespeare.* Reading, PA: The Spencer Press, p. 345.
5. Reder, A., Catalfo, P., and Hamilton, S. (1999). *The Whole Parenting Guide.* New York: Broadway Books, p. 390.
6. Stein, J., ed. (1984). *The Random House College Dictionary*, Revised Edition. New York: Random House, p. 766.
7. Kabat Zinn, M. and Kabat Zinn, J. (1997). *Everyday Blessings.* New York: Hyperion, p. 24.

8. Weil, A. (1997). *Eight Weeks to Optimum Health.* New York: Alfred A. Knopf, p. 60, 95.
9. Ibid., p. 41.
10. Ginnott, H. (1956). *Between Parent and Child.* New York: Avon Books, p. 243.
11. Kabat Zinn, op cite, p. 3.
12. Ibid., p. 387.
13. Elkind, op cite, p. 51.

Recommended Readings

Benson, P., Galbraith, J., and Espeland, P. (1998). *What Teens Need to Succeed.* Minneapolis: Free Spirit Publishing.

Boldt, L. (1999). *Zen and the Art of Making a Living.* New York: Penguin/Arkana.

Bolles, R. N. (2000). *What Color Is Your Parachute? 2000.* Berkeley, CA: Ten Speed Press.

Carlson, R. (1998). *Don't Sweat the Small Stuff with Your Family.* New York: Hyperion.

Covey, S. (1997). *The Seven Habits of Highly Effective Families.* New York: St. Martin's Griffin.

Faber, A. and Mazlish, E. (1990). *How to Talk So Kids Will Listen and Listen So Kids Will Talk.* New York: Avon Books.

Ginnott, H. (1956). *Between Parent and Child.* New York: Avon Books.

Kabat Zinn, M. and Kabat Zinn , J. (1997). *Everyday Blessings.* New York: Hyperion.

Reder, A., Catalfo, P., and Hamilton, S. R. (1999). *The Whole Parenting Guide.* New York: Broadway Books.

St. James, E. (1997). *Simplify Your Life with Kids.* Kansas City: Andrews McMeel Publishing.

Schor, E. L., ed. (1999). *Caring for Your School Age Child.* New York: Bantam Books.

Shelov, S., ed. (1998). *Caring for Your Baby and Young Child, Revised Edition.* New York: Bantam Books.

Sinetar, M. (1987). *Do What You Love, the Money Will Follow.* New York: Dell Publishing.

Related Web Sites

Environmental Defense Fund. *www.edf.org*
Mothering. *www.mothering.com*
New Age: The Journal for Holistic Living. *www.newage.com*

CHAPTER 9

THE SPIRITUAL CONNECTION

Objectives

This chapter should enable you to:

- Describe the differences between spirituality and religion
- Describe the process of letting go of preconceived notions
- List two elements of spiritual preparation
- Discuss the healing value of service to others

Since the 1980s you may have seen many people change their diets, begin a regular exercise program, and read a wide range of self-help books as they have become increasingly aware of the impact of healthy living. Even conventional medicine has slowly, yet progressively, incorporated some common sense lifestyle suggestions into patient care. But, health is influenced by more than just the maintenance of the body. Increasingly, research is shedding light on the relationship between spirituality and health.

KEY POINT

Spirituality is not synonymous with religion.

Spirituality and Religion

Looking past the worship practices and belief systems of organized religion, you can move into an integrated dimension of wholeness known as *spirituality*. Being essential to life, spirituality reflects the common threads that flow through all religions and belief systems. Spirituality embraces all aspects of every living thing; it embraces the mind, the body, and the spirit. From this larger perspective in consciousness, you embrace life and life's issues from a place of collective being and knowing. This is different from the choices involved in practicing a religion.

Reflection   How are spirituality and religion viewed and expressed differently in your life?

Spirituality is simply *being*. Religion is like following a map that was charted to keep people on a predetermined single path toward a destination. Spirituality is similar to sitting on top of a mountain where insight is gained from a larger viewpoint, which draws one to the best path. As perspective widens from religion to spirituality people begin to realize the unity and connectedness of all things. This innate state of being is essential to life. It is that place that enables people to know their authentic selves. Spirituality does not negate religion; rather it shows where the commonalties or universal truths among all beliefs are founded.

When comparing spirituality and religion, some interesting differences can be noted. Words defining religion relate to belief systems and practices of worship that can vary from culture to culture. Words used to define spirituality have a wider universal expression that goes beyond religion and opens you to a greater awareness of one's true being (Exhibit 9–1).

Spirituality as a Broader Perspective

From a broader perspective of spirituality, commonalties among all religions and beliefs can be seen. There is a unifying force, a power, a presence, an essence to

EXHIBIT 9–1 COMMON WORDS ASSOCIATED WITH SPIRITUALITY AND RELIGION	
Spirituality	*Religion*
Ethereal	Belief
Airy	Creed
Holy	Faith
Higher power	Church
Sacred	Cult
Essence	Sect
Transcendence	Theology
Being	Doctrine

life that is greater than the individual, yet encompasses all human beings and all living things.

> **KEY POINT**
>
> That which represents the spiritual dimension is represented by many names and ideas such as: God, Chi, Allah, Great Spirit, Infinite Intelligence, Unconditional Love, Goddess, Universal Life Force, Intuition, Higher Power, and, most simply, from India, The Energy.

Spirituality impacts everything people say, think, and do. This ornate tapestry of interconnectedness expands from the individual to other people, places, and things. Seeing a beautiful picture or experiencing great music can fill one with love and rapture of emotions. Still expanding in unity and connectedness, the connection with nature, the planet, and the universe is also realized. One can become lost in a beautiful sunset, enjoying and connecting with it so much that for a few moments the sunset is all there is. This connectedness also means experiencing pain and hurt, as well as beauty and inspiration. Pictures of a war-torn country can cause people to feel the pain, sorrow, and hardship of its victims.

From this place of seeing and experiencing, people begin to comprehend on a deeper level, the spiritual level. Seeing that what happens to one affects everything and what happens to everything affects the one. This often results in a sense of awe or inspiration as people discover this creative force/God in everything.

Planetary Connectedness

In this place of awareness and connectedness, many people are discovering a deep reverence for the planet. There is an awareness that the abuse of the planet not only affects the earth, but each of its inhabitants. The individual affects the planet and the planet affects the individual. The individual's health affects your community and the community's health affects an individual's health. The individual, the community, the nation, and the world are all connected.

Being, Knowing, and Doing

In considering spirituality, *being*, *knowing*, and *doing* take on new meanings. People become more aware of their inner selves and begin to intuitively sense what to do and how to do it. They begin to feel more comfortable acting on these feelings. Herein lies the essence of the spiritual connection and the beginning of healing.

Being is the art, the awareness of the here and now, or the present. There are no thoughts—only stillness—and, with stillness comes awareness through all the senses. The mind becomes quiet and just *is*. This stillness heightens the awareness of each of the senses even more. This place of stillness with self, others, and the environment enables one to experience the moment on a deeper level. It is as though the body is responding to observations from all of the senses. This state is often referred to as being *centered* or *balanced*; yet, it is more.

Reflection

Experience Being:
   Take a deep breath and gently release it.
   Feel how the mind releases with the body.
   Take another deep breath and another.
   Notice how each breath permits the body and mind to relax even further
   Now take a breath and as you exhale, linger in the exhalation.

From this larger place of being, people begin to express with greater awareness, peace, and connectedness rather than from desires, self-centeredness, or envy. It is in this place of awareness and peace that healing takes place.

Knowing comes from being open to all things, not just the ones we have stored in our memory. There is a deep inner sense of awareness of things and their interactions and effects. This knowing is accompanied with a feeling of openness or lightness in the entire body.

Reflection

Experience Knowing:
   Close your eyes.
   Take some slow, deep breaths with gentle exhalations.
   Scan your body for any tight places.
   Gently breathe into the tight areas.
   Remain in this easy breathing.
   Notice how your body is becoming lighter and lighter.
   Feel the freedom and lightness with each breath.
   Feel the gentle lightness—almost tingling.
   Continue with this breathing.
   Stay in this place of freedom and healing as long as you desire.

Often, people come to recognize that they reach a place of clarity and right thought when the knowing and the light feeling come at the same time. It is like the tingling or lightness is validating or confirming the clarity of the knowing. This is a natural intelligence unrelated to physical memory. This natural intelligence is intuition, one's energy talking. It lets people know what they need to be doing. It tells them what is and isn't supportive, what opens or constricts them, and makes them feel heavy or light. Knowing comes with sensing and feeling this natural intelligence.

From this inner place of being and knowing emerges *doing*. This outward expression is spirituality made visible. Doing starts with individuals taking care of themselves in healthy, loving, life-giving ways. Honoring knowing and being is sometimes a challenge, especially when being and knowing conflict with expectations imposed by self or others.

Learning from Relationships

The ability for people to experience and express themselves from a wider consciousness is an evolving process. Relationships are the school for this growth in spirituality. People are in a relationship with everything in their lives…other people, places, things, themselves, and their higher powers. All desires for fame, fortune, and to get ahead are transient happiness as they are nonrelational. Ultimately, the nonrelational aspects of life increase the hunger for the real relationship, the inner connection, the spiritual connection with a power greater than self.

Some people may spend considerable time trying to fix things on the outside when their need is to respond to their deepest calling. They may want to change jobs, improve their image, live in an upscale community, or lose weight. The changing and fixing of these outer things brings some satisfaction for a brief period, but then the novelty wears off and they must be attended to once again. Striving for satisfaction through outer means is indicative of a need for a deeper inner relationship with being.

The deepest calling, the deepest yearning, is to know and remember one's connectedness and oneness to something greater than oneself. As people begin to realize the power and peace of this unity, this oneness in their lives, they begin to desire and experience connectedness more and more. They begin to realize that this connectedness is almost magical, and most certainly sacred. Seeking this inner light or higher power, individuals find that the unity that feeds the spirit is more important than their physical pleasures or dreams of wealth and prestige. They are able to let go of having to create images and control others and events. And, as they let go, their lives and health begin to change.

KEY POINT

Releasing all need for control, one can move with love, joy, and clarity in the moment.

Abundance is a simple yet profound truth of the universe. When people want and move into the eternal more than the ephemeral, they begin to experience a peace that surpasses all understanding. They discover the unconditional love that sees beyond all outward appearances and behaviors. They feel the inner joy that is always there, independent of what is happening in their lives.

How people deal with outer relationships reflects their state of consciousness and inner awareness of who they really are. The emotional personality, that constricted ego place in consciousness, is like blinders on a horse that keep it looking and moving only in one direction while ignoring many of the things nearby. Living without blinders allows people to experience the expansive spiritual place and see the joy and beauty of everything around them. Spirituality assists in examining emotions, behaviors, and attitudes. Without the blinders, individuals can see more clearly the limitations that constrain them in self-serving, destructive thinking. The individual can be his or her own best teacher. By observing how they respond to others and their deeper motivations, people can begin to understand the purposes behind their actions. This insight can guide them in discovering the blocks and hindrances to healthy, joyous relationships. They begin to identify the ideas that keep them locked in limitation, disease, and imbalance.

KEY POINT

Native Americans instruct their youth to look beyond to discover truth. Once that truth has been discovered, one looks beyond, again and again until one has reached the essence of universal truth.

Individuals' relationships with others demonstrate the limitations that they hold in their minds. Their judgments and pronouncements only lead to a frustrating cycle of trying to fix someone else. Rather than thinking and acting in a limiting and tightening manner, they need to loosen up and allow themselves to be open, accepting, and free. When they release the preconceived notions of how things should work or how others should act, life begins to flow easily. The mind and body respond by being in balance; this is health.

Reflection

Experience Letting Go:
  Consider a recent situation that caused you to become unsettled.
  Look at the reason for the emotion.
  Now look beyond that reason to the underlying reason.
  Keep looking beyond to the next reason and the next until you reach the core reason
    and can go no further.
  Take slow deep breaths and gently release them.
  Remain in this place of peace and ease as long as you like.

Being Honest

Being honest with oneself is an important part of healthy living. Honestly going within may reveal things that people may not feel comfortable discovering; but, this process could help them to discover the blinders and falsehoods that have been accepted as being real. Take this example:

A college administrator was sitting at her desk perplexed at the response she was receiving from her faculty regarding the proposed curriculum changes. She kept attempting to figure out how to present the curriculum so that the changes would be accepted. In her silence and quiet breathing, she realized that she was manipulating the faculty to do things "her way," rather than being open to their recommendations for changes. It felt awful to see herself in the role of a manipulator when she had thought of herself as an empowering leader. Releasing this, she stayed with her breathing and went deeper. She realized that she needed to present the facts as clearly as possible and allow the faculty to make decisions. The administrator "let go" of any need to have the curriculum changes fit her preconceived idea and opened herself to the faculty's suggestions. The faculty moved together and improved the curriculum beyond everyone's expectations.

When issues are seen for what they really are, people are in a better position to release them. These issues no longer have control and people can move deeper into a place of clarity, healing, and being.

There is a saying that insanity is doing the same thing and expecting different results. Stopping the insanity is paramount to being honest. If a person's joints are stiff each morning after drinking wine the previous evening, why does he keep drinking the wine and expecting different results? If life is not working, if a person is not healthy and not moving in a healthy direction, it is time to do something different. Often, insights and guidance provided by a healthcare professional can help individuals clarify unhealthy habits and initiate actions to change them.

Gratitude

Gratitude comes in continually larger and larger doses as one takes the time to go within and be quiet. The vicious cycles of anger, fear, and resentment are replaced with love, knowing, being, and increasing awareness. Spirituality soon permeates every part of life, giving guidance, comfort, healing, purpose, and direction. The body and mind are taken to new levels of connectedness and a person is able to see the unity and beauty in everything.

KEY POINT

As spiritual awareness is heightened, a person begins to feel thankful for the ordinary—a new day, the ability to get out of bed independently, a job that can provide the means to keep a roof over one's head and food in one's stomach, the support of loved ones—these aspects of everyday life that often are taken for granted can, instead, be appreciated as special gifts.

Prayer is an expression of gratitude. People can express appreciation that they are being protected and blessed as they face that which is before them, and also give thanks for the protection and blessings that have been experienced. Prayers of thanksgiving reflect a connection with a higher power and contribute to feelings of abundance.

Spirituality as Lived Experience

Spirituality is a daily experience highlighted with some peak experiences. Within the unity and connectedness there is a sense of order and natural balance in life and in the world. One discovers that there is no single path to spirituality, no road map. Spirituality simply *is*. This is a lived experience and a moment-by-moment awakening and discovering of one's true being. Things that used to baffle a person in the past, become understood and manageable. Problems are viewed as opportunities to learn and grow. Unhealthy habits begin to melt away. An individual begins to respond from a different place in consciousness.

Reflection You have probably heard of situations in which people risked their lives to help others in emergency situations. They immediately responded and did what was necessary at the time without consideration of the personal risks and dangers. Can you think of a time when you or someone close to you took this type of risk?

When guided by spirit, there is no fear but rather, being, knowing, and doing. Fear enters when the mind leads. Being is a place of no fear—no peripheral thoughts or emotions—just total presence in the moment. Fear comes from one's memory of personal experiences or what others have led him or her to fear (e.g., warnings from persons in authority, situations described in the media). The memory collects everything that is happening in the environment whether a person is aware of it or not. This collection of memory is what is used as a standard against which current situations are measured. This memory, although helpful at times, can keep a person locked into certain beliefs, ideas, and concepts.

Resisting the temptation to be limited by the memories that have guided their actions in the past, people can face the present without fear. They will learn to trust that they will not be harmed or overwhelmed, which can help them to discover happiness, joy, and spontaneity unlike anything experienced before.

Moving to Solutions

Throughout life people experience many challenges in their relationships, health, work, and family lives. When challenges continue beyond what people feel is reasonable they may begin to get concerned, worried, and fearful. Prayers do not seem to be answered and they may begin to question, usually silently, whether there really is a God, an infinite intelligence. At these times it feels as if they will never be free of the challenge. These experiences offer an opportunity to either be part of the solution or part of the problem. Moving to solutions expands and opens people to positive ideas, thoughts, and a way through the situation; whereas, remaining in the problem keeps them locked in the role of victim. Helping people to move to solutions empowers them to act, change, and discover the path to effectively managing the situation.

Complaining is an example of an activity that causes people to remain in their problems. For example, a person may telephone several friends complaining about a situation, repeating the same story each time. She may be so consumed with complaining that she doesn't take the time to reflect and consider possibilities for changing the situation, somewhat like a person who complains about being hot and thirsty, but fails to take a drink of water! It is when the person is willing to let go of the problem, that she can move into the solution.

When people have a challenge or a health problem in their lives they need to take the time to be quiet and still, and go within. In this place of stillness there is no talking, just quiet. Focusing on their breathing they become peaceful and let go of the fear, the judgments, the blame, and all the defenses that may contribute to this challenge.

Reflection

Moving to Solutions:
  Close your eyes and begin to take long, slow breaths.
  Gently allow the exhalations to become longer than the inhalations.
  Focus on your breathing. If necessary say, "breathe in, breathe out."
  Feel the tension, fear, judgments, and blame leaving.
  Accept and know that peace and harmony are filling you.
  Remain in this place of peace until you naturally come back.

Simply feeling the experience of peace and harmony is a very powerful type of prayer, a very powerful healing process. It is this feeling of peace that works the magic.

There was a woman who was clearing an overgrown garden and contracted poison ivy. She was very allergic not only to poison ivy, but also to the steroids and other conventional treatments for poison ivy. In the ensuing days it slowly spread across her arms and legs. She had a choice; she either could complain and become the victim of the poison ivy or she could move toward solutions. She chose the latter. First she became quiet and still and gently released all the anger and frustration that had been building up in her life. She moved into a consciousness of knowing that the healing was taking place. Whenever that knowing became shaken by how the poison ivy was spreading or by what someone said to her, she returned to that place of peace and quiet until that knowing returned. She began to find natural ways to alleviate the symptoms, such as cool Epsom salts, lavender baths and soaks, drinking large amounts of water, and homeopathic remedies. She talked only of health, healing, and solutions. She let go of any negative thoughts or words. In addition, she found one person who would really support her through this healing process. She talked to him each day and shared her triumphs and her places still needing solutions. The other person was genuinely positive and knew that the healing was taking place and supported her in consciousness. She listened to tapes at night set low, on continuous play that talked about connectedness and healing ability. She woke knowing and feeling the peace, connection, and healing—and she kept her sense of humor! She had wet T-shirt contests when she was soaking in the Epsom salts. She found that there was a map of the Aleutian Islands on her inner thigh and Asia was spreading across her abdomen. She changed her name depending on the symptoms: Columbus as she discovered new sites, Red Hot Mama as the poison ivy became inflamed, and Itchy, Scratchy, and Lumpy. Each morning she did a body search as she looked for the progress of the healing. Soon over 40 percent of her body was covered with the poison ivy. Still she persisted. After four weeks she awoke one morning with no new sites. She was ecstatic! Over the next three weeks the poison ivy dried up and receded while she continued moving to solutions. Rather than just trying to change the condition, this woman changed her reaction to the condition.

KEY POINT

Life is about expanding. People become small when they remain in the problem. As they become still and peaceful, inner knowing emerges and they become whole again. Wholeness begins in thought and then is expressed in the physical.

Spiritual Preparation for Health and Healing

Increasing time in conscious connection and stillness brings people into a place of expanding peace, love, and healing. They begin to feel extremely positive and safe, as though nothing can go wrong. However, their comfort can cause them to be surprised and taken off guard when difficulties arise.

Pilots take time before each flight to do a preflight check of the craft and its instrumentation. They know that this preparation helps to ensure a smooth flight because problems are handled before the plane leaves the ground. Like the pilot, people can spare themselves some problems and function more smoothly by starting each day with a check of their minds, bodies, and spirits.

When individuals have had negative experiences that have not been worked through, they accumulate and find expression in various aspects of life. A daily time of quiet reflection can clarify the challenges that are present and assist in resolving issues. This time of daily reflection—sometimes called prayer, personal private time, getting quiet, meditation—is a time of being reflective and honest with the self. It gives one the opportunity to work on unresolved emotional issues.

Life can be categorized into five universal areas: personal relations, sexual relations, financial security, emotional security, and self esteem (1). Everything in life fits into one or more of these areas. When people begin to see the areas of life that are being threatened, then they are able to determine how these threats repeatedly appear in different forms. Once they identify the blocks to health, peace, and love, they can turn these blocks over to a Higher Power and continue with living and being. They are taking action to control their threats rather than be controlled by them.

Reflection

Identifying Patterns:
   With paper and pencil in hand find a quiet place.
   Review your day.
   Select a current issue or problem.
   In two or three words state why it is a problem.
   Ask what area or areas of your life is being threatened: personal relations, sexual
      relations, financial security, emotional security, and self-esteem.
   Select another issue and repeat the process.
   Continue repeating the process until all of the day's issues have been identified.
   Look for similarities in causes among the issues.
   These are the patterns that restrict your life.

Imagine that you have a very special friend whom you hold in great esteem. This wonderful and fantastic friend takes care of your requests. After you tell this friend about whatever areas of your life are being threatened, you immediately feel secure, light, and free. Wouldn't it be great to have a friend like this? People do. This friend goes by many names: *Higher Power, Infinite Intelligence, God, the Absolute, or Creator.*

The second part of spiritual preparation is having faith that every thing is being taken care of and that there is nothing more that one needs to do. When you instruct the computer with a series of commands, you often get a please wait comment on the screen while the computer is working on the instructions. Likewise, when things are turned over to God or a higher power, people often get a "please wait" message, although this response may not be communicated as obviously as the message on a computer screen. Individuals must go about their lives and trust that the higher power is in charge and taking care of everything. When worry is released to a higher power it is no longer necessary to think or obsess over it. This also means that not only is the outcome out of one's control, but that it also may not be what one envisioned. Sometimes what we want isn't what we really need.

Service as Healing

In the process of healing people can become quite absorbed in changing the effects or symptoms in their lives. It soon becomes clear that as long as they stay focused on themselves, they will not be fully connected to the whole. In truth, they are part of every-thing: the planet, the universe, and the situations happening around them. All of these effect reality. When people personalize illness, it keeps them separated from the whole; they can blame others, their situations, and themselves. When they move illness from a personal to a larger perspective it changes their primary consciousness—a change out of the blaming, self-serving ego into the expanded awareness of the unity and con-nectedness of all things.

From this larger perspective people can begin to realize that a critical part of heal-ing is being of service to others. As long as they are focused on themselves, people can never truly heal. They need to discover that to receive they must give; to be loved, they must be loving; and to heal, they must be healing to others. There can be no re-ceiving without giving.

KEY POINT

The universal law of giving and receiving is interactive and circular: One cannot occur without the other.

Being of service comes in all shapes and forms—offering a glass of water to a thirsty traveler, paying the difference at the cash register for some one who is short of cash, calling someone who is feeling isolated and down, washing a daughter's new dress by hand, volunteering to clean the gutters of a neighbor's home. Service without motive creates an atmosphere of love and joy. The only reason for doing is the pure act of love and connectedness. In order to be healed one must be in the place of service to others, to administer to others without any motive except to give.

Health Benefits of Faith

Faith has been accepted and recognized as very powerful through the ages. This includes faith in oneself, in what one is doing, in friends, and in God. Faith is much more than just the religious experience of faith, although the highest expression of faith is in the spiritual attitude.

Frequently, the main element lacking in prayer life and daily life is faith. People pray, turn things over to a higher power, then dig them up to see if they have sprouted or taken root.

Reflection How often do you ask for assistance and then take your troubles back and worry about them, rather than trusting that help will be provided?

Faith establishes a rapport with the infinite. There is the realization that whatever is causing the stress and the imbalance—a higher power, God—is in complete charge. Every thing is moving in divine concert for the highest and best. Faith opens people not only to healing, but to all the activities that support that healing process—diet, exercise, environment, and thinking patterns.

Faith means a conviction that all is well. People must nurture faith and release thoughts that would in any way weaken this conviction. The attitudes of belief, acceptance, and trust build and nourish faith. Any thoughts that threaten or weaken any of these attitudes, even in the slightest, also weaken faith. When thinking is in line, then the healing process is accelerated.

Attention, Attitudes, and Healing

Attention, attitudes, and healing are invisible, yet their effects are constantly producing visible forms in life. If this thought life is not aligned and in balance, there will be painful consequences. Where individuals place their attention is what they bring into their lives. When they focus on problems, they potentially are inviting more problems. By focusing on pain, they experience more pain; by focusing on the relief of the pain they experience comfort.

Reflection

Where Is Your Attention?
  Wait until you are thirsty.
  Fill a glass half full with water.
  Observe your thoughts.
  Are you seeing the glass half empty or half full?
  Are you thinking about how good the water will taste or that it won't be enough?
  Are you thinking about how your thirst will be quenched or that you will still be thirsty?
  Where is your attention?

Simply observing breathing will reveal much about how individuals are responding to a situation. When people become constricted in their thinking or are becoming fearful about something, their breathing becomes shallow. People need to be taught that when this change in breathing is observed, they need to breathe deeply and remind themselves that their higher power is in charge, not the fear or the doubts of the life situation.

People are living an endless and ever-expanding experience. Only by expanding the mind and spirit can one evolve, grow, and heal. When bound by the past with all its constrictions and predetermined ways to do things, people are contracting. When they breathe deeply and allow themselves to move past this, they expand consciousness and enter into new understandings of unity and connectedness with a Higher Power.

People have the opportunity to begin life anew—to have the opportunity to set into motion the deeper positive attitudes that heal. They can either stay where they are and repeat their mistakes of the past in different forms, or change their attitudes and the attention of their thoughts. Through attention and the observation of their thoughts, they come into alignment with awareness and its health and healing properties. They become where they place their attention.

Reflection

Read this story and consider if you have witnessed similar experiences in your life. Think about what a health professional could do to lead more people to behave like Beth.

There were three women who all lived in the same town; they all had the same type of breast cancer in the same location at the same time. They all went to the same doctor. When Sally heard the diagnosis she cried and felt her life had ended. She could think of nothing else but the dreaded course of the disease and how she was going to die. She was dead within six months. June received the news with mixed emotions and vacillated between being dreadfully depressed and feeling rather well about the prognosis and treatment. She had treatment on and off for three years, gradually going down hill and finally dying. Beth was shocked to hear the news of her breast cancer and went home and shared it with her husband. She spent time getting quiet, reading about the symptoms, and finding the treatment that felt the best for her. She discovered tapes, books, and friends that talked and worked in positive thinking. Her attention was on healing—herself, her family, and others. Twenty years later she is doing well, still focusing on healing—herself, her family and others.

When attention is coupled with an attitude of healing, movement can begin toward new solutions. People will begin to feel and know that healing is taking place in every aspect of their lives. Every time they realize they strayed from this place of high watch they can return. The art of realization is enough to take them out of the negative thoughts. It is as though they have become the watcher of their thoughts rather than being their thoughts. They can move back into the center of all life and allow peace to substitute for judgment, anger, and impatience. Being here in the present moment is the place of peace, healing, truth, and oneness with the Infinite.

KEY POINT

Be *here* NOW.

The Spiritual Connection

We came from a perfect creator. Our essence is whole, perfect, and complete. We are our creator in microcosm. Health, healing, and balance are already present.

The task of every person is to know wholeness, health, perfection, and completeness in his or her mind and heart right now; to recognize his or her perfection as a spiritual being. No doubts, no disbeliefs, no maybes—simply assurance in knowing. Any beliefs that do not support this must be released. As the mind becomes cleared from doubt and limitation, one is able to discover radiant health and healing.

Chapter Summary

Although spirituality is a thread within religion, it is a broader concept than religion. It entails the relationship with a higher power that can be identified by various names by different people. It is important to health and healing for individuals to get in touch with their spirituality. This can be facilitated by establishing a daily quiet time for reflection, letting go of preconceived notions of how things should go and people should act, turning things over to a higher power, and serving others.

Reference

1. A. A. World Services, Inc. (1955). *Alcoholics Anonymous*. New York: Alcoholics Anonymous.

Suggested Readings

Aresvik, S. (1995). *An Adult Primer for a Happy Life*. Seattle: Aresvik, S.

Bailey, J. V. (1990). *The Serenity Principle*. San Francisco: Harper.

Barnum, B. S. (2003). *Spirituality in Nursing*. 2nd ed. New York: Springer Publishing Company.

Carlson, R. (1992). *You Can Be Happy No Matter What*. San Rafael, CA: New World Library.

Chopra, D. (1995). *The Seven Spiritual Laws of Success*. California: Amber-Allen.

Clark, G. (1989). *The Man Who Tapped the Secrets of the Universe*. Waynesboro, VA: The Walter Russell Foundation.

Dass, R. (2002). *One-Liners: A Mini Manual for a Spiritual Life*. New York: Bell Tower.

Dossey. L. (2003). *Healing the Body: Medicine and the Infinite Reach of the Mind*. London: Random House.

Dossey, L. (1999). *Reinventing Medicine: Beyond Mind-Body to a New Era of Healing*. San Francisco: Harper.

Dossey, L. (1997). *Prayer Is Good Medicine*. New York: HarperCollins.

Furtado, T. (1992, January/February). The listening cure. *Utne Reader*, 89–96.

Hillman, J. (1999). *The Force of Character and the Lasting Life*. New York: Random House.

Hirshberg, C. and Barasch, M. (1995). *Remarkable Recovery: What Extraordinary Healings Tell Us about Getting Well and Staying Well*. New York: Riverhead Books.

Kimble, M. A., McFadden, S. H., Ellor, J. W., and Seeber, J. J., eds. (1995). *Aging, Spirituality, and Religion*. Minneapolis: Fortress Press.

Krishnamurti, J. (1989). *Think on These Things*. London: Perennial Library.

Krishnamurti, J. (1975). *Freedom from the Known*. New York: Harper & Row.

Larson, D. B., Sawyers, J. P., and McCullough, M. E. eds. (1998). *Scientific Research on Spirituality and Health: A Consensus Report*. Rockville, MD: National Institute for Healthcare Research.

Leder, D. (1997). *Spiritual Passages: Embracing Life's Sacred Journey*. New York: Jeremy P. Tarcher/Putnam.

Lowry, L. E. and Conco, D. (2002). Exploring the meaning of spirituality with aging adults in Appalachia. *Journal of Holistic Nursing, 20*(4):388–402.

Moss, R. (1981). *The I That Is We: Awakening to Higher Energies through Unconditional Love.* New York: Celestial Arts.

Myss, C. (1996). *Anatomy of the Spirit.* New York: Three Rivers Press.

Nerburn, K. and Koch, M., eds. (1991). *Native American Wisdom.* California: New World Library.

Pargament, K. I. (1997). *The Psychology of Religion and Coping.* New York: Guilford Press.

Shelly, J. A. and Miller, A. B. (1999). *Called to Care. A Christian Theology of Nursing.* Downers Grove, IL: InterVarsity Press.

Schweitzer, R., Norberg, M., and Larson, L. (2002). The parish nurse coordinator: A bridge to spiritual health care leadership for the future. *Journal of Holistic Nursing, 20*(3):212–231.

Stanley, C. (1997). *The Blessings of Brokenness.* Grand Rapids, MI: Zondervan Publishing House.

Thomas, E. L. and Eisenhandler, S. A. (1999). *Religion, Belief, and Spirituality in Late Life.* New York: Springer.

Tolle, E. (1999). *The Power of NOW: A Guide to Spiritual Enlightenment.* California: New World Library.

Tsai, C. C. (1994). *Zen Speaks: Shouts of Nothingness,* B. Bruya, Trans. New York: Anchor Books, Doubleday.

Wallace, S. (2000). Rx RN: A spiritual approach to aging. *Alternative and Complementary Therapies, 6*(1):47–48.

Walters, D. (2000). *Marrow of Flame: Poems of the Spiritual Journey.* Arizona: Hohm Press.

Weber, E. B. (1983). *Quiet Talks with the Master.* California: DeVorss.

Weil, A. (2000). *Spontaneous Healing.* New York: Knopf.

Wilt, D. L. and Smucker, C. J. (2001). *Nursing the Spirit.* Washington, D.C.: American Nurses Publishing.

Related Web Sites

www.livingthepresence.org
www.spiritualityhealth.com
www.wellbeingranch.org

CHAPTER 10

BALANCING WORK AND LIFE

Objectives

This chapter should enable you to:

- Define *work*
- List three purposes of work
- Describe at least eight characteristics of a positive work attitude
- List three negative work experiences
- Describe at least three measures to convert negative work experiences into positive work experiences

"Good living and good work go together. Life and livelihood ought not to be separated but to flow from the same source, which is Spirit, for both life and livelihood are about Spirit" (1). Life and work are about living with meaning, intention, joy, and a sense of contributing to the order and harmony of the family, community, and the universe.

Meanings of Work

Work is defined as "exertion or effort directed to produce or accomplish something" (2). We work to provide ourselves with goods and services needed for life. Work is simply part of life. However, work is not a simple term. Work has different meanings for different people, often as a result of their experiences with work.

Some people say they are lucky because work does not feel like work to them. They claim their work is enjoyable and satisfying regardless of the monetary reward. One wonders why these people are reluctant to identify work as work. What does the word *work* mean to these people? Why do they associate the term *work* with something undesirable?

Others connect work only with drudgery, toil, travail, and slavery. They consider work as something to be avoided as much as possible. They may say, "If I could only win the sweepstakes, I would never work again." One wonders if they would really be satisfied to live the rest of their lives in total leisure. Is it really work they abhor or the work in which they are currently engaged that they abhor?

Many people associate work with earning money and consider any activity for which they receive pay work. Yet, not all work is paid work. Those who devote their time to rearing children and caring for the sick and elderly in their homes, for example, are often considered unemployed even though they are surely working. As caretakers they use their talents to provide service to others and may even be aware of the purposes of their service in the universe. Their work is sometimes fascinating, delightful, and joyful but also demanding, distressing, frustrating, sad mysterious, and even frightening. Although caretaking may not be acknowledged as work, most people do understand that it is important and contributes to the good of society.

Reflection   What does work mean to you? What has influenced your thoughts about what constitutes work?

Work contributes to self-development, thereby serving a purpose greater than the production of goods and services (3). Work causes most people to feel productive, satisfied, and worthwhile. Therefore, the need to work remains even when sufficient goods and services can be produced with ease, as is witnessed in technologically advanced societies. Work, moreover, is essential to our well-being as humans.

A survey of older Americans showed that 40 percent of men and women between the ages of 50 and 75 were working or planned to work in retirement (4). Another 40 percent served as volunteers or planned to volunteer when they retired. They did not want a full-time job, but they wanted to work and make a contribution in the larger scheme of society. Apparently, for many, the need to work does not automatically disappear at the age of retirement. They may quit their jobs, but they do not stop working.

KEY POINT

Work serves many purposes, among them providing necessary and useful materials and services, an opportunity for service, and—in cooperation with others—an opportunity to build community, and a means to use and develop individual gifts and talents.

Positive Work Experiences

You probably have experienced the joys of work at one time or another, whether in a job for which you receive wages or in doing a household chore, such as cleaning your house or raking the yard. You drew satisfaction not just from the results of the work (a job well done or a clean house or yard), but also from the process. You inherently know what work is good regardless of what others may think.

Perhaps your work is not separated from the rest of life, but permeates your entire manner of living. You see work a useful endeavor that is satisfying in itself and brings significant pleasure. Such work is an important part of a harmonious life and is not viewed as a duty or an obsession.

A positive attitude toward work contributes to a harmonious life–work spirit state. Some of the qualities that contribute to a positive work attitude are described in Exhibit 10–1. People who display these qualities consider whatever work they are engaged in to be part of a greater whole. Their sense of purpose is not obscured by a particular task so they can shift their thinking and actions as needed. In the interests of furthering a project, they will put aside what they are doing to help a co-worker when necessary.

- They see the unifying patterns and common threads, not just the conflicts and contradictions.
- They perceive the possibilities and draw on varied resources instead of becoming mired in old mind sets.

EXHIBIT 10–1 QUALITIES CONSISTENT WITH A POSITIVE WORK ATTITUDE

A person with a positive work attitude:

- Is rejuvenated rather than depleted by work
- Gives full attention given to the effort
- Experiences an altered sense of time
- Displays a creative and nurturing outlook
- Is optimistic
- Demonstrates open-mindedness
- Has abundant energy
- Feels a sense of purpose
- Sees self as an important contributor to a great order
- Appreciates the contribution of others

- They recognize and appreciate the contributions and talents of their co-workers.
- They measure their effectiveness by the quality of their relationships.
- They delight in the work process as well as the product.
- They possess an enthusiasm in the work setting that suggests harmony of spirit and optimum balance of life and work.

Negative Work Experiences

Not everyone in today's society experiences harmony in their life and work. Job stress seems to be a common problem in all industrialized societies. Unemployment, underemployment, and overwork are major problems.

Work is commonly seen in negative terms in our modern industrial society. In the interests of efficiency, jobs sometimes are limited to a small segment of a task that does not afford us a sense of the whole. Our language reflects this idea. The term *job* once meant *lump* and was used to refer to insignificant, trifling work (5). People are called "cogs in the wheels of industry" or a "minor functionary in the machinery of an organization," and compared to computers with their effectiveness measured by their ability to multitask. Work becomes misdirected and no longer serves our purposes. Instead, work creates undue stress and absorbs an undue portion of our attention.

Unemployment

For those who are unemployed, the lack of work can have profound emotional and spiritual effects. These people are deprived of an opportunity to realize their unique talents, contribute to the welfare of their families, and to pay taxes that will service the greater community. When they are forced to depend on public assistance for extended periods of time their pride is further undermined. They receive the message that they are not needed or valued and in some measure almost become invisible.

Unemployment certainly affects society in more than an economic sense. The unemployed are unable to fully participate in the community. Is it in any wonder that people who are not able contribute through working turn to violence, drugs, and other modes of self hatred as a way of announcing their presence? Everyone needs a sense of feeling needed and making a contribution to the welfare of others within the scope of their capability.

Underemployment

Underemployment, though perhaps not as clearly harmful as unemployment, also takes a toll on the persons affected. The message for the underemployed, though more subtle, is the same as for the unemployed. Some may derive limited satisfaction from being gainfully occupied and perhaps being able to pay bills. They often work in part-time jobs or only part of the year when they want full-time employment year round. They believe they have no options, so they stay in their jobs. Still others remain in jobs that do not truly engage them simply because they earn high wages. They turn to activities other than work for fulfillment or seek pleasure in what their wages can buy them. They may work in jobs that require little skill and afford almost no chance to develop any of their special talents or realize personal achievements.

Overwork

Overwork is an increasing problem. Sometimes this addiction to work is driven by the desire for consumer goods. Nothing is good enough; there is always a better appliance or gadget to lure us, and these new and improved objects cost money. It is easy to get caught in the wheel of earning and spending. As we increase the time devoted to work, we often sacrifice health, relationships, and other important areas of our lives. We spend so much time earning money to buy things that we seldom get to enjoy what we've bought.

KEY POINT

There is a perception that "people are killing themselves with work, busyness, rushing, caring, and rescuing. Work addiction is a modern epidemic and it is sweeping our land" (6).

Some of us become workaholics whereby our fundamental identities are equated with our work; we see ourselves only in terms of our jobs: "I am an accountant"; "I am a lawyer." Success is solely measured by the number of clients or cases and/or the amount of money earned. Workaholics have difficulty relaxing. There is a persistent need to complete a few more tasks before they can feel good and allow themselves a break. At the same time, they often feel resentful about their need to continue their frantic, compulsive working. If anything happens to prevent them from continuing this pattern, their basic identity is threatened. Being is completely absorbed by doing.

Even when performing acts of charity, workaholics press on to do more and more. Guilt drives them on, never allowing them to rest.

KEY POINT

Overwork is toxic, whatever the goal, because it separates us from our deeper selves and unbalances us.

Many people have separated their lives from their work and endure work in order to satisfy materialistic needs and desires. They dream of retirement when they can be free of the burden of work. Work is not a natural part of their lives.

Work for many is experienced in jobs that mostly consist of mindless and repetitive tasks for which they have little interest that are designed to produce profits for which they have little shares. Discontent, passiveness, boredom, lack of joy, a sense of hopelessness, and a vague feeling that life is meaningless permeates these situations.

Organizational Changes

Fortunately, there is emerging awareness that job situations that are fragmented and disconnected from a sense of the whole are not only disadvantageous for the workers, but not good for the bottom line either. Flexible hours, child care, parent leave, and job sharing are helpful in some cases, but do not serve most workers. Current trends of increasing burnout, decreased employee satisfaction, and rising healthcare costs are spurring changes in work settings. Greater attention is being paid to how an organization can improve the quality of work for employees, not just how employees can benefit the organization. New models for organizations that emphasize balance are being tried.

KEY POINT

Organizations, like individuals, need to achieve a balance between input and output. Like fossil fuels, individuals and organizations need to be replenished.

What Is to Be Done?

The problems associated with work in today's society are very complex. So, what can be done? The achievement of harmony and balance in work and life occurs when life and livelihood are reunited. People need to search for ways to convert negative work experiences into positive ones. This begins with them taking the first step by changing their image of work.

Some people may have given little thought to the full impact and image of work in their lives. They may think of work in terms of a paycheck and benefits and productivity for the employer. In order for them to achieve a healthier work life, they need to reflect on the quality of their work experience. Exhibit 10–2 offers a Spirituality of Work Questionnaire that can be used to guide people through this process. The response can be used as a springboard for discussion leading to a deeper exploration of the meaning of work.

What Our Language Tells Us

Our language reflects the time pressure many of us feel on a regular basis. Phrases, such as *time savers, fast food, express lane, rapid transit, overnight delivery,* and *instant*

EXHIBIT 10–2 SPIRITUALITY OF WORK QUESTIONNAIRE

1. Do you feel drawn to the work you do? If yes, why did you choose this work? Has this feeling increased or decreased over time? Why?

2. Do you have a sense of purpose in the work you do?

3. Do you experience your work as a part of a greater whole?

4. What are the unifying patterns in your work?

5. Do you experience enthusiasm for your work? If so, under what circumstances? How frequently? What increases your enthusiasm? What dampers it?

6. How does your work enhance or interfere with your creative expression?

7. Do you continue to learn from your work? Why or why not?

8. How does your work affect others?

9. Who benefits from your work?

10. In what ways does your work distress others?

11. How do you recognize the talents and contributions of others in your work setting?

12. What is the quality of your relationship with coworkers?

13. How does your work affect the environment?

14. Is your work in harmony with the environment?

15. How does your work contribute to caring for the environment?

16. How will your work affect future generations?

17. What are the long-term effects of the work you do?

18. What are the unintended consequences of the work you do?

19. Would you continue to work if you suddenly became independently wealthy? What would you do instead of the work you are now doing? How would you use the money?

20. How do you rest from work and renew yourself?

21. What do you do with your leisure time?

22. What would you do if you had a sabbatical year?

23. What is sacred about the work you do?

24. What is your philosophy of work?

25. What do you value about your work?

message control our lives. Colleges and universities have created accelerated programs so students can complete the requirements for a baccalaureate in three rather than four years and even begin working for a graduate degree while still an undergraduate. Young children are pressured to get a head start in our highly competitive world. Parents rush around shuttling their children to gymnastics, soccer games, computer classes, and other assorted activities to ensure their admission to the better colleges. Free play is almost a thing of the past. We even have an expression for this need to hurry; we say we are experiencing a "time crunch." It is as though things are out of control and we are all traveling at warp speed.

Reflection Notice how your life is affected by the messages that link a fast pace and busyness with importance. What do they do to you? Uncover, accept, and understand the patterns that influence your life. As you increase your awareness of these patterns, you will be in a better position to correct the imbalances you find.

The popular press offers many articles on how to cope with our accelerated pace and be more efficient. We are inundated with suggestions for setting goals, improving organization, and increasing efficiency. We are told, for example, to handle each piece of mail only once; to make lists and prioritize tasks and to reduce the time in meetings by allotting specific, limited times for each item on the agenda. We are encouraged to speed read and are inundated with periodicals that provide digests of the literature of journals in our fields.

The motto in many work settings is, "Do more with less and do it faster." Workers sometimes feel that they are treated like parts of a machine, and they must maintain the expected pace or be discarded as obsolete. Although some of the ideas can be helpful, there is the danger of over-planning and structuring life at the expense of living life.

The material and psychological rewards people receive from their increased efficiency, may simply prompt them to invest more time and energy into work at the expense of their health, family, and community. They may end up working more efficiently, but also longer hours. Workers in the United States already work more hours than workers in other industrialized countries. (7) It is easier to become psychologically trapped by success as success begets greater expectations for performance.

Reflection Reflect on your own work situation and consider what you can change to promote balance. Reestablish control of your life and schedule. You may need to review your spending habits and eliminate expenses that are not essential in order to reduce the amount of time you spend working. Avoid turning to shopping as therapy. Consider decommercializing holiday festivities and creating simpler but meaningful holiday rituals. Find ways of sharing with your neighbors through borrowing and lending. Practice saying "no." Restore the practice of providing Sabbath time for your-self. You may discover increased life satisfaction!

Balancing Work and Life

People are encouraged to live a balanced life, but what is a *balanced life*? *Balance* means the harmonious ratio between all parts, not necessarily equally divided parts (8). Just as people need to balance the time they devote to sleep with the time they are awake, they need to balance the time spent in work with the time spent in other activities. Individuals determine this balance for themselves. The ratio of time spent in each activity creates a harmonious whole for them and fosters their well-being.

People need to be challenged with the question: "Why do you work?" All activities—sleeping, eating, playing, and working—are part of living. Work is not something done merely to acquire something else. Work should be connected to one's being and be its expression; it is a *spiritual activity*. Work that is externally driven interferes with that connection.

KEY POINT

Work should serve a higher purpose than merely as the means to acquiring material goods.

Converting Negative into Positive Work Experiences

There is much talk about stress and its effects on health. Some believe stress causes illness and should be decreased, if not totally eliminated. This is an oversimplification of the notion of stress. Stress is inevitable and can be a positive force. Stress, for example, can prompt you to look for solutions and solve problems.

Any number of events that people experience as normal—changes in living conditions, work, relationships, even ordinarily joyous occasions such as marriage or the birth of a child—can be stressful. These stressors, however, do not inevitably cause illness. People can learn to manage them by finding balance with nutrition, exercise, play, and relaxation.

KEY POINT

Humans have varied natural, biologic rhythms like those found in nature (9). One of the important rhythms humans experience during one 24-hour period is known as the *ultradian rhythm*. The general pattern of this rhythm is 90-to-120 minutes of activity, followed by a 20-minute recovery period. Periods of higher energy regularly alternate with signals suggesting a need for rest. Ignoring signals calling for rest while continuing to work will upset the ultradian rhythm and lead to stress. Responding appropriately to the call for rest supports the normal pattern and allows for recovery and renewal. Even a small change in activity may be beneficial. Planning your work so that after approximately 90 minutes of concentration on a project, you take a stretch break or engage in a different activity will help. A play break during work may help to restore us. An egg of silly putty in your pocket may be all that is needed to shift focus and provide the needed relief (10).

Life-Balancing Skills

Although major problems associated with work can only be addressed on a societal level, there are some things that can be done to manage many of the problems on an individual basis. Individuals have inner resources that can be drawn upon to cope with daily stresses. Researchers have found that certain personality traits help people cope effectively with emotional wear and tear. These traits prevent people from breaking down emotionally and physically in the face of life crises.

The capacity to *Attend, Connect,* and *Express* (ACE factor) feelings can help people to maintain physical and mental health. Feelings (emotions) are gifts that provide people with information about the effects of what is happening at that moment. When people attend to those feelings, connect them to consciousness, and express them appropriately, they are able to successfully cope with stress and restore balance to their systems. For instance, when you notice a dull, aching pain in your right shoulder, you draw your attention to the pain (attend) rather than simply try to mask the pain with medication. You ask yourself questions to connect the pain with what is happening to you. When did the pain start? Can the pain be associated with a particular activity or movement? Is the pain worse at the end of the work day or work month; when the weather is cold or damp? What is the character of the pain? Does it come on suddenly or does it build up gradually over time? You may immediately recognize that the pain is related to the increased time you spend at the computer doing billing before the end of the month. A closer look at how you arrange your work area may suggest that you are stressing your right shoulder. You notice that you are repeatedly twisting your right shoulder as you do this monthly task. You are now in the position to look for creative solutions to your problem. You may realize that you can rearrange your work station to avoid the stress on your right shoulder. By doing so, you eliminate the source of your pain and still fulfill your job responsibilities.

Other troubles in the workplace can occur. Work can be a place of misunderstanding or undue competition that threatens well-being. Perhaps your work situation causes irritation or even anxiety. Skill in using the ACE factor can be helpful in such situations. For example, you notice that you tend to make mistakes when you are assigned to work with a particular coworker. The same thing doesn't happen when you work with others. You feel that this one person doesn't like you; he acts unfriendly and seems to be impatient when things do not go smoothly. You notice that as soon as you receive your assignment to this coworker, your stomach seems to get tied up in knots and you already sense things will not go well. You may get stuck in blaming this coworker for your difficulties, complain to your supervisor or union, and/or do all in your power to discredit this person. You may be successful in changing the situation; you or the targeted coworker may be reassigned. You may find you are forced to work with someone who is even more difficult and the situation may grow worse. Now you are faced with an even bigger problem. You are reluctant to call attention to the problem for fear of being labeled "difficult." Your anxiety increases and you find that your health deteriorates as a result. The ACE factor can be applied in this circumstance as well. You start to attend to the signs that your anxiety level is increasing. You connect the increased anxiety to your tendency to make errors. You acknowledge (express) the link between your anxiety and errors. Your awareness allows you to take steps to reduce your anxiety (take a few deep breaths, for example). You may further consider the link and discover the underlying source of the anxiety. This coworker works at a faster speed than you do and your anxiety increases when you cannot match his speed. You ask your coworker for help and you work together to find a solution to the problem.

KEY POINT

The ACE factor can be good for your health. Research shows that people who lack the ACE factor have weaker immune systems, which results in less ability to defend against infectious diseases and cancer (11). Persons who have greater ACE abilities have stronger immune systems. Quite simply, neither the presence or absence of anxiety, nor the degrees of anxiety are the deciding factors. Rather it is how the person deals with the anxiety that makes the difference.

You cannot ignore feelings, disregard their meanings, and repress expression without adverse consequences to your health. Anxiety, like pain, is a signal that tells us something is wrong and needs our attention.

People who are psychologically hardy have been found to have certain characteristics referred to as the three Cs: *commitment, control,* and *challenge* (12). People who are strong in commitment find meaning and purpose in their work as long as the work is useful and not harmful. They are wholeheartedly involved in whatever work they do. A person who works as a garbage collector, by knowing the meaning of his or her work and appreciating its contribution to society, has commitment. Drudgery may be part of the work, but drudgery does not negate its purpose or value. When we are committed, the meaning of our work will be present to us even when it is obscured by routine and only breaks through to our awareness from time to time.

Reflection Do you feel you have control over your work activities, are committed to them, and are able to framework problems as challenges to overcome rather than threats?

People who believe and behave as though they have influence over life circumstances demonstrate control. These people have a sense of mastery and confidence in their ability to deal with the challenges of life even when faced with limitations in external freedom. Their sense of control is healthy and should be distinguished from unhealthy attempts to control others' behavior and reactions. People who demonstrate control respond to reports that there will be major layoffs in their plant with plans for dealing with that possibility. They begin to make immediate changes in their lifestyles to set aside extra money in the event they are among those laid off. They do not spend their energy railing against events over which they have no control.

People who are high in challenge view problems resulting from change as trials to overcome and not as threats. These people recognize that change also represents opportunities for growth and not just loss of comfort and security. They creatively adapt to the fact that they may lose their job by exploring other employment possibilities. These are the people who usually have an exit plan in place before they receive their pink slip.

Commitment, control, and challenge, often referred to as the hardiness factors, are the building blocks of healthy coping. Healthy copers respond to loss, instability, and change by drawing on their own inner resources. Those who have the hardiness factor are not necessarily younger, wealthier, better educated, or in possession of greater social support (13).

People ought not to postpone living because of their work or because of their plans to buy something with the money they make. It is easy to become absorbed in acquiring more and more money and lose sight of the original goal. Exhibit 10–3 lists questions that people can use to gain insight into their work/life balance. It can prove useful for people to discuss their responses with significant others in their lives or a professional who can assist them in making changes.

> ### EXHIBIT 10–3 QUESTIONS TO USE IN GUIDING ASSESSMENT OF LIFE/WORK BALANCE
>
> - Are you doing that which energizes and renews you?
> - What gives you the greatest joy?
> - Do you continue to expand your business in response to the opportunity to make more money to the detriment of your health and personal life?
> - Do you devote more time to work in order to escape problems at home?
> - Do you spend wastefully and then work overtime to pay your bills?
> - How would you really like to spend your time?
> - What are the things you always wanted to do but do not because of lack of time? How can you find the time to do these things?

Downshifting is one response to these daily realities. People find that by working less, they are able to do something more meaningful with their lives, including spending more time with their children. This requires a change in their basic thinking. A common tendency is to acquire things that allow us to live more luxuriously, but that do not necessarily enhance our lives. These possessions can become anchors that hold us down rather than free us. A person may buy a boat with the dream of spending sunny days relaxing on the water. However, the reality of the attention a boat needs may soon hit. The person will either have to invest time and energy to maintain the boat or spend money for someone else to do so; either option could impose a burden sufficient to dilute the joy of boat ownership. People need to ask themselves if their purchases will enhance the quality of their lives or be added burdens. Perhaps trips to the local public beach with family and friends could provide equal or greater pleasure than owning a boat.

It is difficult, however, for people to resist the predominant culture on their own. Adjusting to a reduced income requires adjusting to decreased spending. One needn't drop out of society to achieve the goal of simplicity. Refusing to buy name brand clothes for their children can initially create conflict for parents. Deciding to reduce spending on holiday presents and celebrations takes courage. Joining a group with similar goals can provide much needed support in efforts to downshift. Newsletters, Web sites, and study circles are springing up around the country to help those interested in transforming their work lives, spending habits, and values to create life/work balance. A list of suggested Web sites is provided at the end of this chapter.

Work is part of your life, but people should not live to work. They need to be careful not to postpone living in order to work. Work life needs to be in balance with personal life in a way that causes people to experience a unity that celebrates their personhood. Current lifestyle habits need not be permanent. People need to ask the critical questions that will help them to create a harmonious life-work balance in their lives.

Chapter Summary

Work serves many purposes, including providing materials and services, offering services to others for the purpose of building community, and enabling people to use and develop their gifts and talents. A positive work attitude contributes to a harmonious life–work spirit state and is reflected by being rejuvenated rather than depleted by work, giving full attention to the effort, experiencing an altered sense of time, displaying a creative and nurturing outlook, showing optimism, having abundant energy, demonstrating open-mindedness, feeling a sense of purpose, seeing self as an important contributor to a greater order, and appreciating the contributions of others.

Negative work experiences include unemployment, underemployment, and overwork. Some ways to convert negative work experiences into positive ones include re-arranging work schedules to coincide with ultradian rhythm, being attentive to feelings, developing psychological hardiness, and downshifting. People can achieve a higher quality of life by making work a meaningful, but not all-consuming experience.

Exploring the Web

For ideas about simplyfying your life, go to
http://www.tedtanaka.com/ted/workmgmt/keepsimp.htm

Find the latest publications in mental health related to work at
http://healthway.hypermart.net/mental8.htm.

To see an example of time management software go to
http://www.llamagraphics.com/LB/LifeBalanceTop.html.

To join a discussion on career and workplace issues go to
http://www.nytimes.com/library/financial/082299.html.

For ideas about downshifting go to the following sites:
www.adbusters.org
www.coopamerica.org
www.worktoliveinfo/poen_vaca.html

References

1. Fox, M. (1995). *The Reinvention of Work*. San Francisco: Harper, p. 1.

2. Random House. (1993). *Unabridged Dictionary*, 2nd ed., p. 2188.

3. Harman, W. (1998). *Global Mind Change. The Promise of the 21st Century*. 2nd ed. San Francisco: Berrett-Koehler, p. 170.

4. Older Adults Do Not Want "Golden Pond." (1999, September 11) *News and Record*, Greensboro, NC, A12.

5. Fox, M. (1995). *The Reinvention of Work*. San Francisco: Harper, p. 6.

6. Fassel, D. (2000). *Working Ourselves to Death. The High Cost of Workaholism and the Rewards of Recovery*. Lincoln, NE: iUniverse.com.

7. Swenson, R. A. (1998). *The Overload Syndrome*. Colorado Springs: VAV Press, p. 171.

8. Muller, W. (1999). *Sabbath. Restoring the Sacred Rhythm of Rest*. New York: Bantam Books, p. 97.

9. Bartol, G. M. and Courts, N.F. (2000). The Psychophysiology of Bodymind Healing. In Dossey, B. M., Keegan, L., Guzzetta, C. E., eds., *Holistic Nursing*, 3rd ed. Gaithersburg, MD: Aspen Publishers, pp. 77–78.

10. Kolkmeier, L. G. (2000). Play and Laughter: Moving toward Harmony. In Dossey, B. M., Keegan, L., Guzzetta, C. E., eds., *Holistic Nursing*, 3rd ed. Gaithersburg, MD: Aspen Publishers, p. 321.

11. Dreher, H. (1995). *The Immune Power Personality*. New York: Penguin Books, p. 51.

12. Ibid., p. 52.

13. Ibid., pp. 125, 128, 167.

Suggested Readings

Aron, C. S. (1999). *Working at Play*. New York: Oxford University Press.

Bolles, R. N. (2002). *What Color Is Your Parachute*. New York: Barnes & Noble.

Briggs, J. and Peat, D. (2000). *Seven Life Lessons of Chaos*. New York: Harper-Perennial.

Caproni, P. J. (2000). *The Practical Coach: Management Skills for Everyday Life*. New York: Pearson Education.

Damasio, A. (1999). *The Feeling of What Happens*. New York: Harcourt, Brace.

Davidson, J. and Dreher, H. (2003). *The Anxiety Book.* New York: Penguin Putnam.

Dossey, B. M., Keegan, L., and Guzzetta, C. E. (2000). *Holistic Nursing*, 3rd ed. Gaithersburg, MD: Aspen Publications.

Fassel, D. (2000). *Working Ourselves to Death. The High Cost of Workaholism. The Rewards of Recovery.* San Francisco: iUniverse.

Fox, M. (1994). *The Reinvention of Work.* San Francisco: Harper.

Harman, W. (1998). *Global Mind Change. The Promise of the 21st Century*, 2nd ed. San Francisco: Berrett-Koehler.

Post, N. S. (1995). Bringing Your Body to Work: The Five Element System in Organizational Life. *Dissertation Abstracts International: Section B: The Sciences & Engineering, 55*(11–B):5113.

Robinson, J. (2003). *Work to Live: The Guide to Getting a Life.* New York: Perigee.

Rutledge, T. (1998). *Earning Your Own Respect.* Oakland, CA: New Harbinger Publications.

Rutledge, T. (2002). *Embracing Fear.* New York: HarperCollins.

Schor, J. B. (1999). *The Overspent American.* New York: HarperCollins.

Schumacher, E. F. (1989). *Small Is Beautiful. Economics as if People Mattered.* New York: HarperCollins.

Swenson, R. and Margin, A. (1998). *The Overload Syndrome.* Colorado Springs: NAV Press.

Wheatley, M. J. (2001). *Leadership and the New Science.* San Francisco: Berrett-Koehler.

Wheately, M. and Kellner-Rogers, M. A. (1999). *A Simpler Way.* San Francisco: Berrett-Koehler.

CHAPTER 11

CREATIVE FINANCIAL HEALTH

Objectives

This chapter should enable you to:

- Define *money*
- Discuss the energetic principles of money
- Describe the universal laws that apply to money
- Discuss the difference between a *mechanistic* and *holistic* perspective on money
- List at least six measures that can promote harmony of body, mind, and spirit in achieving financial goals

Except for the payment of services, the area of finances is rarely regarded a consideration in health care, yet it can significantly influence health status. Money affects all areas of life, including where you live, your education, the types of food you eat, and the amount of stress in your life.

It seems that everywhere you turn you are faced with television programs, articles, and seminars that correlate money with health and happiness. In actuality, there is truth to this. The emerging medical specialty of *psychoneuroimmunology* is confirming that positive emotions and happiness result in a higher-functioning immune system and, consequently, better health. If the amount of money you have is responsible for your level of happiness and contentment in life, then you could surmise that money is an important factor in promoting health.

KEY POINT

Minted coins first appeared about 650 B.C. in Asia Minor. The neighboring Greeks began minting coins soon thereafter and within a few centuries developed a system of banking that included borrowing and lending money.

What Is Money?

Money is defined as standard pieces of gold, silver, copper, and nickel used as a medium of exchange. The word *money* is derived from the Latin word *moneta*, which means mint. One of the definitions of *mint* is to create, so you could reason that money serves to create. Money often is referred to as *currency* in which it shares a definition with *electricity*.

You may think of money in terms of paper and coins that carry value, but it is more than that. Money is an energy that is neutral. Your consciousness gives money the charge, either negative or positive, resulting in how it serves your life. Just as your mind can affect your physical health, it also can affect your financial health.

KEY POINT

There is a common view among spiritual and conscious prosperity coaches that suggests if all of the wealth in the world were distributed evenly to every man and woman, within a short time period the rich would be rich and the poor would be poor again.

Beliefs About Money

What is *wealth*? Who is rich? How do you determine financial security? The answers are based on perceptions, and your belief system creates your perceptual field. Beliefs are derived from a variety of sources, such as societal and cultural influences, religious background, ancestral heritage, educational systems, and the mind set of the adult household in which you were raised. Beliefs about money influence how you manage and use it, and how much you have. For example, many people who carry negative beliefs about money find themselves in states of financial deficit and struggle.

Many cultural influences shape beliefs about money. For example, your work ethic conveys the message that "you have to work very hard and struggle for all your money." Certain religious views imply that "to be spiritual one must live in poverty." These views are very old and embedded into masses of minds and consciousness. What messages have influenced your views about money? An awakening moment can come when you gain an understanding of the factors that have contributed to the beliefs you hold about money.

Reflection   What does financial security mean to you? How did you develop your beliefs about this?

It may be difficult to identify your true beliefs about money. A good way to discover your beliefs is to observe your thoughts, feelings, emotions, and desires when in the act of a financial exchange. For example, when writing a check to pay a bill or giving a donation, what are your thoughts and feelings? People who see the glass as half empty often find themselves with ongoing thoughts, such as "I can't really afford this." or "I wish I had more." Emotions that often accompany these thoughts can be anger, fear, or guilt; they come from a negative perspective. The good news is that it is possible to change beliefs to heal the wounds of *scarcity consciousness* and move into a more positive place by acquiring *abundance consciousness*.

Energetic Principles of Money

As mentioned earlier, money often is identified as currency, representing an avenue in which electricity or energy flows. Currency also carries a charge (another electrical/energetic term that has been adapted in our monetary transactions) that is given to it by the substance through which it is flowing. The way this applies to the way you deal with money is that the charge comes from your beliefs and attitudes (negative or positive). This charge magnetizes your energy field (through which you view the world) and consequently, through the use of universal law (definition and description to follow), you can put an energetic charge on money with your intentions and thoughts.

Become aware of the thoughts and intentions you have while you are handling money. If you note that they are negative, plan to create a change in your mind set. One suggestion is to have a positive thought or consider your blessings each time money passes through your hands. Gratitude is always a good energy to instill into money.

Energy masters from the East (who work with energy for healing) teach their students how to handle the physical aspects of money (bills, coins, checks, etc.). They instruct the handling of money to be done with energetic regard to help it flow more easily in one's life. For example, they advise that money should not be folded or stuffed in one's pocket or wallet, but placed properly in order with the bills facing in the same direction.

Money as Spiritual Energy

Money's spiritual roots are represented in its physical form of the dollar bill. On the dollar bill is an eagle that holds in its beak a scroll that reads *E pluribus unum*, which in Latin means *From many, one*. Also pictured on the bill is a pyramid, which is a noted spiritual geometric structure that has a truncated tip that holds the all-seeing eye of the Divine Providence, the guiding power of the universe, and the motto *Annuit coeptis,* which means *He has smiled on our undertakings.* Below the pyramid is a scroll that bears the inscription *Novus ordo seclorum* translated as *new order of the ages*. On every bill we read *In God We Trust.*

Many people who are seeking ways to develop an abundance consciousness utilize the affirmations, prayers, and other wisdom offered in ancient religious texts. For example, an ancient Hebrew prosperity affirmation is *Jehovah-Jireh, the Lord now richly provides*. In Deuteronomy 8:18, the insight that God is the source of prosperity is conveyed in the words *You shall remember the Lord your God, for it is he who gives you your power to get wealth.* The biblical admonition that *the love of money is the root of all evil* doesn't imply that money in itself is bad and harmful, but that the *love* or *worship* of money is. It is how people use money that matters. A healthy spiritual perspective realizes that money has its place and that it should not be idolized or used to harm others.

Reflection   Money can represent many things in a person's life. What does it mean to you?

Money as Metaphor

As money is a formless substance, it can take on various meanings in your life and represent different things. To many people, the degree to which one is loved and cared for is demonstrated with money. Money can represent something that has authority over you, or that can be used as a means to control others. Also, the way in which you deal with your money is a reflection of how you take care of yourself. Money is an extension of who you are in all areas of your life, therefore it is important when taking a holistic view of self and others that money be an integral consideration. The more ways in which this aspect is integrated and seen as a metaphor for different parts of yourself, the more you can come into your wholeness.

Universal Laws

Universal laws are unbreakable, unchangeable principles that operate in all phases of our lives and existence, for all people everywhere all the time; they are impartial, irrefutable, and unavoidable.

Universal laws are the framework in which you can operate as you change the perspective of money in your life, especially if there is an interest in working on the co-creative process of manifesting more money in your life. In actuality, universal laws exist whether you know about them or not—or whether you choose to work with them or not. They are similar to many physical laws that operate in your daily life of which you may not be aware—such as the law of gravity. Universal laws are nonphysical in nature, but are fundamental laws of mind and spirit. Everyday life is based on these laws, much like physical laws and laws of nature (changing of seasons, the sun shining, turning on a light switch, taking a shower, listening to the radio). As you rely on these laws in the physical world, so can you rely on universal laws of mind and spirit. People who consciously work in harmony with these laws find a high degree of fulfillment because they begin to align their actions with their purpose in life.

Florence Nightingale wrote extensively about universal law in an attempt to unify science and religion in a way that would bring order, meaning, and purpose to human life. She was motivated to use this information to help the working class people of England who wanted and needed an alternative to atheism. Nightingale said that universal laws are expressions of God's thoughts and law is a continuous manifestation of God's presence.

How Universal Laws Work

Universal laws work on an energetic premise with simple, subtle energy principles. There are two energetic fields in operation, co-existing and intermingling: the universal energy field and the human energy field. The divine order of energy is often referred to as God and is fixed. The human energy field, resulting from beliefs, thoughts, and attitudes, is a mutable force that can be created and formed (the free will aspect). That which you carry in your human energy field in the form of beliefs, attitudes, and thoughts will create an energetic charge that will incur a response according to universal laws. You can charge your field with new beliefs, attitudes, and thoughts simply by bringing in new input in the form of thoughts, much like one would program information into a computer. The following examples of universal laws will help to further explain how they work.

The Law of Expectancy

The Law of Expectancy suggests that *whatever you expect you will receive*. This is not the same as wishful thinking, but rather something that is expected with certainty, much like a pregnant woman is expecting a baby. The degree of expectancy that is maintained in your consciousness is vital. What is it that you are expecting? Do you expect to go to work tomorrow? Do you expect to make a certain amount of money? Expectations can limit you, even when you learn to temper your expectations. It is suggested that when working with the Law of Expectancy an open-ended thought should always be maintained; for example, "this or something better," "this or something more."

Faith is an important element in the Law of Expectancy. This wisdom is reflected in Matthew 9:29 where it is said *according to your faith be it done unto you*. In working with this law it is important not to limit expectations. Imagination helps with that. That is why Einstein said that *imagination is more powerful than knowledge*.

KEY POINT

Working with the Law of Expectancy is similar to working with principles of the reemerging ancient art of Chinese placement called *Feng Shui*. Feng Shui is an energetic approach to improving all aspects of one's life by working with the physical space in which people spend most of their time—either at home or in their offices. In Feng Shui, a *BaGua* is a map utilized of physical space. The BaGua is a standard template that has in it all areas of one's life and the location in their physical space that is connected to these areas of life. The section of the BaGua that is connected to money is in the Fortunate Blessings location. If there is junk, clutter, or physical discord in this area of someone's home or office, then that may impede the flow of financial energy in one's life. A way to enhance financial abundance in one's life is to clear the physical space in this area of their home according to the BaGua so as to prepare for the flow of blessings and prosperity.

The Law of Preparation

When you prepare for something you often get it, and that includes negative things as well positive ones. Do you know people who have put money away for a rainy day or an emergency? In a sense they are preparing for these negative experiences. The energy can be shifted and instead, they could consider preparing for abundance and success. It is important to prepare for something in your consciousness and then take action to achieve it.

The Law of Forgiveness

Energetically, forgiveness helps to remove blocks to receiving. It releases negative experiences in your consciousness and creates space that allows the entrance of divine consciousness in the form of abundance. One of the country's leading prosperity coaches, Edwene Gaines (1), believes that all financial debt is about unforgiveness of past issues and, mostly, not forgiving ourselves. She teaches that one of the fastest ways to prosperity and abundance is forgiving on a daily basis. Everyone and everything in the past should be forgiven so as to move forward in one's life abundantly.

Reflection Who and what do you need to forgive?

The Law of Tithing

The word *tithe* means *one-tenth* and usually is related to offering a portion of income to spiritual or sacred purposes. A tithe is usually given to a person, place, or institution that contributes to one's spiritual nourishment and growth. Tithing is one of the fundamental laws of life and a powerful prospering exercise. It is an ancient, spiritual practice mentioned throughout the Bible. In Genesis 28:20 Jacob said *of all that Thou shalt give me, I will surely give one tenth unto Thee.* Tithing can be seen as simple as the inflow/outflow principle. As with breathing where it is necessary to regularly rid yourself of air in order to receive fresh air into the lungs, so it is necessary to give regularly if you wish to receive regularly. "Whatsoever a man soweth, that shall he also reap." If you do not sow, you do not reap.

KEY POINT

The intent with tithing is to plant a seed. A farmer tithes in order to reap harvest, returning one-tenth of the grain to the soil.

Your Mission Becomes Your Money

Every person on this planet has a mission and a purpose in this lifetime. In order to fulfill your destiny, this work (*work* in the sense of contribution to the world not the source of a paycheck, although it may be delivered in that form) needs to be carried out. Too often, people are not connected to their purpose in life and, consequently, many imbalances may appear, including physical ailments, relationship disputes, and financial difficulties. Financial fulfillment can be derived through the process of following your own heart to perform the work of your dreams. More importantly, by tapping into and executing the right livelihood, spiritual aspects of life can be fulfilled.

The process of discovering your life mission can be a very challenging one. Often, people find themselves going through the motions of a job that not only is ill-suited for them, but may go against many of their natural energetic rhythms. However, the fear of not having enough and not being able to survive compel many to go against their natural flow and tolerate ill-suited work.

Reflection In what ways is your attitude about work different and similar to that of your parents and grandparents?

Discovering your mission in life is a spiritual and creative process. The approach to this process is very simple and begins by exploring your desires. It is that which is your greatest longing that takes you to your mission. Some people spend years not knowing what their purpose in life is, while others seem to know their purpose the moment they arrive on the planet. Many job opportunities in our society are focused on the needs of the employer, rather than being designed to fill people's needs of expressing their creative essence and offering their God-given gifts to the world. The system is created in such a way that people end up redesigning themselves to fit the system's needs. This, combined with fears about survival, results in stifled missions. Fear drives people to be stuck in containers (i.e., jobs) that aren't made for them.

KEY POINT

A mid-life crisis can occur when people feel they are limited by their jobs and not fulfilling their missions. In this awakening, there is a yearning to follow one's longing. The crisis can result in some unfortunate consequences, such as divorce and unsound business ventures, or in new opportunities that realign with values and life purpose.

Passion Creates Magnetism

There is a vital force connected with fulfilling life purpose and mission. Think of the vitality that people have when they are excited about what they are doing, even if it is interpreted as a mundane act to others. When one is excited, passionate, and satisfied with fulfilling an act of life there is a certain charge that is being created in the vital force field (energy; electro-magnetic field) of the individual. This energy creates magnetism and this magnetism draws in universal energy, which manifests abundance.

Fulfilling Mission versus Collecting a Paycheck

Identifying your mission is integral to the process of attaining financial balance that leads to wealth and abundance, but equally important are the implementation and action. There is a popular confusion with work being defined as paid employment. By expanding your thinking to defining work as any activity from which you derive purpose, fulfillment, and meaning—rather than limiting the view of work to paid employment—you can begin to value your activities and yourself differently.

Being limited in your ability to express your mission because of needing to meet the employer's agenda potentially can be disempowering to you. It is important to recognize this and allow your own mission to be expressed—even if it is through a hobby or volunteer activity rather than formal employment.

Reflection It is possible that one's mission may not be expressed regularly in the daily place of employment. What are your avenues to expressing your purpose and mission?

From a Mechanistic to a Holistic Perspective on Money

Dealing with money from a physical perspective keeps it in the mechanistic model, which implies that money is a separate entity in and of itself. The making and utilization of money are confined to the physical realm. This suggests that there are no other influences on money other than cause and effect from the physical perspective—work, investments, savings, and budgeting increase available money.

There is another way to view money, however, involving a more holistic view. A crucial principle involved in the holistic paradigm is that nonphysical substance (thought, intention, requests) results in physical matter (physical manifestation of the request). In other words, belief that a goal can be fulfilled can bring about desired results. Spiritual masters have promoted similar beliefs, including Jesus who said "All things whatsoever ye shall ask in prayer, believing, ye shall receive," (Matthew 21:22).

KEY POINT

The scientific arena of quantum physics aids in understanding how the mind's creative force can manifest itself in the physical world by explaining that rapidly spinning atomic particles are invisible, but slower ones exist in the form of physical matter. Faster spinning particles can slow down and create physical forms. Consistent with this theory, thoughts can be manifested as physical matter.

The nonphysical substance used in this holistic paradigm is a creative force that allows individuals to produce in the physical world that which they are thinking. The creative force within people is not connected to personality or ego. However, it is important to identify the belief systems and perceptions under which personality operates to be aware of barriers that could impede the creative force.

After aligning with purpose, the next step is to focus on the request, desire, or goal that one wants to manifest. It is important to remember to leave results open-ended by adding the words *or something better* to requests. At this point is can be helpful to visualize what the end result may look like. For example, if you desire a specific amount of money, visualize a bank statement that shows that particular amount as your savings account balance or the exact item you wish to purchase with that amount of money.

As it is important to visualize and see in the mind's eye what is desired (Exhibit 11–1), at the same time it is important to let go of the process and outcome. Releasing is the last and possibly the most difficult step in the creative manifestation process. The act of releasing the whole process and letting go of the outcome calls one to progress in faith and trust that a greater power will be in control.

We live in a time in which the ways we perceive the world and our lives are changing. We can access information from higher places and pay more attention to the higher senses of our being, such as intuition and belief in the nonphysical world. With this heightening in perspective comes more options and approaches for accessing creative

---

EXHIBIT 11–1 ACHIEVING MIND, BODY, AND SPIRIT HARMONY IN ACHIEVING FINANCIAL GOALS

- Recognize that there is a power greater than yourself that can affect your outcomes.
- Quiet your mind, and connect to the creative force of the universe.
- Clarify and align with your purpose and mission in life.
- Consider the ways in which you can share and use your money to benefit other people and purposes.
- State and visualize your desire and specific goal.
- Be aware of emotions connected to financial goals and actions.
- Release preconceived notions of the ways in which resources will be delivered and the forms in which they will come.
- Trust and have faith that your results will be achieved.
- Express gratitude for what you receive.

solutions. Money is a representative energy through which we can demonstrate the ability to affect forces in our life and create something out of nothing.

Chapter Summary

From a mechanistic view, money is viewed in terms of its physical characteristics. However, from a holistic view, money is more than a medium of exchange to purchase goods and services; it represents an avenue through which energy flows. People's attitudes and beliefs about money and their financial well-being can influence the amount of money they receive and its use. To successfully obtain financial goals, people must have harmony of body, mind, and spirit.

Reference

1. Gaines, E. (2003). *Riches and Honor.* Audiocassette. Valley Head, AL: Prosperity Products, *www.prosperityproducts.com.*

Suggested Readings

Barnett, E. W., Gordon, L. S., and Hendrix, M. A. (2001). *The Big Book of Presbyterian Stewardship.* Louisville, KY: Geneva Press.

Blomberg, C. (1999). *Neither Poverty or Riches: A Biblical Theology of Possessions.* Grand Rapids, MI: Eerdmans.

Chopra, D. (1994). *The Seven Spiritual Laws of Success.* Novato, CA: New World Library.

Chopra, D. (1998). *Creating Affluence: The A to Z Steps to a Richer Life.* Novato, CA: New World Library.

Dunham, L. (2002). *Graceful Living: Your Faith, Values, and Money in Changing Times.* New York: Reformed Church in America Press.

Forward, S. (1995). *Money Demons: Keep Them Away from Sabotaging Your Relationship and Your Life.* New York: Bantam.

Gawain, S. (1997). *Creating True Prosperity.* Novato, CA: New World Library.

Haughey, J. C. (1997). *Virtue and Affluence: The Challenge of Wealth.* Kansas City: Sheed & Ward.

Horton, C. (2002). *Consciously Creating Wealth.* Higher Self Workshops.

Murphy, L. and Nagel, T. (2002). *The Myth of Ownership: Taxes and Justice.* New York: Oxford University Press.

Ponder, C. (2003). *A Prosperity Love Story: Rags to Enrichment*. Camarillo, CA: DeVorss & Co.

Ponder, C. (1983). *The Prospering Power of Prayer*. Camarillo, CA: DeVorss & Co.

Sinetar, M. (1989). *Do What You Love, The Money Will Follow: Discovering Your Right Livelihood*. New York: Bantam Doubleday.

Walters, D. J. (2000). *Money Magnetism: How to Attract What You Need When You Need It*. California: Crystal Clarity Publishers.

CHAPTER 12

ENVIRONMENTAL EFFECTS ON THE IMMUNE SYSTEM

Objectives

This chapter should enable you to:

- List at least six symptoms of toxicity
- List six sources of toxic substances
- Describe at least four ways that people can reduce environmental risks to the immune system
- Outline guidelines for detoxification

Everything in the environment—the food that you eat, the air you breathe, the sensations you experience—effects your immune system in a positive or a negative way. When environmental elements enhance the immune system, you function well and feel healthy, however, when environmental pollutants weaken the function of the immune system, you feel below par or become sick. Maximizing the benefits of the environment on the immune system, while reducing the negative impact is important to promoting good health.

Internal and External Environments

You are affected by two types of environments: external and internal. External environment implies anything that is outside your body, such as the weather, elements in the air, food, sounds, and interactions with other people. Major environmental crises such as catastrophic floods, fires, and hurricanes affect you, as do the minor daily crises, such as waiting in long lines at the supermarket or getting stuck in traffic.

Internal environment pertains to that which is inside you. All that you encounter in your daily living is experienced within you and influences your thinking, feelings, and behavior. Often, these events produce some degree of stress that you deal with uniquely based on your sensitivity, perception, awareness, flexibility, and adaptability. You use many skills and resources to balance the stressors from your external and internal environments and stay healthy.

Reflection Think about times in your life when your stress levels have been unusually high. Did you find that you had a higher incidence of illness or injury during or after those times?

Immune System

The immune system's primary purpose is to offer protection from infections or illnesses, and to fight disease-producing microorganisms, such as bacteria, viruses, and fungi. In other words, the immune system helps to maximize your health potential as well as to maintain your health. The weakening of the immune system frequently results in an increased susceptibility to unpleasant symptoms, illnesses, and diseases. If the immune system is severely weakened or suppressed, it cannot destroy or reprogram the cells in the body (1). Environmental conditions influence the normal function of the immune system and can threaten its optimum function. (See Chapter 5 for a discussion of the immune system.)

Toxicity

KEY POINT

The word *toxicity* generally refers to a poisonous, disease-producing substance that is produced by a microorganism.

Toxicity can result from environmental agents that produce poisonous substances that cause an unhealthy environment within the body, leading to physiological or psychological problems. The accumulation of toxins weakens the immune system. Initially, mild symptoms affecting the body organs, such as a headache, sneezing, swollen eyelids, or irritability may be experienced. Other physical symptoms often include fatigue, restlessness, insomnia, difficulty breathing, and confusion. At first, these symptoms are faint and may be missed or minimized, however, when such symptoms continue over an extended period of time, they are difficult to ignore. Toxicity that continues for a long time begins to impede the normal functions of the body's organs and systems. This results in an imbalance, leading to impairments in normal digestion, walking, and thinking.

Heavy Metals

In your daily environment, you are constantly exposed to environmental factors that lead to the development of toxicity in your body. Of these, the major category of toxic substances is heavy metals.

KEY POINT

Toxic substances can be found in a variety of sources, such as heavy metals, chemicals, parasites, pesticides, and radiation.

Aluminum, arsenic, cadmium, lead, and mercury are examples of heavy metals. They are found in air, food, and water, and have no function in the human body. Over a long period of time, these heavy metals accumulate in the body and reach toxic levels (2). Heavy metals tend to accumulate in the brain, kidneys, and immune system where they can severely disrupt normal functioning (3). Heavy metal toxicity causes unusual symptoms and ailments that tend to linger for an extraordinary length of time. People with symptoms related to this toxicity may visit several medical doctors to find out what is wrong, but often, physicians are unable to identify and treat the problem. Frequently medications are prescribed for symptomatic relief, but may provide minimal to no relief.

Transportation companies, waste management companies, and manufacturers have been major sources of heavy metal pollution. For example, many manufacturing plants throughout the United States have polluted the air with poisonous toxins, particularly lead, from their industrial processes and productivity. Exhibit 12–1 lists the common sources of the five heavy metals—aluminum, arsenic, cadmium, lead, and mercury.

KEY POINT

Overall the heavy metals tend to (4):

- Decrease the function of the immune system
- Increase allergic reactions
- Alter genetic mutation

- Increase acidity of the blood
- Increase inflammation of arteries and tissues
- Increase hardening of artery walls
- Increase progressive blockage of arteries

EXHIBIT 12–1 COMMON SOURCES OF HEAVY METAL TOXINS			
Type of Toxin	*Source*	*Type of Toxin*	*Source*
Aluminum	Aluminum cookware		Dolomite
	Aluminum foil		Drinking water
	Antacids		Drying agents for cotton
	Antiperspirants		Fish
	Baking powder (containing aluminum)		Herbicides
	Bleached flour		Insecticides
	Buffered aspirin		Kelp
	Canned acidic foods		Laundry aids
	Cooking utensils		Meats (from commercially raised poultry
	Cookware		and cattle)
	Dental amalgrams		Metal ore
	Foil		Pesticides
	Food additives		Seafood (fish, mussels, oysters)
	Medications-Drugs		Smelting
	Antidiarrheal agents		Smog
	Antiinflammatory agents		Smoke
	Hemorrhoid medications		Specialty glass
	Vaginal douches		Table salt
	Processed cheese		Tap water
	"Softened" water		Tobacco
	Table salt		Wood preservatives
	Tap water	**Cadmium**	Air pollution
	Toothpaste		Art supplies
Arsenic	Air pollution		Bone meal
	Antibiotics (given to commercial livestock)		Cigarette smoke
	Bone meal		Fertilizers
	Certain marine plants		Food (coffee, tea, fruits, and vegetables
	Chemical processing		grown in cadmium-laden soil)
	Coal-fired power plants		Freshwater fish
	Defoliants		Fungicides

Exhibit 12-1 Common Sources of Heavy Metal Toxins *(continued)*			
Type of Toxin	*Source*	*Type of Toxin*	*Source*
	Highway dust		Batteries
	Incinerators		Canned foods
	Meats (kidneys, liver, poultry)		Ceramics
	Mining		Chemical fertilizers
	Nickel-cadmium batteries		Colored advertisements
	Oxide dusts		Cosmetics
	Paint		Dolomite
	Pesticides		Dust
	Phosphate fertilizers		Food grown near industrial areas
	Plastics		Gasoline
	Power plants		Hair dyes and rinses
	Refined foods		Leaded glass
	Refined grains		Newsprint
	Seafood (crab, flounder, mussels, oysters, scallops)		Paints
			Pesticides
	Secondhand smoke		Pewter
	Sewage sludge		Pottery
	Soft drinks		Rubber toys
	Soil		"Softened" water
	"Softened" water		Solder in tin cans
	Smelting plants		Tap water
	Welding fumes		Tobacco smoke
Lead	Air pollution	Mercury	Contaminated fish
	Ammunition (shot and bullets)		Cosmetics
	Bathtubs (cast iron, porcelain steel)		Dental fillings

Sources: Adapted from Balch and Balch (1997), Marti (1995), Post-Gazette (10/14/99), Pouls (1999), Ronzio (1999).

Aluminum

The average person ingests between 3 and 10 milligrams of aluminum each day (5). Of the various sources of aluminum, the highest exposure comes from the chronic consumption of aluminum-containing antacid products. It is primarily absorbed through the digestive tract as well as through the other organs, such as the lungs and skin. Research has shown that at least 10 human neurological conditions have been linked to toxic concentrations of aluminum (6). Other study results suggest that the heavy metal aluminum contributes to neurological disorders such as Parkinson's disease, dementia, clumsiness of movements, staggering when walking, and the inability to pronounce words properly (4). Findings also show a relationship between elevated levels of aluminum and other heavy metals with behavioral difficulties exhibited among school children (7). Children suffering from learning disorders or hyperactivity were found to have elevated aluminum levels in the blood (8). Aluminum tends to accumulate in the brain, bones, kidneys, and stomach tissues. Consequently, the common health problems caused by aluminum are colic, irritation of the esophagus, gastroenteritis, kidney damage, liver dysfunction, loss of appetite, loss of balance, muscle pain, dementia, psychosis, seizures, shortness of breath, and general weakness (4, 5, 9).

Arsenic

Arsenic is another highly toxic substance. It has an affinity for most of the bodily organs, especially the gastrointestinal system, lungs, skin, hair, and nails (4). In acute arsenic poisoning, nausea and vomiting, bloody urine, muscle cramps, fatigue, hair loss, and convulsions are noted. Headaches, confusion, abdominal pain, burning of the mouth and throat, diarrhea, and drowsiness may occur in chronic arsenic poisoning. Arsenic toxicity can contribute to the development of cancer (lung and skin), coma, neuritis, peripheral vascular (vessels of the extremities) problems, and collapse of blood vessels (4, 5, 9) .

Cadmium

Cadmium is also considered an extremely poisonous heavy metal. Inhaling cadmium fumes causes pulmonary edema, followed by pneumonia and various degrees of lung damage. Another way that a person can acquire cadmium poisoning is by ingesting foods contaminated by cadmium-plated containers; these cause violent gastrointestinal symptoms. Cadmium levels also arise in individuals who have zinc deficiencies (5).

KEY POINT

The health problems that can arise from cadmium toxicity are: anemia, cancer, depressed immune system response, dry and scaly skin, emphysema, eye damage, fatigue, hair loss, heart disease, hypertension, increased risk of cataract formation, joint pain, kidney stones or damage, liver dysfunction or damage, loss of appetite, loss of sense of smell, pain in the back and legs, and yellow discoloration of the teeth. These problems occur because cadmium tends to gravitate to tissues of specific body organs, including the brain and its pain centers, the heart and its blood vessels, the kidneys, and the lungs, as well as the tissues that influence the appetite (4, 5, 9).

Lead

Of all the common heavy metals, lead has attracted public attention since the early 1900s. At the turn of the twentieth century, paint companies knew that lead was a serious factor in the health of consumers, however, they continued to produce building paints that contained a lead base. These paints were used in homes and commercial buildings. In addition, the Environmental Protection Agency (EPA) estimated that drinking water accounts for approximately 20 percent of young children's lead exposure (10). Consequently, children were seriously affected by lead poisoning. Health problems in children caused by lead poisoning include: attention deficit disorder (ADD), hyperactivity syndromes, learning disabilities, loss of appetite, low achievement scores, low intelligent quotients, seizures, and, on occasion, death. Due to public outcry against lead-based paint it was banned in 1978. At the same time, the government issued regulations cutting out lead in gasoline.

KEY POINT

In 1999, Rhode Island became ". . . the first state to sue the makers of lead paint, seeking millions to pay for removing the paint from homes and caring for poisoned children" (11). Rhode Island was among the states with the highest lead poisoning rates, having greater than three times the national average.

Lead poisoning affects cognitive (intellectual) function. Studies have revealed that low-level lead exposure impairs children's IQ (7). In addition to the danger for young children, there was also a great risk of harm from lead exposure for infants and pregnant women. In pregnant women, lead toxicity may cause premature birth, miscarriage, and birth defects. Lead toxicity may produce a variety of additional symptoms, including abdominal pain, anemia, anorexia, anxiety, bone pain, brain damage, coma, confusion, constipation, convulsions, dizziness, drowsiness, fatigue, heart attack, headaches, high blood pressure, inability to concentrate, indigestion, irritability, kidney disease, loss of muscle coordination, memory difficulties, mental depression, mental damage, muscle pain, nervous system, neurological damage, pallor, and vomiting (1, 4, 9).

Mercury

As Exhibit 12–1 shows, mercury is found in many sources that we use in our daily life. This toxic metal accumulates in the bones, brain, heart, kidneys, liver, nervous system, and pancreas. Several dental studies have shown a relationship between unusual symptoms and mercury exposure from silver fillings, finding that a major source of mercury toxicity in the human body was the dental filling (12). When mercury fillings were removed, the symptoms and related health problems disappeared (12). The safety of the silver filling is being challenged. Currently ongoing studies are investigating the effects of mercury not only on the immune system, but also on the central nervous system, the renal system, and the reproductive system (13).

Reducing Environmental Risks to Health

Assess

To begin helping yourself, you need to take an objective look at yourself. One method of self-assessment is The Toxicity Self-Test (TST) shown in Exhibit 12–2. It involves checking off symptoms frequently experienced within 15 common areas and the degree to which each symptom has been noticed; then the score is totaled. The final score may fall in the mild, moderate, or severe range as indicated at the end of the TST checklist. Once this assessment is completed, you can explore ways of reducing the toxicity that exists in your body.

There are daily positive actions that you can take to reduce or prevent the accumulation of toxins in the body.

Attend to the Basics

With the fast pace of life and all the demands of family and work, it is easy to neglect yourself. This negligence affects your sleep, rest, relaxation, and leisure. Reflect on your daily activities and ask: Am I getting adequate rest? Do I awaken feeling refreshed? Am I taking time to relax and enjoy the simple pleasures of life?

It is important to make sure you are getting sufficient water in order to flush toxins from the body. Be sure to drink at least eight glasses of chemical-free water daily.

Reflection Are you drinking at least eight glasses of water daily to flush toxins from your body? How can you assure the water you drink is free from contamination by lead and other chemicals?

It could be useful to avoid using aluminum cookware. Some experts believe that foods cooked or stored in aluminum containers produce a substance that neutralizes digestive juices, leading to acidosis and ulcers; worse, the aluminum in cookware can leach from the pot into the food (5).

Relax

Relaxation can be achieved by using a variety of techniques.

Guided imagery: Investigative findings have revealed a relationship between lowered immune function and health problems. Guided imagery is done by creating mental scenes in one's mind and has been shown helpful in strengthening the immune system. This imagery technique, also known as *mental imagery* or *visual imagery*, uses the body–mind connection to alleviate energy imbalance in the body.

Meditation: Meditation is the practice and system of thought that incorporates exercises to attain bodily or mental control and well-being as well as enlightenment.

EXHIBIT 12–2 TOXICITY SELF-TEST

Rate each of the following symptoms based upon your health profile for the past 30 days.

POINT SCALE:

0 = *never* or *almost never* have the symptom

1 = *occasionally* have the symptom; effect is *not severe*

2 = *occasionally* have the symptom; effect is *severe*

3 = *frequently* have the symptom; effect is *not severe*

4 = *frequently* have the symptom; effect is *severe*

1. Digestive Function

_____ Nausea or vomiting

_____ Diarrhea

_____ Constipation

_____ Bloated feeling

_____ Belching, passing gas

_____ Heartburn

_____ TOTAL

2. Ears

_____ Itchy ears

_____ Earaches, ear infection

_____ Drainage from ear

_____ Ringing in ears, hearing loss

_____ TOTAL

3. Emotions

_____ Mood swings

_____ Anxiety, fear, nervousness

_____ Anger, irritability

_____ Depression

_____ TOTAL

EXHIBIT 12–2 TOXICITY SELF-TEST *(continued)*

4. Energy/Activity

_____ Fatigue, sluggishness

_____ Apathy, lethargy

_____ Hyperactivity

_____ Restlessness

_____ TOTAL

5. Eyes

_____ Watery, itchy eyes

_____ Swollen, reddened, or sticky eyelids

_____ Dark circles under eyes

_____ Blurred vision/tunnel vision

_____ TOTAL

6. Head

_____ Headache

_____ Faintness

_____ Dizziness

_____ Insomnia

_____ TOTAL

7. Lungs

_____ Chest congestion

_____ Asthma, bronchitis

_____ Shortness of breath

_____ Difficulty breathing

_____ TOTAL

8. Mind

_____ Poor memory

_____ Confusion

_____ Poor concentration

_____ Poor coordination

EXHIBIT 12–2 TOXICITY SELF-TEST *(continued)*

_____ Difficulty making decisions

_____ Stuttering, stammering

_____ Slurred speech

_____ Learning disabilities

_____ TOTAL

9. Mouth/Throat

_____ Chronic coughing

_____ Gagging, frequent need to clear throat

_____ Sore throat, hoarse

_____ Swollen or discolored tongue, gums, lips

_____ Canker sores

_____ TOTAL

10. Nose

_____ Stuffy nose

_____ Sinus problems

_____ Hay fever

_____ Sneezing attacks

_____ Excessive mucus

_____ TOTAL

11. Skin

_____ Acne

_____ Hives, rash, dry skin

_____ Hair loss

_____ Flushing or hot flashes

_____ Excessive sweating

_____ TOTAL

12. Heart

_____ Skipped heartbeats

_____ Rapid heartbeat

EXHIBIT 12–2 TOXICITY SELF-TEST *(continued)*

_____ Chest pains

_____ TOTAL

13. Joints/Muscles

_____ Pain or aches in muscles

_____ Arthritis

_____ Stiffness, limited movement

_____ Pain or aches in muscles

_____ Feelings of weakness or tiredness

_____ TOTAL

14. Weight

_____ Binge eating/drinking

_____ Craving certain foods

_____ Excessive weight

_____ Compulsive eating

_____ Water retention

_____ Underweight

_____ TOTAL

15. Other

_____ Frequent illness

_____ Frequent or urgent urination

_____ Genital itch and/or discharge

_____ TOTAL

Add the numbers to arrive at a total for each section. Add the totals for each section to arrive at the grand total.

Mild toxicity   =   0–96 Grand total score

Moderate toxicity = 97–168 Grand total score

Severe toxicity   = 169–240 Grand total score

Studies have shown that a relationship exists between meditation and increased immunity. There are several ways to meditate. One person may prefer to meditate to a particular sound while another may focus on breathing. You may need to try a few styles to determine your personal preference.

Deep breathing: Deep breathing or belly breathing can promote relaxation. This method is described in Chapter 4.

Get a Massage

Deep tissue massages or lymph massages are helpful for the release of toxicity and balancing energy. In deep tissue massage, the therapist applies greater pressure and focuses on deeper muscles than in the Swedish massage, which primarily aims to promote relaxation. The purpose of lymph massage is to increase the circulation throughout the lymphatic system. Through massage of deeper tissues and increased circulation, toxins are mobilized, released, and eventually eliminated from the body. Beware that deep tissue massage is not recommended for individuals who have high blood pressure, a history of inflammation of the veins, or any other circulatory problem.

Sweat It Out

Engaging in regular saunas can help relieve the body of toxins through the skin. If you choose to use a sauna, it is best to avoid eating within one hour prior to the sauna to avoid nausea.

Brush Your Skin

Another valuable technique is brushing the skin with a dry brush that has firm natural bristles. The purpose of skin brushing is to rid the body of the poisonous substances that are excreted through perspiration.

Use Nutritional Supplements

There are specific nutrient supplements that can be taken when you are trying to combat heavy metal toxicity:

- Multivitamin supplement
- Vitamin C
- B-complex vitamins
- Mineral supplements, especially calcium, chromium, copper, iron, magnesium, and zinc
- Sulfur-containing amino acids, including cysteine, methionine, and taurine

Detoxify

Another simple method for the general elimination of toxins is cleansing the bowel (15). This is a form of detoxification therapy.

KEY POINT

Detoxification was strongly recommended by pioneers in nutritional and natural medicine, including Bernard Jensen, John H. Kellogg, Max Gerson, and John Tilden.

Detoxification, a noninvasive process, has been quite popular in many healthcare systems around the world, especially Europe—to a much greater extent than in the United States. Detoxification is essential as a first step in clearing the body of toxicity because a person cannot rebuild nor maintain health if the toxins remain stored in the body. The majority of toxins tend to accumulate in the bowel where waste matter in the intestines remains for lengthy periods of time. This allows the toxins to be absorbed into the bloodstream throughout the body, causing health problems. Once the toxins are cleansed out of the bowel, the body can begin to heal itself. Typically, a fiber substance, such as ground flaxseeds or psyllium husks in powdered form is taken to aid the body in eliminating the toxins. Exhibit 12–3 shows the effect of toxins on unhealthy and healthy functions within the body.

EXHIBIT 12–3 IMPACT OF TOXINS ON UNHEALTHY AND HEALTHY FUNCTIONS IN THE BODY

Unhealthy

- Toxins form internally, leak through the unhealthy intestine, and flow to the liver.
- Toxins are not completely detoxified in the unhealthy liver.
- Unchanged toxins leave the liver and are stored in tissues, such as fat, the brain, and the nervous system.

Healthy

- Few toxins are formed and most of the them are excreted, with only a small amount naturally transported to the liver.
- Toxins are transformed to an intermediate substance.
- The intermediate substance is transformed to a more water soluble substance and released to the kidneys.
- The water soluble substance is excreted via the urine.

Source: *Detoxification*, San Clemente, CA: Metagenics, Inc. August, 1994.

KEY POINT

General Guidelines for Detoxification

In using the detoxification process, be aware that it must be done slowly. The reason for this is that the body must adapt to the changes that are occurring. If the detoxification occurs rapidly, unusual symptoms can develop due to the bodily changes that are causing an imbalance. If the detoxification is performed at a slower pace, the body develops its equilibrium while it is eliminating the toxins. Following the detoxification, it is generally recommended that you:

* Drink at least eight ounces of water each day. Water helps the body to get rid of the debris and also provides sufficient liquid to help with elimination.

* Begin eating raw food, including vegetables. This provides fiber, a natural substance, that helps with rebuilding tissue in the body.

* Continue to avoid eating the foods listed in Exhibit 12–4. The avoidance of the suggested foods will decrease the faulty bowel function that occurs with an imbalanced diet.

Chelation Therapy

Chelation therapy, approved by the federal drug agency (FDA), is another modality primarily used to detoxify the body of heavy metals. Research findings have shown that chelation therapy is highly effective for eliminating heavy metals and for treating arteriosclerosis as well (14). Additional benefits of chelation therapy are listed in Exhibit 12–5.

The word *chelation* is derived from the Greek word *chela*, meaning *claw*, and implies that heavy metals and excess calcium bind to carrier molecules after they are picked up in a pincer-like fashion (14). Chelation therapy is an intravenous solution that removes toxins from the bloodstream. Specifically, the solution involving an amino acid compound formulation called ethylene diamine tetra-acetic acid—commonly known as EDTA—and various nutrients, is administered slowly for approximately three hours, two or three times a week. EDTA was first used in medicine in 1941 for lead poisoning and later for heavy metal toxicity (15). Initially EDTA was patented in Germany in 1930.

Today, chelation therapy is becoming well known among clients as well as healthcare professionals. Chelation is used to treat symptoms related to heavy metal intoxication, cardiovascular problems, peripheral vascular problems, diabetes, memory loss, and strokes. The program plan typically calls for the client to receive a course of 20-to-30

EXHIBIT 12–4 RECOMMENDED NUTRITIONAL CHANGES TO REDUCE TOXICITY

Avoid the following:

- Alcohol, drugs, cigarettes
- Caffeinated drinks
- Chlorinated (tap) water
- Commercially prepared foods
- Fats
- Foods high in additives and preservatives
- Hydrogenated and partially hydrogenated oils
- Fried foods
- Heated polyunsaturated fats (fast food oils, theater popcorn oil)
- Monosodium glutamate (MSG)
- Refined sugars
- Soft drinks
- Softened tap water
- Topical oils (cottonseed, palm)
- White flour foods

EXHIBIT 12–5 CHELATION THERAPY: SUMMARY OF BENEFITS

Chelation therapy:

- Eliminates heavy metals
- Removes calcium deposits from blood, arterial plaque, and arterial walls
- Strengthens blood vessels
- Improves blood circulation
- Absorbs the fatty deposits in the veins and arteries
- Provides oxygenation to the heart
- Improves the immune function
- Improves function of cell function

treatments depending upon one's condition. Thereafter, a maintenance program is strongly recommended consisting of a smaller number of sessions given each year (14). The maintenance program will vary depending on the client's state of health and other related health problems.

Chelation also is effective in removing calcium deposits from the body. In the process of chelation, the EDTA passes through veins and arteries and absorbs the plaque, which is then flushed through the kidneys and excreted in the urine. This process improves

---

EXHIBIT 12–6 SUMMARY OF COMMON INGREDIENTS FOR ORAL CHELATION

Ingredients	Action
Amino acids (L-cysteine, L-methionine, and others)	• Serve as detoxifiers and antioxidants • Aids in prevention of fat buildup in the liver and arteries
Copper	• Assists in formation of hemoglobin, elastin, and red blood cells
Magnesium (often taken with calcium)	• Assists in calcium and potassium uptake • Protects the arterial lining
Pectin	• Helps fight free radicals • Removes unwanted toxins • Lowers cholesterol
Vitamin A	• Promotes growth and repairs damaged cell membranes
Vitamins B1, B3, B6, B12	• Promotes red blood cell formation and metabolism • Lowers serum cholesterol levels • Neutralizes free radicals
Vitamin E	• Prevents oxidation of fat compounds • Serves as an anticoagulant

Note: Other ingredients in chelation formulas include: adrenal, brometain, choline, chromium, co-enzyme Q10, flax powder, folic acid, gentian, iodine, inositol, PABA, thymus, and selenium.

Source: Hawkens, C. (1977). *Chelation Therapy.* Pleasant Grove, UT: Woodland Publishing, pp. 10–11.

blood circulation. Toxins exit the body through the kidneys, preventing the formation of stones and hardened tissues.

Chelation therapy is considered a safe, effective alternative to coronary bypass surgery and angioplasty (14). It is recommended that chelation therapy be used in conjunction with exercise, and proper nutrition, including consuming less saturated fat and more plant food, such as vegetables and fruits, and mineral and vitamin supplements (16).

Recently an oral form of chelation has been produced, providing the client convenience of travel and time. Walker defines the oral chelation process as "a prolonged process of chemical detoxification of the most inner recesses of one's physiology" (17). The chelating product in liquid form is mixed in juice and taken orally, digested, and assimilated so that the chelating affects the entire body—its systems, organs, tissues, cells (18). Oral chelation contains EDTA, the most well-known chelator, in addition to several vitamins and minerals (see Exhibit 12–6).

Reflection   What can you do to reduce exposure to toxins?

EXHIBIT 12–7 BASIC SUGGESTIONS TO MINIMIZE TOXICITY IN THE WORKPLACE, HOME, AND COMMUNITY ENVIRONMENTS

- Remove, if possible, the source of any toxic materials:
  - Acid
  - Cleaning agents
  - Dyes
  - Glues
  - Insecticides
  - Paints
  - Solvents
- Use an air-purification system in the home if materials cannot be removed
- Wear protective clothing and/or breathing apparatus when using any toxic materials
- Replace furnace and air-conditioning filters in the home on a regular basis
- Eat fresh, wholesome foods, including fruits, vegetables, grains
- Avoid using pesticides and herbicides
- Do not smoke cigarettes

Contact with environmental pollutants is a reality of daily life. You come in contact with them in the air you breathe, the foods you eat, and the water you drink. These toxic substances can threaten your health in several ways and lead to major health problems such as lung damage, mood changes, neurological dysfunction, tissue damage, and visual disturbances. By avoiding exposure as much as possible and minimizing or eliminating the build up of toxins within your tissues and organs, you can protect your health and enjoy maximum function. Exhibit 12–7 gives specific suggestions to help avoid exposure to toxicity in our work, homes, and community environments.

Chapter Summary

Internal and external environments affect the health of the immune system. The accumulation of toxins can weaken the immune system and cause a wide range of dysfunctions of the body and mind. In normal daily life, exposure to heavy metals, parasites, pesticides, radiation, and geopathic stress can lead to toxicity and cause serious health consequences. It is important to identify symptoms associated with toxicity and implement measures to reduce it. The approaches to reduce or prevent the accumulation of toxins in the body include good basic health practices, relaxation techniques, deep tissue massage, sauna, skin brushing, consumption of nutritional supplements, detoxification, and chelation. Because exposure to toxins is a reality of life for the average person, active steps must be taken to prevent exposure and strengthen the body's ability to resist the ill effects of toxins.

References

1. Marti, J. (1995). *The Alternative Health Medicine Encyclopedia*. Detroit: Visible Ink Press, p. 116.

2. Kellas, B. and Dworkin, A. (1996). *Surviving the Toxic Crisis*. Olivenhain, CA: Professional Preference Publishing, p. 186.

3. Marti, J. (1995). *The Alternative Health Medicine Encyclopedia*. Detroit: Visible Ink Press, p. 115.

4. Pouls, M. (1999). "Oral Chelation and Nutritional Replacement Therapy for Chemical & Heavy Metal Toxicity and Cardiovascular Disease." *Townsend Letter for Doctors & Patients*, (192)84.

5. Balch, J. and Balch, P. (1997). *Prescription for Nutritional Healing*. Garden City, NY: Avery Publishing.

6. Gasdorph, H. and Walker, M. (1995). *Toxic Mental Syndrome*. Garden City Park, NY: Avery Publishing, p. 120.

7. Needleman, H. and Gatsonis, C. (1990). "Low-level Lead Exposure and the IQ of Children. A Meta-Analysis of Modern Studies," *Journal of the American Medical Association*, 263:673–678.

8. Howard, J. (1984). "Clinical Import of Small Increases in Serum Aluminum." *Clin. Chem.*, 30:1722–1723.

9. Ronzio, R. (1999). "Antioxidants, Nutraceuticals, and Functional Foods." *Townsend Letter for Doctors & Patients*, 192:50–51.

10. Alleger, I. (1999) "Healing from the Inside Out," *Townsend Letter for Doctors and Patients*, 192:124–125.

11. "Local Groups Seek EPA Help Over Coke Plant Emissions." *Pittsburgh Post-Gazette*, July 16, 1999, B–3.

12. Lorscheider, F., Vimy, M., and Summers, A. (1995). "Mercury Exposure from 'Silver' Tooth Fillings: Emerging Evidence Questions a Traditional Dental Paradigm." *The FASEB Journal*, 9:504–508.

13. Pendergrass, J., Haley, B., Vimy, M., Winfield, S., and Lorscheider, F. (1997). "Mercury Vapor Inhalation Inhibits Binding of GTP to Tubulin in Rat Brain: Similarity to a Molecular Lesion in Alzheimer Diseased Brain." *NeuroToxicology*, 18:315–324.

14. Null, G. (1998). *The Complete Encyclopedia of Natural Healing*. New York: Kensington Publishing Corp.

15. Hawkens, C. (1997). *Chelation Therapy*. Pleasant Grove, UT: Woodland Publishing, p. 18.

16. Salaman, M. (1998). *All Your Health Questions Answered Naturally*. Mountain View, CA: MKS, Inc., pp. 3, 7.

17. Walker, M. (1977). *Everything You Should Know About Chelation Therapy*. New Canaan, CT: Keats, p. 152.

18. Salaman, M. (1998). *All Your Health Questions Answered Naturally*. Mountain View, CA: MKS, Inc., p. 9.

Suggested Readings

Bennett, P. (1999). *7-Day Detox Miracle*. Rocklin, CA: Prima Publishing.

Fitzgerald, P. (2001). *The Detox Solution.* Santa Monica, CA: Illumination Press.

Jensen, B. (1999). *Dr. Jensen's Guide to Better Bowel Care.* Garden City Park, NY: Avery Publishing Group.

Krohn, J. and Taylor, F. (2002). *Natural Detoxification*, 2nd ed. Point Roberts, WA: Hartley and Marks Publishers, Inc.

Slaga, T. (2003). *The Detox Revolution.* New York: Contemporary Books/McGraw Hill Co.

CHAPTER 13

PROMOTING A HEALING ENVIRONMENT

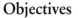

Objectives

This chapter should enable you to:

- Explain *electromagnetic field*
- Describe *chakras*
- Describe energy associated with different colors
- List five factors that can influence the vibrational fields

Life is a perpetual cycle as revealed in the constant changes that occur in nature: the changing tides, the seasons, the weather patterns, and the circadian rhythm of day and night followed by the final cycle of life and death. Being part of nature, all human beings are influenced by energy cycles within the physical body as well as the vibrational or universal body that corresponds to the electromagnetic field. The electromagnetic field is multidimensional and ranges from radio waves to gamma waves. The visible spectrum of the electromagnetic field ranges from infrared to ultraviolet.

KEY POINT

During the twentieth century, theorists such as Albert Einstein and Martha Rogers emerged with scientific theories that revealed man as an energy being. These theories challenged man's relationship with nature and the universe.

The electromagnetic field is referred to as the vibrational field and an individual's energy body as the vibrational body. The field that surrounds the dense physical body is known by the scientific term *electromagnetic* or *bioenergy field*. This field is depicted by ancient Christian artisans who showed the presence of a light or halo emanating from the head or crown of religious men and women. The vibrational field is comprised of at least seven layers that correspond to the physical, intellectual, and spiritual components of the visible body. Thus, both positive and negative external stimuli can have a profound impact on the body, mind, and spirit of an individual.

KEY POINT

People are more than skin and bones, thoughts and feelings. They are spectacular vibrational beings who resonate with the full-spectrum rays of the sun.

The vibrational field is hypothesized to be made of seven major *chakras*. A *chakra* (coming from the Sanskrit for *wheel of light*) is a spinning wheel or energy vortex that acts as a vibrational transformer within the field that extends outside the body. Although the chakra energy system is just now gaining recognition in the United States, ancient Indian Yogi literature described chakras approximately 5,000 years ago.

The vibrational body is in part also comprised of seven major chakras, each of which connects with a nerve plexus, endocrine gland, and specific physiology and anatomy within a specific area of the body. The first five chakras extend from the base of the spinal column to the cervical spine; the sixth chakra to the pituitary gland; and the seventh chakra to the pineal gland. The seven major chakras resonate with the full spectrum rays from red to violet. (For a fuller discussion of chakras see the *Symptoms and Chakras* chapter.)

Each chakra resonates with a musical note, as well as the sequence of the seven colors in the rainbow from infrared to ultraviolet. The chakra energy system energetically connects with the associated endocrine glands, nerve plexus, and anatomy and physiology at the individual points of origin. For example, the fourth chakra—the heart chakra—is located mid-chest and corresponds to the thymus gland, cardiac nerve plexus, heart, and lungs.

KEY POINT

The environment consists of the objects, conditions, and situations that surround us.

Sunlight

Sunlight provides a complement of the full-spectrum rays that correlate with the vibration of the seven major chakras. Although artificial light does allow us to partake in life after dark, artificial light does not resonate with the colors of the chakras. A means to correct inadequate natural sunlight or poor artificial lighting is the use of a full-spectrum lightbulb in primary rooms. These are not essential in every light source.

KEY POINT

Seasonal affective disorder (SAD) is a severe form of winter depression. It is characterized by lethargy, boredom, lack of joy, hopelessness, increased sleeping, and overeating. The primary factor responsible for this is the lack of natural sunlight. Natural sunlight affects the pineal gland (seventh chakra) to reduce its release of melatonin, which controls the circadian rhythm of the sleep–wake cycle. Although artificial light allows us to partake in life after dark, it does not resonate with the colors of the chakras.

Color

Color is a vibration that resonates with the chakra energy system, and it can influence the sense of well-being. The vibration flows in accordance with the full spectrum of colors of the rainbow: red, orange, yellow, green, blue, indigo, and violet. Even visually impaired people are influenced by color because of its vibrational quality.

KEY POINT

Various colors are associated with different types of energy.

Violet: spiritual energy connected to universal power and healing

Indigo: a blend of red and violet, stimulates intuition or the third eye

Blue: invokes a sense of calm

Green: a healing quality, the color of nature that supports the heart chakra

Yellow: associated with solar energy, power, and intellect

Orange: a nurturing energy related to creation, sunrise, and sunset

Red: invigorating life force in small amounts, can be energetically overwhelming with large or continual exposure

It is useful for people to determine their favorite color. After the favorite color has been identified, people should determine how much this color appears in their personal environments. It is important that the favorite color be in the immediate environment either as an accent or as a primary color. With some planning, the color can be incorporated into the environment while respecting others who share the same space. For example, a bowl of fresh oranges could be sufficient to incorporate a favorite color of orange into an area rather than painting an entire room that color. Fresh flowers, plants, fruit bowls, pillows, jewelry, and clothing of the favorite color are useful vibrational remedies that can be incorporated into daily life. People also may want to pay attention to their life's circumstances to see if their favorite color changes as result of their experiences.

KEY POINT

Color Therapy's Struggle for Acceptance

The history of color therapy dates from 1550 B.C. when Egyptian priests left papyrus manuscripts showing their use of color science in their healing temples. A renewed interest in color therapy developed over the past two centuries, but was met with skepticism. For example, in 1878 Edwin Babbitt wrote a book that is referred to as the *Materia Medica* for color therapy or chromotherapy, yet during his lifetime his thoughts and views were equally praised and criticized by his peers (1). In the early part of the twentieth century Dinshah Ghadiali developed *spectro chrome tonation*, which was a system of attuned color waves that struggled for 40 years to gain acceptance from the American Medical Association. Roland Hunt promoted the meditative approach of color breathing and color visualization in his 1971 book, *The Seven Keys to Color Healing* (2), however, this had little impact in mainstream healthcare circles.

Clutter

Clutter is a major stress factor that potentially irritates the nervous system. It not only disturbs the visual field, but the vibrational field as well. This is due to the fact that the vibrational field exists beyond the skin, therefore clutter in a space can cause a restriction of that field.

Vibrational remedies for clutter begin with the simple act of examining the environment with a critical eye. People can be challenged to consider how they would like their homes to look if a special guest was visiting. They can be encouraged to begin the habit of not bringing a new item into their homes without discarding or giving away something in return. Reorganizing living space and donating unnecessary belongings can be beneficial, as can recycling (which not only reduces clutter, but helps to protect the earth). In addition to the reward of a more harmonious environment, people most likely will discover more floor space to use for relaxing or exercising.

Sound

Reflection   Try closing your eyes and noticing the sounds in your immediate environment. List three pleasant sounds, for example the voices of loved ones, sounds of nature, even the absence of sound (peace and quiet). Now, list all the negative sounds in your home or office: unpleasant verbal interactions, loud music, machinery, persistent phone ringing, household appliances, etc. Be aware that noise pollution can disturb the nervous system, creating an increase in stress levels. Compare your lists and try to make adjustments to reduce auditory overload and enhance positive aspects of sound in your environment.

The link between music and health is ancient and elemental. Music therapy influences the chakra energy system according to vibration and tone. The natural rhythm of the ocean, raindrops, wind-ruffled leaves, and birds chirping universally promote relaxation. Manmade music dates to the ancient cultures and mythology. Apollo, known as the god of medicine, also was the god of music. Drumming correlates to the human heartbeat. New Age music with synthesizers and string instruments connects with the higher vibrations of the chakra energy system. Today, classical music is incorporated into surgical suites, dentists' offices, and hospice facilities as a holistic, stress-reducing measure.

KEY POINT

The vibrational body can be soothed through the sound of a water fountain. People can create their own fountains with a fish tank, water pump, deep pottery bowl, and imagination.

Scents

It is interesting to note that the vibrational body adapts to most situations over time. The sense of smell is an ideal example of this. Normally the sense of smell is keen when a scent or odor is first detected, but it then becomes less acute with continued exposure. This can create a problem in that toxic substances can permeate living areas without detection. Toxic chemicals found in the home or workplace can lead to a host of symptoms, such as headaches, nasal stuffiness, and shortness of breath, related to chemical sensitivity.

KEY POINT

Radon is an inert radioactive gas that is the natural radioactive decay of radium and uranium found in the soil. Excessive levels of radon have been linked to an increased lung cancer risk. (There is a very high incidence of lung cancer in uranium miners.) There are many factors that determine the amount of radon that escapes from the soil to enter a house: weather, soil porosity, soil moisture, granite, and ledge. The incidence of radon is greater from water supplied from a well versus city water. (Call the EPA hotline to learn more about this problem at 1-800-SOS-RADON.)

Aromatherapy is a holistic approach that utilizes the essential oils extracted from plants, flowers, resins, and roots for therapeutic effects. It has an important role in promoting a healing environment. (To learn more, please refer to Chapter 23.)

To promote a healthy sense of smell, people should use all-natural cleaning agents and scents. It is important for people to learn to be wise consumers by reading labels looking for toxins in all products that contain artificial chemicals. Less is better when aromatics are used in the home.

> **KEY POINT**
>
> The basic ingredients for natural cleaning agents are white vinegar and baking soda. Essential oils such as eucalyptus, lemon, lavender, and tea tree can be added to these agents to offer antibacterial and antiviral effects.

Feng Shui

Feng shui, which grew out of Chinese astrology, is the Chinese art of arranging the environment to positively affect a person's internal state. It offers ways to align pieces of furniture that are said to promote better health, prosperity, and overall well-being (3). The attributes of the five elements—water, wood, fire, earth, and metal—are considered in planning an environment that is best suited for an individual.

Flavors

Food preparation is one of the greatest expressions of love. Love and caring is especially evident when an effort is made to maintain the integrity, quality, and nutritional value of all the foods that are served. Good old homecooking can do wonders to restore the body, mind, and spirit.

A rainbow diet satisfies nutritional needs as well as the vibration of the seven chakras. To follow a rainbow diet people need to eat as many colors in natural foods (fruits and vegetables) as there are in the rainbow. Examples of this could include red apples, orange squash, yellow lemons, green broccoli, blueberries, indigo eggplant, and purple potatoes. The rainbow diet also provides a variety of flavors, which enhances food consumption.

Touch

Touch is imperative in the development of a healthy life, yet the advent of technology has contributed to an era of touch deprivation. The ease of computer communications reduces personal interactions, such as a friendly handshake or a hearty hug. Studies have revealed that babies in hospitals or orphanages who were not picked up or nurtured suffered from a potentially life-threatening syndrome, "Failure to Thrive."

Reflection   Consider the amount of touch in your own life and how you can increase opportunities for touch, such as classic hugs and handshakes.

A mere touch on the hand with the intention to send healing love to someone can make a world of difference. Pets provide opportunities to touch and be touched in return. Remember the value of touch is vital to life enhancement.

Intuition or higher sense perception is accessible to every one. It is that small inner voice—a knowing without knowing how or why—that nudges you along to pay attention to positive and negative aspects of daily life. Pay attention to caustic or harmful situations in your environment. Invite your intuitive thoughts to surface regularly as a barometer of your personal healing environment.

Chapter Summary

The body is more than physical substance. An electromagnetic field that offers energy to promote health surrounds the body. It is theorized that the body also has a vibrational field made of seven chakras, which are spinning wheels of energy. Each chakra resonates with a musical tone and represents colors in the rainbow from infrared to ultraviolet. Various colors are associated with different types of energy. The vibrational fields are influenced by color, clutter, sound, scents, flavors, and touch. People can influence their health and well-being by selecting colors that promote the desired feeling, reducing clutter, controlling noise, selecting music that is soothing, using scents therapeutically, and increasing touch contact with other people and pets. People need to develop sensitivity to the reality that positive and negative external stimuli can have a profound impact on the body, mind, and spirit.

References

1. Babbitt, E. (1976). *The Principles of Light and Color.* Secaucus: The Citadel Press.

2. Hunt, R. (1971). *The Seven Keys to Color Therapy.* San Francisco: Harper & Row Publishers.

3. Simons, T. R. (1996). *Feng Shui, Step-by-Step.* New York: Crown Trade Paperbacks.

Suggested Readings

Bassano, M. (1992). *Healing with Music and Color.* New York: Samuel Weiser, Inc.

Cass, H. (2001). Update on seasonal affective disorder: Light therapy and herbs relieve many symptoms. *Alternative and Complementary Therapies,* 7(1):5–7.

Demarco, A. and Clarke, N. (2001). An interview with Alison Demarco and Nichol Clarke: Light and Colour Therapy Explained. *Complementary Therapies in Nurse Midwifery,* 7(2):95–103.

Klotsche, C. (No year of publication given.) *Color Medicine. The Secrets of Color/ Vibrational Healing.* Sedona, AZ: Light Technology.

Liberman, J. (1991). *Light: Medicine of the Future.* Santa Fe: Bear & Co.

Wong, E. (2001). *A Master Course in Feng Shui.* Boston: Shambhala Press.

Web Resources

Ecopsychology
www.ecopsych.com

Encyclopedia of Environmental Contaminants
www.aqd.nps.gov/toxic/index.html

Health and Light
www.ottbiolight.com

CHAPTER 14

THE POWER OF TOUCH

Objectives

This chapter should enable you to:

- Describe the way touch has been used for healing throughout history
- Describe at least five touch therapies
- Discuss factors that promote healing benefit from touch
- Describe three techniques that can be used to become self-aware and have a centered heart while practicing touch

There is a mysterious healing power in touch that is beyond words and beyond our ideas about it.

— Aileen Crow

Touch … something we are all born to receive and to give to others. As you came into the world you felt the touch of hands welcoming you, be it from a midwife, doctor, mother, or father. You may not remember that touch, but it was a very important one. It provided you with an initial sense of safety, security, and love. When you were given to your mother to be cradled in her arms, that sense of security and love grew. You began learning the power of touch.

Touch is important in every aspect of life. It helps define who someone is as a person—in his or her family and in society. All races, cultures, and religions have spoken and unspoken rules regarding touch. People learn to know when touch is and isn't appropriate, to differentiate types of touch, and evaluate if a touch was good or bad.

In the Beginning, There Was Touch

Since the beginning of time, touch has had an important part in healing and survival. Almost instinctively, people physically reach out to those in pain, those who are suffering, those who are injured or sick, and those they love. Touch provides a soothing comfort and security.

Before the era of modern medicine as we know it, touch was a basic therapy used to compress a wound to stop it from bleeding, to caress the dying, and to welcome the newborn. Although other components of healing grew throughout time, touch remains constant.

Ancient Societies

Ancient carvings and pictures have been found throughout the world that show touch as a part of healing. In Egypt, rock carvings show hands-on healing for illness. All the ancient societies—Indian, Egyptian, Greek, Chinese, and Hebrew—used touch as part of the healing provided to their people (1).

The Egyptians learned much of their healing techniques from the Yogis. The Greeks, in turn, learned from the Egyptians and the Indians. In ancient Athens, Aristophanes details the use of laying on of hands to heal blindness in a man and infertility in a woman (2). In addition, the Greek priests used their hands to heal as did the physicians. As each society learned from the other, new healing modalities were added.

Native American Indians also used touch, with direct and nondirect body contact, as a method of healing. In nondirect body contact, healers hold their hands about six inches above the body or on opposite sides of the area needing healing. They incorporate ritual, such as cleansing the body, prayer, song, and dance, with the touch to promote healing. The Native American Indians brought to the healing process the sense of spirituality (3).

KEY POINT

Hands-on healing, or the laying on of hands, can be found in all major religions.

Religious Stronghold

Accounts of the laying on of hands for healing can be seen in both the old and new Judeo-Christian texts. For centuries, average people have been using this type of healing with their families, friends, and others in their community. Unfortunately, the works of Plato in the early second century helped stir the thinking of separating the spirit from the body. As this common belief took hold, the church also followed in its thinking of the spirit and body as separate. Touch healing came under the domain of the religious leaders or the political leaders of that particular society. Because the political leaders had such a strong association with religion, it was natural for them to assume the same or better position of authority than the religious leaders (4).

There are many references to hands-on healing by religious and political figures. Ancient Druid priests were said to breathe on body parts and touch certain body areas in conjunction with prayer and ritual. St. Patrick helped to heal the blind and St. Bernard healed the deaf and lame. Emperor Vespasian, Emperor Hadrian, and King Olaf were also said to have the ability to heal by touch. In fact some of the early kings in England and France performed touch healings, which became known as the "King's touch" (5).

This power of hands-on healing began to lay solely with the priests and monarchs. Touch for healing soon began to disappear among the lay people. Unfortunately, those lay persons who continued to do hands-on healing were often labeled as pretenders to the throne or witches. Women often were targeted as witches because they made up the majority of the healers.

> ### KEY POINT
>
> The power of healing by women held religious, political, and sexual threats to both the ruling and religious states. From some religious viewpoints, women were considered evil due to their association with sex, so it was not much of a stretch for women to be suspected of practicing witchcraft when they demonstrated their healing powers. Politically women were viewed to be organized and hold certain power because they were the healers in their communities. By eliminating female healers, the ruling class created chaos and gained control. Sadly, it is estimated that millions of women and girls were executed in the Middle Ages under the guise of witchcraft (6).

Science and Medicine

Medicine began with the priests and philosophers of early Egyptian and Greek thinking. Over the centuries, medicine became the domain of men and women who were excluded from the profession. As medical science developed, touch as a healing act became viewed as within the domain of the church or monarchy.

Medicine considered touch to be within the realm of superstition rather than something with any scientific basis for healing. There was no hard proof that touch did anything, therefore no touching of patients was needed other than that involved in performing a task. As the Age of Science developed, healing techniques and medicine became empirically based (proved by experiments). It was believed that if something could not be proved by science, it did not or could not work and had to be superstition or sorcery. Touch as a healing tool could not be proved. This same thinking continued into the twentieth century and only recently has gained new awareness within the medical community.

We Have Come Full Circle

With the massive amount of information available in the last several years, new knowledge has been gained about old methods of healing. With the world becoming smaller due to the mingling of cultures, computer networks, and advances in education, the old is being rediscovered. As more people turn to complementary and alternative therapies, mainstream medicine is forced to acknowledge the power of touch in healing.

The United States government, through the National Institute of Health's National Center for Complementary and Alternative Medicine (NCCAM), is conducting research on many types of healing. One aspect of healing they are examining is the power of touch to heal. Among the touch therapies they recognize are Healing Touch, Therapeutic Touch, and massage.

Some major medical teaching institutions are also researching touch therapies as complements to traditional western medicine. More than 150 schools of medicine now incorporate complementary therapies as part of their physician education program. Columbia Presbyterian Medical Center in Manhattan has established a center for patients to receive touch therapy as part of a research study. The University of Miami/Jackson Memorial Hospital has a Touch for Health affiliation that is studying the effects of infant massage. In addition, their Women's Hospital Center has developed a program for staff and patients that includes several types of touch therapy, such as Healing Touch and Qigong. These are used in conjunction with music, aromatherapy, and guided imagery, and with other hospital services that include psychosocial oncology, pastoral care, and certified music therapy.

The Jackson Memorial Hospital program is looking at the effect of touch therapy in relation to pain, anxiety, and depression in women with gynecologic problems, surgery, and cancer. Unofficial data is revealing a significant impact on the perception and reduction of pain, anxiety, and depression as noted by pre- and posttreatment measurements using visual analogue scales. Formal research involving this population is presently being considered.

Will Science Prove It Works?

Research indicates that touch may be so much more than the physical contact between individuals. Nursing has led the way in this research with the earliest studies from the 1970s. Dr. Delores Krieger, a nurse scientist and professor at New York University, began studying touch as therapy with the help of Dora Kunz and Oskar Estebany. Kunz was not someone who would be considered a healthcare provider based on the standards of having a license to heal someone. Rather, she was born with the ability to perceive energy around living things and describe them as accurately as a medical reference book.

Estebany was a retired colonel in the Hungarian Calvary who found he could heal animals. He was able to heal his own horse by spending the night in his stable, stroking and caressing the animal, talking and praying over it. By the next day, the horse was better. Soon people brought other sick animals for him to heal, and then children. He became known in his country as a hands-on healer. He decided to offer his services for research and moved to Canada where he met and joined Dora Kunz.

Dr. Krieger met the two of them and decided to do research after watching them in a healing session. She observed Estebany laying hands on people wherever he sensed they were needed. He would mostly sit in silence during the 20-to-25 minute sessions. Kunz would observe him and redirect him to another area if she perceived another area needing treatment. Dr. Krieger found that most people reported being relaxed and that most felt better. He treated those with emphysema, brain tumors, rheumatoid arthritis, and congestive heart disease (7).

Estebany did not think hands-on healing could be taught to other people, but that it was a gift that one has. Kunz disagreed and decided to begin workshops to teach people how to do hands-on healing. Dr. Krieger joined her in these workshops and learned how to do hands-on healing, too. Together they developed *Therapeutic Touch*, and began an interesting trend in research and healing. As the research developed and the outcomes began to show significant responses, the power of touch was revealed. In the past 20 years, Therapeutic Touch has been offered in classes and workshops in more than 80 colleges and universities in the United States and over 70 countries worldwide (8).

KEY POINT

Therapeutic Touch is based on the principle that people are energy fields who can transfer energy to one another to potentiate healing. The practitioner's hands do not directly touch the client, but are held several inches above the body surface within the energy field and positioned in purposeful ways. A core element of Therapeutic Touch is the mind set or intent of the practitioner to help.

Another method of hands-on healing called *Healing Touch* was developed by nurse Janet Mentgen. This modality was inspired in part from Therapeutic Touch, the work of Brugh Joy, and energy and philosophical concepts from Rosalyn Bruyere and Barbara Brennan. It began as a pilot project at the University of Tennessee and in Gainesville, Florida, in 1989. By 1990, it became a certificate program with certification beginning in 1993. This multilevel program combines healing techniques from various healers throughout the world.

KEY POINT

Healing Touch is an energy-based therapy, which assists in healing the body-emotion-mind-spirit component of the self.

Healing Touch is done through a centered heart, bringing to it a spiritual aspect. There is no affiliation with any one religious belief and it can be used by those of any religion. It complements traditional healing through modern medicine and psychotherapy, but is not used as a substitute for them. Many hospitals are now incorporating Healing Touch as part of patient services through specific areas within the hospital and the use of Healing Touch is being studied in people with cancer, pain, depression, HIV, cardiac problems, and diabetes.

Another form of hands-on healing is Reiki. This Japanese derived therapy means *universal life energy* (9). Reiki was developed by Dr. Mikao Usui, a Christian minister, in the middle of the nineteenth century. It is comprised of laying hands on the body or leaving them above the body and channeling energy to the recipient.

KEY POINT

Reiki is a form of healing in which the Reiki master channels energy to another individual.

Reiki is learned through a series of intensive sessions whereby a Reiki master passes on the knowledge to others by way of *attunements*. These attunements permit the new practitioner to be able to perform healings by touch. There is no formal certification process in the Usui system of Reiki. A student is deemed competent when a Reiki master decides so. Several forms of healing have been derived from Reiki, such as MariEl by Reiki master Ethel Lombardi (10).

There are additional kinds of hands-on healing, with more being developed all the time. Examples of others include craniosacral therapy, polarity, chakra balancing, acupressure, and shiatsu. Some involve tissue or muscle manipulation, such as neuromuscular release, Rolfing, Trager, massage therapy, and reflexology (Exhibit 14–1). While they all have a slightly different belief or philosophy, they share the common denominator of touch.

Exhibit 14-1 Types of Touch Therapy

Therapy	Purpose
Acupressure	Used to stimulate the body's natural self-healing ability and to allow chi to flow, the life energy of the body. The hands apply pressure to specific acupoints on the body similar to acupuncture.
Craniosacral Therapy	Started in the early 1900s by Dr. William Sutherland, an osteopathic physician. He determined that the skull bones move under direct pressure. By working the skull, spine, and sacrum with gentle compression, the therapist aligns the bones and stretches underlying tissue to create balance and allow the spinal fluid to flow freely. This helps the body self-adjust.
Polarity	Created by Randolph Stone, polarity combines pressure-point therapy, diet, exercise, and self-awareness. Based on the body having positive and negative charges. By varying hand pressure and rocking movements, the energy can be rebalanced.
Chakra Balancing	An energy based modality using the hands to balance the energy centers, or chakras, of the body.
Neuromuscular Release	The goal is to assist the person in letting go by moving the limbs into and away from the body. It helps with circulation and emotional release.
Rolfing	By manipulation of muscle and connective tissue in a systematic way, the therapist helps the body readjust structurally to allow proper alignment of body segments.
Trager	Rhythmic rocking of limbs or whole body to aid in relaxing of muscles. This promotes optimal flow of blood, lymph fluid, nerve impulses, and energy.
Massage	Various types of light touch, percussion, and deep-tissue pressure by hands to assist in muscle relaxation, improved blood and lymph flow, and release of helpful chemicals naturally occurring in the body, such as endorphins.
Reflexology	By applying pressure to specific points on the body, energy movement to corresponding parts of the body are activated to clear and restore normal functioning. It can be done on the feet, hands, or ears.

Energy as a Component of Touch

There is considerable discussion today about *energy*. People state, "I don't have any energy today," "I feel energized," or " I have a lot of energy." You may have experienced these feelings and know there is a difference between having high and low energy. After listening to an uplifting speech and hearing the thunderous applause, one may say the room was "energized" or "electrified." But what is this energy we are talking about?

Reflection Do you have sensitivity to your body's energy? Are there particular experiences or people that seem to energize you and others that drain your energy?

The terms for energy date back to the older traditions of ancient cultures. Every society had a term for the life force. For some cultures, caring for this energy influenced health and wellness; by blocking or disrupting energy, disease or death could result. Other societies merely referred to it in reference to religious or spiritual beliefs. For examples of these terms, see Exhibit 14–2 (11).

The Role of Chi

The Chinese culture has used the idea of energy for thousands of years through the philosophy of *chi (qi)*, or life force, which is an energetic substance that flows from

EXHIBIT 14–2 CULTURAL NAMES FOR ENERGY	
Culture	*Energy Name*
Aborigine	Arunquiltha
Ancient Egypt	Ankh
Ancient Greece	Pneuma
China	Chi (Qi)
General Usage	Life Force
India	Prana
Japan	Ki
Polynesia	Mana
US	Bioenergy, Biomagnetism, Subtle Energy

the environment into the body. The chi flows through the body by means of 12 pairs of meridians (energy pathways to provide life-nourishing and sustaining energy). The organs of the body are affected by pairs of meridians. There needs to be a balance of chi flowing through each side of the paired meridian in order for balance to occur and health to be attained and/or maintained (12).

Science is beginning to get a better understanding of this energy, what it is, and how it functions. Some researchers have developed machinery to try to detect this energy. While success has been limited for some, others have been more successful.

KEY POINT
_____

Motoyama, a Japanese researcher, developed a machine to assist in the detection of meridian lines within the tissues of humans. He found that these meridians do exist and that an energy flow, he calls *ki*, travels through the body. Motoyama states that a center in the brain controls the movement of ki (13). In addition, these meridians feed the different organ systems of the body. By using his machine, called the *AMI machine*, he has been able to detect strong correlations between meridians that have energy imbalances to organs systems, which have diseases present (14). His machine is being used in the research of Parkinson's disease at the Bob Hope Parkinson Research Institute in Florida.

The Energy Fields or Auras

In addition to the seven chakras (see Chapter 20, Symptoms and Chakras, for an explanation of chakras), there exist seven layers of energy fields, or auric fields, around the body. These energy fields surround all living and nonliving matter (15). Science has begun to study and explain these fields over the last several years. The science of physics has done the most extensive work in explaining energy fields. Through Newtonian physics, field theory, and Einstein's theory of relativity, a better understanding of how energy works has been acquired. But it is quantum physics that has really helped explain the characteristics and behaviors of energy (16). Since then, many scientists have begun looking at things as a *hologram* (a multidimensional piece of something whole) (17). The discussion of specifics is beyond this chapter, however, it is intended to show that science is now rethinking some of its early and persistent cause and effect notions.

One way energy fields have been viewed is through *Kirlian photography*. This form of photography was created in the 1940s by a Russian researcher, Semyon Kirlian. By using this form of photography, he was able to measure changes in the energy fields of living systems. He found that cancer causes significant changes in the electromagnetic field around the body. One of the best known experiments is that of the Phantom Leaf Effect whereby a portion of a leaf was cut away and Kirlian photography done on the amputated leaf. Amazingly, the leaf still appeared whole with an energy field present in the form and space of the cut away portion (18).

In other important work, a Japanese researcher named Motoyama, has developed a number of electrode devices to measure the human energy field at various distances from the body (19). So it is now possible to measure the excess or lack of energy around the body and determine a person's health status. Future technology advances may allow a body to be scanned and the beginnings of disease detected prior to symptoms appearing in the physical body. In fact, a new CT scan is being used for this very reason to detect early onset of heart disease and cancer.

But where exactly are these fields? As stated previously, there are seven energy fields that are generally accepted by most energy workers. Each field corresponds to a specific chakra, for example the first energy field with the first chakra and so on. However, the fields lie one on top of another yet do not interfere with each other's functions. These fields interconnect yet maintain their own separateness (20).

KEY POINT

Energy fields of the body work similar to a television. When you change channels, you get a different picture. All the pictures do not end up on the same channel, but they do come through one television set. Likewise, when listening to a radio, you change stations to hear different music, but you still have one radio. The same idea works for the energy fields of the body.

When two people interact, their energy fields connect and they can pick up information about each other. For example, you are riding on an elevator and a stranger gets on. You do not say anything to the person, but you feel safe and secure. At another floor, a second person gets on. Immediately you feel uncomfortable with this person even though you have not spoken to him either. What is occurring is the intermixing of energy fields, which is giving you subconscious information about these people. It has nothing to do with what they are wearing or how they look.

One of the leading causes of illness in our society is stress, yet stress is not internal. Stress occurs outside the body and works its way inward through the energy fields and chakras. It is a well-known fact that long-term stress can weaken the immune system's response, cause heart attacks, high blood pressure, and depression. Of course there are physical evidences for each of these, but the process starts long before any physical evidence is detected. How does this occur? Long-term stress causes changes in the energy fields and chakras that over time repattern themselves and begin to affect the cells of the body. Depending on the severity of the repatterning, illness and disease can occur. By addressing the stressors, one is able to fix or heal any changes made in the energy field or chakras.

Humans as Multidimensional Beings

This concept of energy fields and chakras intermixing contributes to humans being multidimensional. In other words, you are made up of more than just your parts. You not only contain energy, but you are energy that is constantly changing. The body uses energy to perform its functions: for nerves to stimulate muscles, for the beating of the heart, for lungs to exchange air, for cells to digest nutrients, and for the creation of an idea. There is nothing in the body that is not involved in some form of energy. When the normal energy flow is interrupted or destroyed, the body is unable to function to its fullest capacity and illness, disease, and disability can develop. When all of the energy workings cease, death occurs.

Yet, quantum physics has shown us that energy cannot be destroyed. So when we die, it is just the physical part of ourselves that dies. The energy that aided us in our physical form transforms and is released into the environment. Therefore, one doesn't die, the physical body is just transformed.

Touch Is Powerful

With this discussion of the energy systems of the body, you can see that a touch is not just a simple physical act. Something happens human to human, human to animal, human to plant, and animal to animal when touch occurs. This exchange of energy affects not only the one receiving the touch, but also the one giving the touch.

KEY POINT

One of the most important aspects of touch is its intention.

There are neutral touches, such as tapping someone on the arm to get their attention. In addition, there are those touches out of anger that are meant to hurt someone, like a slap or kick. Then there are the loving touches of a hug or caress. The intention is what differentiates.

The way to obtain the power of touch for healing is through a centered heart. This is done in several ways. It occurs spontaneously for those in love or the love that a parent feels toward a child. One can feel the heart open and a strong connection to the other, even when they are not physically present. Another way to obtain this power is through the intention of helping someone. This can be spontaneous as in an accident or planned as in changing someone's wound dressing after surgery.

A third way is through inner focus and awareness in order to become calm and in a state of balance. You probably have experienced times when you are not in balance. Things around you are chaotic, you stumble and cannot seem to get anything done. Yet, in a state of balance you are able to accomplish many tasks regardless of what goes on around you.

KEY POINT

Belly breathing, sounds, and imagery can be used to help you center and focus.

You can learn to have a centered heart using several methods, one of which is belly breathing. Taking slow breaths in through the nose and out through the mouth allows you to become present in the moment. By having a rhythmic pattern of breathing, you become still and calm. In addition, belly breathing can help reduce your stress. To belly breathe, move your belly or abdomen outward on inspiration (the in breath) and retract inward on expiration (the out breath). Counting numbers during the in breath and out breath, along with belly breathing, helps quiet the mind and focus the awareness inward.

Another method of becoming more self aware is through the use of sound. By focusing on a sound externally, like the sound of a bell chime, or one that is self created, like *om*, you may be able to quickly focus and center. Some people find it easy to learn how to center by listening to quiet music, whether it be classical music, jazz, nature sounds set to music, religious music, or new age music. There is no one type of music that is perfect for all people. Generally, it is whatever you need to listen to in order to help you attain a sense of focus.

The third method that can be used to center is imagery. The mind is a powerful tool that can be used to create anything you want. You can use it to create a center of focus. The exercise in Exhibit 14–3 is an example of a way to use imagery to focus.

With practice, you will be able to get into a centered state within a few seconds by using your breath, a sound, or imagery. You can combine any of these and see what works best for you. These techniques can be used in conjunction with touch healing or as a method to reduce stress at any time.

Reflection When providing assistance or care to another person, do you give the person your undivided attention? Do you need to adopt a technique to help you get into a centered state?

EXHIBIT 14–3 USING IMAGERY TO CENTER OR FOCUS

1. First, find a quiet place to sit without distractions. Loosen clothes if necessary. Sit upright with back supported, feet flat on the ground, and hands in a comfortable position on your lap or the arms of a chair.

2. Close your eyes, and begin to breathe in through your nose allowing your stomach to move outward, then exhale slowly, allowing your stomach to retract naturally. Try to have the in breath equal the out breath and let this become a cycle. If you have difficulty, just keep practicing. There is no wrong way to do this.

3. Imagine your feet on the ground growing roots downward through the floor, like a tree. With each breath, allow the roots to move further and further into the earth until it reaches the center of the earth. Feel the warmth of the earth on your roots.

4. Using your breath, have the warmth move upward through the roots and into your feet. Feel the warmth. Continue moving this energy higher into your legs, hips, back, and stomach, into your chest and shoulders, your neck, your face, your head, and out the top of your head up to the sky.

5. Imagine a ball of white light way above your head shining downward. Using your breath, help this light come down and touch the top of your head. You may feel some pressure or heaviness on your head. This is normal.

6. Now using the breath, allow this white light to move through the center of your body, out the base of your spine, and down your legs, through your feet and into your roots. Let the energy go down your roots to the center of the earth.

7. Leaving these images there, focus on your heart center in the middle of your chest. Imagine a pink, light, fluffy ball of light like cotton candy. With each breath, allow the ball to become bigger and bigger. Feel how warm and light this is.

8. Imagine a white or pink light coming from your heart center and running down your arms into your hands and fingers. Some of the sensations you may feel are warm, cold, tingly, prickly, vibration, or any other sensation special to you. You may not even feel anything at all. It doesn't matter, just know it is there.

9. You are now centered. At this point, you can either stay in this state and just enjoy it, or if there is someone who you are going to do touch healing on open your eyes and begin.

The Practice of Touch

While centering is one of the most important aspects to any touch healing, intuition is another one. Intuition often is a heart felt feeling of certainty. All people have intuition, but may ignore it or not identify it as such. At one point or another, many people have said "I knew that would happen." Some people can tell who is on the other end of the phone before or at the moment it rings. Others know when loved ones are in trouble or hurt. This is intuition. It is something often used in touch healing in order to allow for the best outcome for that person. You just seem to know where to place your hands.

> ### KEY POINT
>
> Intuition is the internal knowing of something, often without any external or visible means of proving its existence. One just knows.

When you get a burn on your finger, the first reaction is to pull away from the source of the burn and the second to place your hand over the spot that is burned. The covering hand helps reduce the pain. You know what to do. You don't even think about it. This is intuition.

The same thing happens in touch healing. Of course there are many distinct techniques one can learn step by step, but often this is not necessary. If you allow yourself to follow your intuition, you will know where to place your hands. It may be on the body in a specific area, it may be out in the field away from the body, you may use one hand, two hands together, or two hands in different places. Sometimes your hand may start to do a movement over an area for no particular reason. You may feel things while your hands are placed on the body or off the body, such as temperature, texture, vibration, density, or contour (shape). Just let go and allow the energy of touch to work. You do not need to do anything else. And, when it's time to finish, you will just know to stop.

If the power of touch sounds easy, that's because it is. As long as you prevent yourself from thinking about what you are doing and allow the centered heart and energy to do its work, it happens naturally. The centered heart, with the intention of healing, is the greatest gift you can give anyone, including yourself. The energy used to help someone else benefits you, too. It is like you are a hose watering flowers. The flowers receive the water to drink and live and the hose stays wet inside; both benefit.

The way to master touch healing is to practice, practice, practice. In addition, there are many schools and programs that teach the various forms of touch healing for those interested in learning more specific techniques. For more information on various programs, see Exhibit 14–4.

EXHIBIT 14–4 EDUCATIONAL PROGRAMS FOR TOUCH HEALERS	
Healing Touch International, Inc.	12477 W. Cedar Drive, Suite 202 Lakewood, Colorado 80228 (303) 989-7982 E-mail: HTIheal@aol.com *http://healingtouch.net*
Nurse Healers and Professional Associates Therapeutic Touch	11250-8 Roger Bacon Drive, Suite 8 Reston, Virginia 20190 (703) 234-4149 *http://www.therapeutic-touch.org*
American Chiropractic Association	1701 Clarendon Blvd. Arlington, Virginia 22209 (800) 986-4636 *http://www.amerchiro.org*
International Center for Reiki Training	21421 Hilltop St. Unit #28 Southfield, Michigan 48034 (800) 332-8112 *http://www.reiki.org*

The power of touch is a natural gift, ready to be developed. Some people are using it without knowing what they are really accomplishing. They just *know* it is a good thing. Others recognize this ability and use it help others heal and feel better. And some are afraid of the power their touch has on others. Just know that whenever touch is used with a centered heart and the intention to heal or help, it will not hurt anyone. It is a wonderful, loving act you are able to share with others or do for yourself. Touch has a powerful capacity to heal through a centered heart filled with love.

Chapter Summary

All major religions have used some form of laying on of hands for healing, as have most ancient cultures. Therapeutic Touch, Healing Touch, and Reiki are practices in which energy from one person transfer to another to stimulate healing. Other touch therapies include acupressure, craniosacral therapy, polarity, chakra balancing, neuromuscular release, Rolfing, Trager, massage, and reflexology. To obtain the most healing benefit from touch, one needs to have an intention to do good for the person being touched, have a centered heart, and be focused and aware. Self-awareness can be enhanced through belly breathing, focusing on a sound, and the use of imagery. Practice and experience enhance skill in using touch for healing.

References

1. Graham, R., Litt, F., and Irwin, W. (1998). *Healing from the Heart.* Winfield, BC Canada: Wood Lake Books Publishing, p. 41.

2. Sayre-Adams, J., and Wright, S. (1995). *The Theory and Practice of Therapeutic Touch.* New York: Churchill Livingstone, p. 3.

3. Graham, et al.: pp. 48–49.

4. Ibid., pp. 43–44.

5. Krieger, D. (1992). *The Therapeutic Touch: How to Use Your Hands to Help or Heal.* New York: Simon & Schuster, p. 15.

6. Ehrenreich, B. and English, D. (1973). *Witches, Midwives and Nurses: A History of Women Healers.* New York: The Feminist Press, pp. 6–14.

7. Krieger, pp. 4–8.

8. Knaster, M. (1996). *Discovering the Body's Wisdom.* New York: Bantam Books, p. 323.

9. Ibid., p. 324.

10. Ibid., p. 324.

11. Pavek, R. (1994). *Manual Healing Methods: Physical and Biofield* (Report). Washington, DC: National Institute of Health Office of Alternative Medicine.

12. Gerber, R. (1996). *Vibrational Medicine: New Choices for Healing Ourselves.* Santa Fe, NM: Bear & Company, p. 176.

13. Motoyama, H. (1981). *A Biophysical Elucidation of the Meridian and Ki-Energy.* International Association for Religion and Parapsychology, 7(1):1981.

14. Gerber, p. 186.

15. Brennan, B. (1987). *Hands of Light: A Guide to Healing Through the Human Energy Field.* New York: Bantam Books, pp. 42–43.

16. Ibid., pp. 21–25.

17. Ibid., p. 25.

18. Gerber, pp. 53–54.

19. Motoyama, H. (1984). *Theories of the Chakras*. Wheaton, Illinois: Theosophical Publishing House, p. 257.

20. Brennan, p. 43.

Suggested Readings

Courcey, K. (2001). Investigating Therapeutic Touch. *Nurse Practitioner Forum, 26*(11):12–15.

Engle, V. & Graney, M. (2000). Biobehavioral Effects of Therapeutic Touch. *Journal of Nursing Scholarship, 32*(3):287–289.

Halcon, L. (2002). Reiki. In Snyder, M. and Lindquist, R., eds., *Complementary/Alternative Therapies in Nursing*. New York: Springer, pp. 197–203.

Hurwitz, W. (2001). Energy Medicine. In Micozzi, M., ed., *Fundamentals of Complementary and Alternative Medicine*. New York: Churchill Livingstone.

Mentgen, J. (2001). Healing Touch. In Colbath, J. and Prawlucki, P., eds., *Nursing Clinics of North America: Holistic Nursing Care, 36*(1):142–145.

O'Mathuna, D. (2000). Evidence-Based Practice and Review of Therapeutic Touch. *Journal of Nursing Scholarship, 32*(3):277–279.

CHAPTER 15

TAKING LIFE LIGHTLY: HUMOR, THE GREAT ALTERNATIVE

Objectives

This chapter should enable you to:

- Define *gelotology*
- List at least six physiological effects of laughter
- Identify positive from negative humor
- List at least three ways to develop a comic vision
- Describe at least four strategies for adding humor to work and home

Humor adds perspective to life, altering our perception of a potentially negative incident, and providing preventive maintenance against the strain of hard times in personal and professional relationships.

Laughter is the shortest distance between two people.

A humorous perspective about life helps you to deal with stressors in life, from minor irritation to life-threatening illness. Humor can alter the perception of a situation by changing the expectation of a negative result. A man was upset and taking it out on coworkers. A friend thought to query, "What's the matter, John, did you have nails for breakfast?" This quip got John's attention. He realized he was bringing other problems to work and was able to laugh at himself. The nurse leader on a busy hospital unit would walk down the hall wearing a pair of huge sunglasses when staff was rushing and stressed. This was the sign to take a deep breath, have a good laugh, and start again. One long-term patient would tell her, "Lois, get the glasses. We need them today."

Humor and a playful attitude can build relationships at home and at work and prevent negative reactions in stressful times. In an atmosphere of general goodwill, where no one is expected to be perfect at all times, tough times become more manageable. The mother who can make a game out of power outages by roasting hot dogs in the fireplace models a positive coping strategy for unexpected inconveniences. The manager who organizes a baby picture contest for staff mobilizes positive energy, provides something to look forward to at work, and humanizes team members.

Health Benefits of Humor

Gelotology is the physiological study of laughter. This body of knowledge tells us that humor and laughter benefits us in many ways.

- Stimulation of the production of catecholamines and hormones, which enhance feelings of well-being and pain tolerance
- Decrease in anxiety
- Increase in endorphins (natural narcotic-like substances produced in the brain)
- Increase in cardiac and respiratory rates
- Enhancement of metabolism
- Improvement of muscle tone
- Perception of the relief of stress and tension with increased relaxation, which may last up to 45 minutes following laughter (1)
- Increased numbers of NK, natural killer cells, that fight viral infections of cells and some cancer cells
- Increased T cells (T lymphocytes) that fight infection
- Increased antibody IgA (immunoglobulin A) that fights upper-respiratory infections
- Increased gamma interferon, which helps activate the immune system (2)

Laughter exercises the breathing muscles, benefits the cardiovascular system by increasing oxygenation, and promotes relaxation. Laughter helps control pain by distracting one's attention, reducing tension, and changing or reframing one's perspective. During episodes of laughter the blood pressure increases, but then lowers below the initial rate (3). Dr. William Fry, a researcher of the physiology of laughter has called laughter, "internal jogging," giving our internal organs a workout.

Studies have shown that laughter can help in fighting the negative effects of stress. For example, in a study at Loma Linda University School of Medicine, blood samples were drawn after subjects were shown humor videos. Results were compared to those of a control group. The mirthful experience appeared to reduce serum cortisol, dopac, epinephrine, and growth hormone. These changes are related to the reversal of the neuroendocrine and classical stress hormone response (4).

KEY POINT

In times of stress, the adrenal glands release corticosteroids, which are converted to cortisol in the blood. Increased levels of cortisol can suppress the immune system. If laughter reduces serum cortisol, it may diminish the chemical effects of stress on the immune system (5).

Hospitals, long-term care facilities, hospices, and rehabilitation centers have implemented humor programs with a humor cart or designated room equipped with humorous audiocassettes, videos, games, and toys. Staff and residents at one rehabilitation center perform whodunits and conduct their own academy awards to utilize humor as a coping device with loss and stress (6).

KEY POINT

Attention to the role of laughter and healing was profoundly increased when author Norman Cousins shared his personal experience. Trying to cope with pain from the inflammatory disease ankylosing spondylitis, Cousins watched reruns of *Candid Camera*, and old Marx Brothers films, and had people read humorous material to him. He found that 10 minutes of belly laughter gave him two hours of pain-free sleep. Blood studies of his sedimentation rate—a measure of the inflammatory response—which were drawn after his laughter therapy, showed a cumulative positive effect. He had reasoned that if being in a bad mood makes people feel worse, perhaps, being in a good mood would make him feel better! (7)

Positive Versus Negative Humor

Not all humor is positive. Have you ever been on the receiving end of negative humor? Perhaps someone got a laugh at your expense. You feel hurt and angry, and don't see anything funny about the situation. To make matters worse, your reaction may be met with "Can't you take a joke?", making it seem that you are the one with a problem.

Reflection   Negative humor ridicules, belittles, and distances people. It can be sexist, racist, or embarrassing. Have you been the victim of negative humor? If so, how did it make you feel?

Positive humor intends to bring people closer together. It is associated with hope, love, and closeness. It is a gentle banter, not a caustic, sarcastic barb. It is timely and adds perspective.

Consider three criteria for positive uses of humor. Ask yourself:

1. Is the timing right for this quip? When someone is in the middle of a crisis or is in great pain, humor might not be appreciated even though you have often swapped one-liners.

2. Is the other person receptive to humor? Does this person already use humor to cope? Some people do not seem to have or value a sense of humor.

3. Is the content acceptable? Is it in good taste? Does it make light of self, rather than others? Jokes that could help relieve tension in a closely knit work group could be seen as insensitive to outsiders who do not understand the commitment of the group to the service it provides (8, 9).

Develop Your Comic Vision

Sometimes being able to laugh at life and at yourself relieves tension. Consider the mental self-talk that can alter the interpretation of minor irritants in life. How about remembering with a smile, the one-liner from the children's story, *The Little Engine That Could* (10): "I think I can, I think I can," instead of ruminating over such lines as, "I can't do this. It's too hard. It isn't fair." Begin to collect one-liners of your own to share. How about this one?

New clinical studies show there aren't any answers.

— Anonymous

But how do you develop your comic vision? (See Exhibit 15–1, Developing the Comic Vision.) If you think you have no sense of humor or just want more joy in your life, try planning to have fun, looking for humor in your life, and exposing yourself to humorous

---

EXHIBIT 15–1 DEVELOPING YOUR COMIC VISION

1. Start with yourself. Laugh at yourself. Give yourself permission to be human. If you trip, laugh out loud.

2. Read the comics and political cartoons in newspapers as examples of comic vision. Look at local newspapers when you travel to get the community perspective and learn about regional humor.

3. Start an album with cartoons that track current work issues and encourage all team members to contribute.

4. Attend funny movies and comedy clubs. Rent classic comedy videos.

5. Listen to humorous audiocassettes on the way to work to begin your day looking for humor.

6. Collect humorous one-liners that are inside jokes with your work team.

7. Experiment with building a humor kit at work. Start with a few items and encourage participation and a feeling of ownership.

8. Laugh with others for what they do, at the incongruities in life in which we all share.

9. Pay attention to your own self-talk. Replace negative thoughts with positive ones. Focus on being someone others find pleasant company.

10. Share your comic vision to make other people laugh. Laughter is contagious and adds much needed joy in all our lives.

©2000 Julia Balzer Riley. Humor and Health, home study, AKH Consultant, Inc., Orange Park, Florida. Used with permission.

---

stories and other resources. Taking time to read the cartoons along with the front page will help you reframe your day.

Joel Goodman, founder of the Humor Project in New York (11), talks about aikido humor; humor that uses the momentum of the situation to "roll with the punches." Aikido is a form of martial arts that uses the principle of nonresistance rather than pushing forward; it looks like a flowing dance. Goodman exemplified this with the story of an elementary school teacher. Precisely at 10 A.M., while the teacher had her back turned writing on the blackboard, all the students knocked their books from their desks onto the floor. The teacher turned around, looked at the clock, said, "Oh, sorry. I'm late," and swept the books off her desk, too.

Think of things you can use to add a light touch. (See Exhibit 15–2, Building a Humor Kit.) Add colorful confetti, available for all occasions, to letters or memos. Give out

---

EXHIBIT 15–2 BUILDING A HUMOR KIT

Collect these items to use at work or school. Put them in a tote bag or box for easy access by all.

- Bubbles—small bottles, bubble bottles on necklaces, or wands that make giant bubbles. Take a bubble break to give yourself and others a laugh, and to appreciate the small wonders in life.
- Whistles for stress relief
- Funny hats
- Clown noses and other wild noses
- Funny books, audiotapes, videotapes
- Cartoons collected in a photo album or for display on bulletin boards
- Children's games—wooden paddle and ball, pick-up sticks, coloring books and crayons—ahh, that smell! Splurge and get the box of 64 with the sharpener—they even have bigger boxes now!
- A laughter box
- A big teddy bear when a hug is needed
- Lapel buttons with funny one-liners
- A magic wand
- Be on the lookout for funny things. Sources include: toy stores, clown supply stores, party stores, Halloween and other seasonal displays, souvenir shops, teacher/school supply stores, your children's discards, and garage sales.
- Bubble gum for a brief bubble-blowing contest for staff stress relief

Copyright 1996 Julia Balzer Riley, RN, MN, used with permission.

---

stickers at home or at work when someone does something right or just needs a boost. Use a noisemaker to get people's attention when chairing a meeting. The element of surprise can be effective in changing the mood. This is positive humor—when the sound is not an irritating one and is used playfully. It is negative humor if it's used to interrupt someone who is speaking and embarrasses the person. Use toys and props to facilitate teams (12) and to teach important content such as customer service (13). Take a new look at garage sales and your children's cast-off toys. Take a field trip to a toy store or magic shop for props to add to your kit. Purchase inexpensive toys in quantity to use as incentives at work and at home (14).

He who laughs, lasts! — Anonymous

Plan to Laugh

If humor helps you stay healthy, how can you build it into your daily life? Be open to humor and actively pursue it. Remembering jokes and delivering a powerful punch line can be part of a rich sense of humor, but reading jokes or funny greeting cards can do wonders to stimulate laughter, too.

Reflection How long has it been since you have laughed out loud?

Electronic communication can help you find a steady source of laughter. Subscribe to a list of jokes (15). Find a humor buddy online or be one. Remember that not every sense of humor is alike. Try to open yourself to a variety of kinds of humor to see what tickles your funny bone. Exhibit 15–3, PUNs ... Please Forgive Me, offers examples of puns passed around via electronic mail (e-mail). A *pun* is a playful use of words, using words with different meanings that sound alike or similar. It is the stretching that makes these examples funny. If you groan when you read this, consider the comic relief this can offer on a tough day. Exhibit 15–4, OXYMORONS ... Be on the Alert for More, gives examples of oxymorons, also an e-mail gift. An *oxymoron* is an amusing contradiction in language. Trying to construct puns or recognize oxymorons is good practice for creative thinking.

Plan to Play

Evidence of play and toys is found as far back as relics of human existence in ruins of Egypt, Babylonia, China, and Aztec civilizations. Toys were found buried with children and adults (16). Consider the references to play and creativity in our language: "toy with ideas;" "play with possibilities" (17). Corporate consultants help organizations add play at work. Humor can shift our mental paradigms in problem solving to stimulate creative thinking.

To be more open to creativity; plan to play. Put leisure activities on your calendar. Take time to just be and not do; lie on the ground and look at the clouds, fly a kite, take a break to play several games of Solitaire when you have computer fatigue. See Exhibit 15–5, Plan to Play, to get you thinking playfully. This is quite a task for some grown-ups! Take some time now to generate your own list. Ask friends and family

---

EXHIBIT 15–3 PUNS ... PLEASE FORGIVE ME

Middle Age: When actions creak louder than words

Egotist: One who is me-deep in conversation

Income Tax: Capital punishment

Archeologist: A man whose career lies in ruins

California smog test: Can UCLA?

Two Eskimos sitting in a kayak were chilly, but when they lit a fire in the craft, it sank—proving once and for all that you can't have your kayak and heat it, too.

Two boll weevils grew up in South Carolina. One went to Hollywood and became a famous actor. The other stayed behind in the cotton fields and never amounted to much. The second one, naturally, became known as the lesser of two weevils.

A mystic refused his dentist's Novocain during root canal work.

He wanted to transcend dental medication.

A woman has twins, and gives them up for adoption. One of them goes to a family in Egypt and is named "Amal." The other goes to a family in Spain; the name him "Juan." Years later, Juan sends a picture of himself to his mom. Upon receiving the picture, she tells her husband that she wishes she also had a picture of Amal. Her husband responds, "But they are twins—if you've seen Juan, you've seen Amal."

---

members to add to the list. Contract to do one thing just for fun within the next two weeks and develop a plan for increasing the play in your life. (See Exhibit 15–6, Playful Plan of Self-Care.)

Humor and Play at Work

Do you know someone at work who always sees the funny side of life? Think of the popularity of Dilbert® cartoons. How may Farside® cartoons have surfaced in the workplace? Do you have an employee picnic with games? Do you decorate for holidays? Do you celebrate birthdays? How do you feel reading this if your work-

EXHIBIT 15–4 OXYMORONS ... BE ON THE ALERT FOR MORE

Act naturally

Clearly misunderstood

Alone together

Airline food

Found missing

Resident alien

Genuine imitation

Almost exactly

Legally drunk

Small crowd

Taped live

Plastic glasses

Working vacation

Jumbo shrimp

And the number one listing ... Microsoft Works (a little computer humor)

EXHIBIT 15–5 PLAN TO PLAY

1. Find someone to take the children on an outing and have the house to yourself.
2. Go to a museum, a play, or a concert.
3. Look through a catalog and circle all the things you'd buy if you could.
4. Buy a lottery ticket and fantasize how you would spend the winnings.
5. Just move. Turn on music you like and move with the rhythm. You don't have to know how to dance.
6. Go to a travel agency and get some brochures.
7. Go bowling or play miniature golf.
8. Go get an ice cream cone.
9. Take a novel, go to a restaurant, order a drink, and sit and read.
10. Bake bread or prepare your childhood comfort food.
11. Call a local recreation department and sign up for a class.
12. Find a new recipe, buy the ingredients, prepare it, and invite someone to join you for dinner.

EXHIBIT 15-5 PLAN TO PLAY—CONTINUED

13. Go to an arcade and play skee ball. It's like bowling and you earn tickets, which you can exchange for toys.

14. Blow bubbles, buy new crayons and a coloring book and color, jump rope.

15. Buy yourself a flower or pick wildflowers.

16. Buy a wild hat and wear it.

17. Buy a book on Japanese paper folding and practice.

18. Draw something, paint, or make something out of clay.

19. Buy paper dolls and play with them, or cut out snowflakes.

20. Plan a weekend trip. Pack bath gels and books. Order room service. Sit by the pool.

21. Rent three movies and watch them all.

22. Go to the pet store and ask to spend time with one of the dogs or kittens.

23. Go to the driving range and hit golf balls, or actually take time to play a whole game of golf.

24. Sing as loud as you want; shout in the shower as needed.

25. Call someone you'd like to get to know better and ask them to go to a movie.

26. Light lots of candles.

27. Swing on a swing, or rock in a rocking chair.

28. Wander through a beautiful store.

29. Start a joy box. Fill it with cards or notes you have received, a brochure from a tourist attraction you enjoyed, pleasant mementos. Open and go through these things when you need a boost.

30. Drive to a state park and enjoy.

place includes such activities? What if it does not? Some settings do not seem to lend themselves to such formalized play, yet staff appreciate comic relief in meetings. Consider activities that might actually help people to look forward to coming to work. (See Exhibit 15–7, Humor at Work … We Need It!)

KEY POINT

A light touch at work can help staff build team spirit—they who laugh together stay together, manage stress, and tap their creativity.

EXHIBIT 15–6 A PLAYFUL PLAN OF SELF-CARE

Just for fun I can …

1.
2.
3.
4.
5.
6.
7
8.
9.
10.
11.
12.
13.
14.
15.
16.
17.
18.
19.
20.

I, _____ , promise to _____
        print your name   *one fun thing I will do*

by _____ .
        2 weeks from today

_____
                          signature

EXHIBIT 15–7 HUMOR AT WORK ... WE NEED IT

1. Remember to greet staff in person and on the telephone with a smile. Share a joke.
2. Post cartoons that make light of shared concerns at work.
3. Buy a bottle of bubbles. Start building a humor kit for the office.
4. Collect funny Post-it® notes and use with staff. Use stickers and gold stars.
5. Organize a fun activity at work, such as a staff baby picture contest, a pumpkin-carving contest at Halloween, a bowling night, or a funny movie night.

Humor at Home

We take ourselves and our lives so seriously. We need to be perfect and expect others to have a positive attitude at all times and to appreciate our efforts. A helpful principle to remember is that whatever behavior a person offers at any given time, is usually the best he/she can do. We all have grumpy times. Give some thought to the last time you were able to laugh at yourself. Consider how much more peaceful life would be if we could lighten up! (See Exhibit 15–8, Humor at Home.)

Work on keeping a positive attitude. Here are some tips to help keep a positive attitude.

- Focus on positive thoughts, such as "I'm full of energy." "Today is a good day."
- Imagine good things happening to you. If you are trying to lose weight, picture yourself at your ideal weight.
- Stop looking for the negatives or the flaws in situations and people.

EXHIBIT 15–8 HUMOR AT HOME

- Try sharing moments of laughter.
- Learn to laugh at your own seriousness.
- Forgive yourself and others.
- Remember we don't always have to understand each other or even like each other all of the time.
- Lighten up!
- Agree to disagree.
- Don't try to be so perfect and don't expect it of others.
- Add a little humor by intention. Go do something just for fun—get a life!

- Find the humor in a difficult situation.
- Smile. A study showed that using all your facial muscles in a smile can put you in a more cheerful mood.
- Exercise and keep active to keep up the flow of endorphins, a hormone that elevates mood.
- Just do it ... eat right and take care of your body to feel better.

Reflection   What measures do you use to promote a positive attitude in yourself? List a few ways that you can improve this.

Be an Ambassador for Humor

As you search for ways to be healthy, to tap the power of the mind-body-spirit connection, some strategies intuitively feel right. If you are lucky enough to have a sense of humor, a comic vision . . . share it; the world needs you! If humor does not come easily, pursue it. Take life lightly. Humor is a great alternative.

Chapter Summary

Gelotology, the study of the physiology of laughter, reveals that laughter produces many physiological effects, including stimulation of the production of catecholamines, decrease in anxiety, increase in heart and respiratory rate, increase in endorphins, enhancement of metabolism, improvement of muscle tone, increase in natural killer cells, and relief from stress. There are many practical ways that healthcare professionals can implement humor appropriately into healthcare settings; doing so is therapeutic and beneficial to health and healing. In addition, incorporating humor into daily life and work also is an important self-care measure for healthcare professionals.

References

1. Sullivan, J. L. and Deane, D. M. (1988). Humor and health. *Journal of Gerontological Nursing, 14*(1):20–24.
2. Klein, A. (1999). Who says humor heals. *www.allenklein.com/articles/whosays.htm*. Accessed 11/1/03.
3. Scott, C. (1983). Go ahead, laugh. It's good for you! Madison, WI. *Health Notes.*

4. Berk, L., Tan, S. A. Fry, W. F. et al. (1989). Neuroendocrine and stress hormone changes during mirthful laughter. *American Journal Medical Science,* 298(6):390–396.

5. Wooten, P. (1997). The physiology of humor. *Electric Perspectives,* 22(5):72.

6. Foltz-Gray, D. (1998). Make 'em laugh. *Contemporary Longterm Care,* 21(9):44–49.

7. Cousins, N. (1979). *Anatomy of an Illness as Perceived by the Patient.* New York: WW Norton.

8. Leiber, D. (1986). Laughter and humor in critical care. *Dimensions of Critical Care,* 5(3):162–170.

9. Riley, J. B. (2003). *Humor at Work.* Ellenton, FL: Constant Source Seminars.

10. Piper, W. (1978). *The Little Engine That Could.* New York: Grosset & Dunlap.

11. The Humor Project. 480 Broadway, Suite 210, Saratoga Springs, NY 12866-2288. TEL 518-587-8770 FAX 800-600-4242. *http://www.humorproject.com.*

12. Riley, J. B. (1997). *Instant Tools for Healthcare Teams.* St. Louis: Mosby.

13. Riley, J. B. (2003). *Customer Service from A to Z … Making the Connection.* Albuquerque, NM: Hartman Publishers, Inc.

14. Oriental Trading Company, Inc. Call for a catalog. 1-800-228-2269.

15. Send an e-mail to subscribe to a regular list of jokes with *laughalot@listfarm.com.*

16. Kolkmeier, L. G. (2000). Play and laughter: Moving toward harmony. In Dossey, B., Keegan, L., and Guzzetta, C. E. *Holistic Nursing: A Handbook for Practice.* Gaithersburg, MD: Aspen Publishers, Inc.

17. *http://playfair.com*

Humor and Health Resources

Association for Applied and Therapeutic Humor. *www.AATH.org*
The Humor Project. *www.humorproject.com*

PART III

Taking Charge of Challenges to the Mind, Body, and Spirit

CHAPTER 16

UNDERSTANDING THE HIDDEN MEANING OF SYMPTOMS

Objectives

This chapter should enable you to:

- List at least six early warning signs of health problems
- Discuss lessons that can be learned by the choices people make
- Describe the meanings that symptoms can have

Recognizing warning signs is easy when driving a car. The yellow sign with the curved black arrow communicates clearly that the road ahead has a curve, slow down and pay attention. If this warning sign is observed and the driver gives complete attention, the curve in the road makes the journey more interesting. If the warning sign is ignored, the driver could be forced to pay attention to a car accident, a much less pleasant diversion on the journey.

When people experience good health they feel alive, trusting, enthusiastic, and full of expectation. When health is threatened, warning signs can develop that alert them to "watch the curve in the road." A short list of early warning signs of health problems could include:

- A lack of physical vitality
- Symptoms of illness (e.g., pain, rash, abnormal function, shortness of breath, irregular heartbeat, weight loss, discoloration)
- A feeling of isolation or loneliness
- Frequent accidents
- Poor relationships with family, friends, or coworkers
- Inability to concentrate or solve problems
- Absence of meaning in life; feelings of hopelessness
- Having "enough" by the world's standards, but not feeling satisfied

These warning signs first appear as whispers, but, if ignored, may become shouts. A whisper may be a toothache that ignored becomes the shout of an abscess, or a sore knee that unattended gives out and causes you to slip and break a bone. It may be the whisper of a spouse who is unhappy with your behavior and eventually disrupts your life with the shout of a divorce.

Reflection   Would you have the same attention to a whispered message from your own body that you would to an unusual sound from your car?

Purposes of Warning Signs

Warning signs are feedback that signals people to pay attention to the way they are living so their energies won't be diverted to unnecessary complications, expense, and hardship. They remind that "a stitch in time saves nine."

KEY POINT

Warning signs offer important feedback about life choices that affect health.

Warning signs also teach people how to recognize their choices. They do not spell out exactly what people should do, but they give hints as to what a wise decision would be in a particular situation. The warning signs attempt to help people learn how to be healthy and protect themselves. For instance, working-out to stay physically fit is a wonderful way to stay healthy. However, if people try to initiate the same exercise program at age 60 that was used at age 20, they may find themselves frustrated, dreading exercise time, and perhaps, injured—warning signs that their exercise program needs to be adjusted. Warning signs can help individuals to recognize safe limits.

Good Health as a Process

When taking an automobile journey, people usually have some idea of where they are going and when they will arrive at their destination. What about health? How will they know when they have achieved a satisfactory level of health?

Some people have conceived of health as a continuum from 0 to 100 percent, in which 0 is severe sickness and debilitation and 100 is a perfect, disease-free state. This perspective doesn't account for the quality of life, nor does a continuum model address the rewards experienced through living. Individuals can have meaningful, satisfying lives even in the presence of physical illness. There are many people living with chronic illnesses who hold the view that they may have xyz disease, but xyz disease doesn't have them. A continuum doesn't account for this feeling of well-being or enthusiasm for living in the presence of an illness. A continuum doesn't account for the synergy of the physical, mental, emotional, and spiritual aspects of health. Furthermore, a continuum presupposes that death is bad, and by implication that old age is something to be avoided.

KEY POINT

Health involves possessing a greater understanding of self. It means a person feels at peace, whole, alive, and trusting, and that each day is faced with expectation and enthusiasm.

Good health is better conceived of as a process rather than a continuum. What is a process? The *American Heritage Dictionary* defines process as 1) *a series of actions, changes, or functions bringing about a result, for example: the process of digestion and the process of obtaining a driver's license.* Health can be conceived as the process by which people become more aware of themselves. Health, as a process, means one recognizes their level of well-being and acknowledges their ability to respond to their current level of well-being. Once this part of the process is completed, the person will then proceed to either forgive themselves and/or others and change what they need to change, or accept the circumstances in which they find themselves and continue to act in ways that will help them achieve a high level of well-being. Sometimes, people learn to achieve good health by experiencing poor health. If one has always known good health, they may not be aware of what elements make up this experience of well-being, nor are they likely to be aware of how these elements are related. For example, if your computer is working, you may have little interest in what makes it work, but as soon as you can't access your e-mail, you are calling tech support to find out how to fix the problem. Once help is at hand, some people will want to learn more about what caused the problem and how they may be able to to fix it in the future without having to call tech support, while other people may only be interested in having tech support tell them what to do to fix the current problem. Both approaches are valuable because they result in your e-mail being accessible. Likewise, the process of health may lead to a problem being fixed, or it may lead to the problem being fixed and also a greater understanding of what constitutes well-being and what behaviors are likely to sustain it.

If people want to take a vacation and tour the temples of ancient Egypt, they typically hope to enjoy good health on the trip. "Good *enough* health" may be defined in this case as the ability to walk short distances in the hot sun. To achieve their goal of physical endurance they may engage in the behaviors of eating well, exercising, and getting enough rest. These behaviors dynamically interact to produce the experience of physical endurance and health good enough to accomplish their goal of walking short distances in the hot sun. Each time they make choices about food, exercise, and rest, they have the potential to learn more about themselves, such as which attitudes and behaviors support their goal of physical endurance and which do not. They may also become more confident in their ability to recognize choices that result in a feeling of well-being. As individuals make decisions to support their goals, they feel "at one" with themselves. Health is the process of learning how to achieve this sense of wholeness. Health is recognizing, acknowledging, accepting, and continuing the behaviors that lead to a sense of well-being, peace, and wholeness.

People can also learn about themselves by making choices and engaging in behaviors that do not support their goals. When this occurs people feel separated from themselves and conflicted. Health is then the process of recognizing, acknowledging, forgiving, and changing the behaviors that lead us to a sense of separation.

Reflection Choices made about your health can give insight into values; courage and commitment; strengths and weakness; creativity and patience. What do your health-related choices say about you?

In the process of making "bad decisions" there are lessons as well. Here people can touch a part of self that feels cut off. It is a piece of self that is demanding expression, and will most likely sabbatoge them until they either give it their attention or unhappily pay attention to it.

How people choose to give attention and expression to that which seems to be at odds with their goals of good health may, in fact, teach them more about health than their good choices. Forgiveness can be learned and practiced in the presence of bad decisions. Forgiveness has incredible power to help individuals feel whole and at peace.

When people practice forgiving themselves, they find it is only a short step to feeling the forgiveness presented to them as a gift from their creator.

Warning signs are messages of conflicting choices that call for people to make single-minded decisions. When they shrink from the opportunity to examine their choices or see where they have made conflicting decisions, people pass up an opportunity to learn more about themselves. Likewise, when they expect someone else to "fix" them, they forfeit an opportunity to reflect upon their choices, make decisions, and learn. Reflection leads to greater self awareness.

Reflection In what ways does the healthcare system foster consumers' attitudes that someone else needs to fix their health problems?

Warning Signs as Opportunities

Warning signs present at least two opportunities: To ask for help and to have the chance to allow more love into life. In order to ask for help and in order to allow more love into their lives, individuals must recognize the warning signs that are speaking to them; they are in the driver's seat and hold the power. Therefore it makes sense to set aside the temptation to cast blame on self or others for the current situation. The driver is not going to manage a curve in the road by closing his eyes and chanting, "I'm a terrible driver, I shouldn't have started on this journey." Rather, full attention must be given to managing the present reality.

When traveling in a car it would seem rather silly to say, "These yellow signs are distracting my attention from the enjoyment of this trip." If people resent a warning or blame someone else for their experiences, they are being equally absurd and missing the point of a sign that was meant to be of help.

Where does the process of health lead? How will a person know when he or she has arrived at the destination? What is the health destination? The destination is unique for each person. For some, it can be facing death with the assurance that life has been satisfying and meaningful. For others, the experience of health comes in those special and discrete moments when peace with self, others, and God is achieved. Yet for others, health comes in those magic moments when the joy of living is experienced. This view of health does not concern itself with the physical symptoms of an illness because the presence of a disease does not necessarily mean one is not healthy.

KEY POINT

The experience of a physical illness can awaken one to the experience of health, healing, and wholeness.

Symptoms as Teachers

Physical symptoms can be teaching tools to help people learn how to bring more vitality to living and allow more love into their lives. It is possible to learn without experiencing problems, but if problems unfold, then it is a challenge to use them as learning experiences. The presence or absence of physical symptoms may offer feedback about how alive people feel, how trusting, how enthusiastic, and how much expectation they hold. Symptoms can warn people of imbalances and problems that involve more than the body parts in which they are manifested.

Reflection   Symptoms are private and personal messages to you, coded in metaphor. They speak to your uniqueness. How do frequent symptoms that you experience speak to your uniqueness?

In the attempt to decode warning signs, a person may turn to other people—friends, family, and healthcare practitioners—for help. These other people may assist in decoding the messages, but the final interpretation is the person's alone.

These coded messages have the power to bring about change when they are assigned meaning. Decoding the metaphor of a warning sign will have limited power to affect change if it is handled in a cookbook manner that doesn't resonate with the individual. Take for example a problem with your teeth. This problem has many potential interpretations that may have little to do with dental health. It may mean you are afraid to bite into (take on) something, that you are reluctant to chew (reflect) on something, or that you have bitten off more than you can chew. The correct interpretation of the metaphor can only be known by the person experiencing the symptom. It may be helpful to have others suggest possible interpretations of the metaphor. Their suggestions will stimulate you to think, and thinking may promote an insight that, without their suggestion, you may have missed. The power of the metaphor to create change occurs only when the interpretation resonates with you and creates that *aha* feeling.

Warning signs will have different meanings at different times along the life journey. This is not intended to make life more difficult. Life is not a textbook experience. Understanding the variety of possible meanings enables people to learn about themselves more fully and deeply. Furthermore, the many possible interpretations provide the opportunity to choose the specific meaning of a symptom. For example, you have lost a front tooth and while waiting to see the dentist, you reflect on this event. You begin to see a metaphor, and it strikes you that you must be experiencing difficulty "biting into something," or "taking a bite." You could think: "This is another example of how I'm doomed to have one problem after another"; or you could think "This dental problem is an example of how I do not pay ample attention to small matters that eventually accumulate into big problems for me. I need to seek help to do the tasks of daily living that need my attention and action." It is expected that a person would respond to a tooth problem by visiting the dentist. However, the tooth problem holds other meaning. The metaphor, if utilized, can lead to even greater self-knowledge and change. When you manage the physical symptom on more than the surface level (the dentist) and seek to work with the metaphor, you have an opportunity to heal on more than just the physical level. In fact it may be that the physical symptom will not change, but that change will occur on a more profound level, bringing greater happiness, growth, and satisfaction than you could ever experience by simply treating the physical symptom.

KEY POINT

When physical symptoms are addressed on more than the surface level and the other meanings they hold in life are explored, people have an opportunity to heal beyond the physical level.

Chapter Summary

Symptoms involving the mind, body, and spirit can indicate the presence of a health problem. They are warning signs that offer feedback as to the way one is living and lifestyle and health-related choices. Rather than treat or mask their symptoms, people can achieve higher levels of holistic health by exploring their deeper meaning and choosing attitudes and behaviors that will foster health and healing.

Suggested Readings

Bauby, J. (1997). *The Diving Bell and the Butterfly.* New York: Vintage International.

Burkhardt, M. A. and Nagai-Jacobson, M. G. (2002). *Spirituality: Living Our Connectedness.* Albany, NY: Delmar, Thomson Learning.

Cobb, M. and Robshaw, V., eds. (1998). *The Spiritual Challenge of Health Care.* New York: Churchill Livingstone.

Duff, K. (2000). *The Alchemy of Illness.* New York: Random House.

Frank, A. W. (1997). *The Wounded Storyteller: Body, Illness, and Ethics.* Chicago: University of Chicago Press.

McSherry, W. (2000). *Spirituality in Nursing Practice: An Interactive Approach.* New York: Churchill Livingstone.

Morris, D. B. (2000). *Illness and Culture in the Postmodern Age.* Berkeley, CA; University of California Press.

Sacks, O. (1998). *A Leg to Stand On.* New York: Touchstone Books.

CHAPTER 17

WORKING IN PARTNERSHIP WITH YOUR HEALTH PRACTITIONER: ADVOCATING FOR YOURSELF

Objectives

This chapter should enable you to:

- List three responsibilities that consumers have when meeting with their health practitioner
- Describe a consumer's responsibilities when diagnosed with a medical problem, hospitalized, and when facing surgery
- List at least five questions to ask of health insurance plans
- Describe at least six factors to evaluate in a primary healthcare practitioner

A *partnership* implies an active relationship of give and take with a mutual respect between the parties. Of the various partnerships that you may experience in your life, your partnership with your healthcare provider is among the more important ones that you can develop. Yesterday's model of blind obedience and dependency on one's physician or other healthcare provider is no longer appropriate or desirable. People have a right to be informed, to have a variety of healthcare options (conventional and complementary/alternative) made available to them, and to make decisions that are right for them—not only medically, but emotionally, spiritually, and financially as well. They also have the responsibility to take an active role in their health care, educate themselves about health matters, and equip themselves with the necessary information to make sound healthcare decisions. They must be responsible advocates for themselves.

Responsibilities When Seeking Health Care

Choosing a Healthcare Practitioner

Because the relationship with a healthcare practitioner is an important one that should function with the same harmony as a good marriage, people need to choose a primary healthcare practitioner with whom they can communicate. They must feel free to ask questions and expect to get responses they understand.

When making an appointment, if people think they will need more time than usual to talk things over, they should let the office know in advance. The response to this request could offer insight into the type of relationship that can be expected with the healthcare provider. For example, if you ask that you be scheduled for a longer visit because there are some complementary therapies that you want to review with the physician as soon as possible and you are told "Sorry, the doctor only can only spend 10 minutes with each patient," you may need to assess if this is the best source for your primary care.

It is helpful for people to write a list of health concerns or questions they want to discuss before the appointment. They can include information about symptoms, such as when the symptoms started, what they feel like, whether they're constant or they come and go. Records that are kept, such as blood-sugar levels, daily blood pressure, dietary history, and mood changes, should be taken to the appointment. It is important for people to tell their practitioners personal information—even if it feels uncomfortable to do so. Any allergies or reactions experienced in the past to any medicines or foods need to be discussed. Health practitioners need to know as much as possible about their clients.

> **KEY POINT**
>
> People need to prepare for visits to their healthcare practitioners by writing down health history, medications used, symptoms, and other pertinent information that can be shared with the practitioner.

It is helpful for people to compile a written list of the medicines and supplements that are taken, including those that don't require a prescription, such as over-the-counter pain relievers, laxatives, vitamins, herbs, flower essences, or eye drops. Also helpful is a list of the names of other healthcare practitioners visited, including physicians, chiropractors, acupuncturists, massage therapists, nutritionists, and herbalists. People should supply each of their healthcare practitioners with this information. It is useful for people to be open about their reasons for seeing other healthcare practitioners and the care they are receiving from them. If a healthcare practitioner doesn't agree with what is being done, it is useful for people to listen to the reasons. All the facts can be evaluated and decisions made to stay with this practitioner or change to one who is more supportive. Practitioners need to be given permission to contact each other for clarification when necessary.

KEY POINT

It is wise for people to keep their own health file that records their medicines, treatments, surgeries, hospitalizations, and visits to all practitioners.

It is helpful for people to take a notepad to appointments and take notes when given instructions. Most individuals only remember a portion of what they are told and if anxious, they could forget most of the information. In some circumstances, it could be helpful to bring along someone to help ask questions, clarify, and remember responses.

When Diagnosed With a Medical Condition

If diagnosed with a medical condition, people need to ask about the causes. Often, improvements can be made if the reasons are understood. It is beneficial for people to ask for guidelines as to symptoms that should be reported. (For example, if the temperature is over what degree? If the discharge is what color? If the stools are loose for how long? If the coughing persists for how many days? If the pain is not relieved by what time?) Healthcare practitioners may have printed information about conditions (e.g., Diabetes Fact Sheets) that can be given to take home; if not, people should ask where more information can be obtained. People need to be knowledgeable about their conditions. They need to be informed about the tests that are ordered, also (Exhibit 17–1).

EXHIBIT 17–1 QUESTIONS TO ASK WHEN TESTS ARE RECOMMENDED

Why is the test needed?

Does the test require any special preparation?

What are the side effects and risks?

When can the results be expected and how are they obtained?

Will additional testing be required at a later date ?

Does my insurance cover this test?

KEY POINT

It is useful for copies of diagnostic tests to be requested and kept in a personal health record.

It is important for people to learn about the available treatments for their conditions. Some of the questions that need to be answered when treatments are ordered are listed in Exhibit 17–2. People also can check out information in their libraries or on the Internet. Discussing the issue with friends or relatives who are nurses or other healthcare practitioners is beneficial.

After the visit, people need to follow up. Questions should be phoned or e-mailed to the healthcare practitioner. If symptoms worsen or people have problems with what they are asked to do, they need to contact the practitioner. If tests are ordered, arrangements should be made at the lab or other offices to get them done. If tests were completed and people have not been informed of the outcome, they need to call for test results. Some healthcare practitioners' offices call patients to see how everything is going, but in most instances it is up to the individual to do the follow up.

Reflection   How much responsibility do you assume for your personal health care? Do you ask the right questions, demand answers, take action when you think you are not being heard, and follow up as needed? If you do, what has caused you to develop these skills? If you do not, what prohibits you from doing so?

When Hospitalized

Everyone needs to know the physician in charge of their care. This may seem like a ridiculous statement, however, this may be an issue when people go into the hospital for a surgical procedure and have an existing medical problem or several health-related issues. Different doctors may be responsible for different aspects of care. It can be particularly difficult in a teaching hospital where there are several medical residents writing orders. People need to make sure all health professionals know their health history. It is smart for people to keep a brief summary (just a short page) of their condition

EXHIBIT 17–2 QUESTIONS TO ASK WHEN TREATMENTS ARE ORDERED
When should treatment start?
How long will the treatment be needed?
What are the benefits of the treatment and how successful is it usually?
What are the risks and side effects associated with the treatment?
What is the cost of the treatment?

and health history at the bedside. It cannot be assumed that each doctor or resident knows everything about the history. Very likely, they do not.

Protection from errors during hospitalization can be increased when a summary of personal health history is kept by the bedside.

When people have questions about procedures or a medicine and the answer is, "Your doctor ordered it," they need to ask which doctor. If they do not understand the purpose or did not receive an adequate explanation, they are wise to politely refuse. They are not being difficult or uncooperative patients, but rather, informed and responsible patients participating in their own care. They are within their rights to ask their primary doctor to give an explanation. If illness prevents someone from taking on this total responsibility he or she can ask a family member or friend to be an advocate (Exhibit 17–3).

It is helpful for people to learn the names of the hospital staff who do anything to or for them. By having their notebooks handy, they can write down staff names and positions, whether it is the nurse assistant who is responsible for bathing assistance or the anesthesiologist who assists with surgery.

When Surgery Is Recommended

There is information that needs to be considered in order to make an informed decision about surgery. First, people need to ask the doctor the purpose of the procedure. Sometimes, surgery is not the only answer to a medical problem. Nonsurgical treatments, such as a change in diet, special exercises, acupuncture treatments, herbs, or other nonconventional treatments might help just as well, or more. The benefits and risks of these other choices need to be discussed. Individuals can research these on their own.

One approach when surgery is recommended is watchful waiting, in which the doctor and patient monitor the problem to see if it gets better or worse. If it gets worse, surgery may be needed fairly soon. If it gets better, surgery may be able to be postponed, perhaps indefinitely.

There should be a clear understanding of how the proposed operation relates to the diagnosis. It is reasonable for people to ask why a particular surgeon was chosen. When they meet with the surgeon, people should ask for an explanation of the

---

EXHIBIT 17-3 "THE DOCTOR ORDERED IT ..."

An example of what can happen when the only response to your question is "the doctor ordered it" is what happened to a patient who had just gone through a surgical procedure in the hospital to prepare her for kidney dialysis treatments. Early one morning the nurse came in to do a finger stick for a drop of blood. The patient accepted this, assuming that blood tests may be needed. The nurse came in again before lunch to repeat the procedure and the patient asked, "Why are you sticking me again?" The reply was simply, "The doctor ordered it."

Her daughter, a registered nurse, came to visit later in the day just as the nurse was about to do yet another finger stick. Knowing that this type of testing was typically done for persons with diabetes and that her mother wasn't diabetic the daughter asked, "Why are you checking her blood sugar? Is it high?"

"The doctor ordered it," came the reply.

"Well, before you do it, please tell me her blood-sugar level."

With this, the patient said. "Blood sugar! I'm not a diabetic, I don't want you to do this."

The family later learned that one day her blood-sugar level was 147 mg, a little high, but not alarming considering she was receiving intravenous fluids with dextrose (sugar water). An intern had ordered the test.

When the patient told her primary medical doctor he remarked, "The intern was being overly cautious. I'll write an order that they need to check with me before ordering any more tests."

This situation caused the patient unnecessary worry, discomfort, and expense.

---

surgical procedure in detail. They should find out if there are different ways of doing the operation and why the surgeon has chosen the particular procedure. One way may require more extensive surgery than another one and a longer recovery period.

It's important that people know what they will gain by having the operation and how long the benefits are likely to last. For some procedures, the benefits may last only a short time with a need for a second operation at a later date. For other procedures, the benefits may last a lifetime. Published information about the outcomes of the procedure can be reviewed. Because all operations carry some risk, people need to weigh the benefits of the operation against the risks of complications or side effects.

Surgeons should be asked about possible complications and side effects of the surgery. *Complications* are unplanned events, such as infection, too much bleeding, reaction to anesthesia, or accidental injury. Some people have an increased risk of complications because of other medical conditions. *Side effects* are anticipated occurrences, such as swelling and some soreness at the incision site.

There is almost always some pain with surgery. People should ask how much pain can be expected and what the doctors and nurses will do to reduce the pain. Individuals may want to discuss how staff will respond if they want to use nonconventional, alternative methods of pain control. Controlling the pain helps people to be more comfortable while they heal, get well faster, and improve the results of their operation.

It is useful for individuals to find out if the surgeon agrees to their own treatment plans during and after the surgery. For example, what does the physician think about a plan to take higher doses of vitamins and minerals prior to surgery to promote healing afterwards? Will the hospital permit music or guided imagery tapes during the surgery? Can a therapeutic touch practitioner offer treatments after surgery? All desires and suggestions should be openly discussed.

Getting other opinions from a different surgeon and healthcare practitioner of choice is a very good way to make sure having the operation is the best alternative. When people seek second opinions, they can spare themselves unnecessary duplicative testing by obtaining a copy of their records from the first doctor.

Anesthesia is used so that surgery can be performed without unnecessary pain. People should ask to meet with the anesthesiologist to learn about his or her qualifications. The anesthesiologist can explain if the operation calls for local, regional, or general anesthesia, and why this form of anesthesia is recommended for the procedure. Questions about expected side effects and risks of having anesthesia should be asked. Some hospitals are using acupuncture as an adjunct to anesthesia and this may be requested if appropriate.

If surgery is agreed upon, people need to ask if the operation will be done in the hospital or in an outpatient setting. If the doctor recommends inpatient surgery for a procedure that is usually done as outpatient surgery, or just the opposite, the reason should be examined because it is important to be in the most appropriate place for the operation. Until recently, most surgery was performed on an inpatient basis and patients stayed in the hospital for one or more days. Today, many surgeries are done on an outpatient basis in a doctor's office, a special surgical center, or a day surgery unit of a hospital.

People should ask how long they will be in the hospital. The surgeon can describe how people can expect to feel and what they will be able to do or not do the first few days, weeks, or months after surgery. Prior to discharge, individuals should find out what kinds of supplies, equipment, and any other help they will need when they go home. Knowing what to expect can help them better prepare and cope with recovery. They should ask when they can start regular exercise again and return to work. People do not want to do anything that will slow down the recovery process. Lifting a 10-pound bag of onions may not seem to be too much a week after surgery, but it could be.

Choosing an Insurance Health Plan

Selecting a health plan to cover themselves and their families is an important decision many people make every year. Health insurance varies greatly, so, to avoid surprises, it is important for people to find out exactly what their insurance plan covers. Does it allow for any alternative approaches? Many policies now cover acupuncture; and some cover nutrition counseling, massage, and other forms of body work. People need to be informed. Some questions worth asking are offered in Exhibit 17–4.

Health insurance coverage for surgery can vary, and there may be some costs individuals will have to pay. Many health insurance plans require patients to get a second opinion before they have certain nonemergency operations. Even if a plan does not require a second opinion, people may still ask to have one. Before having a test, procedure, or operation, it is advisable for people to call their insurance plan to find out how much of these costs it will pay and how much they will have to pay themselves. They also may be billed by the hospital for inpatient or outpatient care, any doctor who visited, the anesthesiologist, and others providing care related to the operation.

KEY POINT

People have to do their homework to assure they are not surprised by unexpected bills.

The Agency for Health Care Policy and Research, within the Department of Health and Human Services, has excellent information on choosing quality health care. The National Committee for Quality Assurance (NCQA), a nonprofit accrediting agency, has a Health Plan Report Card that shows consumers how well managed health plans are doing. (See Resources at the end of the chapter.)

How to Get Quality Care

From the Primary Healthcare Practitioner

People must decide what they want and need in a healthcare practitioner. What is most important to them in working in partnership? Internists and family physicians

---

EXHIBIT 17–4 QUESTIONS TO ASK OF A HEALTH INSURANCE PLAN

- What benefits and services are covered?
- Is my current doctor in the network?
- How does the plan work?
- How much will it cost me?
- Does the plan have programs in place to assist me in managing chronic conditions?
- Is it evident that qualified healthcare professionals make decisions about medical treatments and services provided to plan members?
- How will I get needed emergency services and procedures that ensure I will get the level of care needed?
- Is the information about member services, benefits, rights, and responsibilities clearly stated?
- Is there easy access to primary care and behavioral health care (mental health services)?
- Does the plan include alternative approaches?
- How prompt are decisions made about coverage of medical treatments and services?
- Are there clear communications from the health plan to members and doctors about reasons for denying medical treatments or services and about the process for appealing decisions to deny treatment or services?

---

are the two largest groups of primary healthcare practitioners for adults. Many women see obstetricians/gynecologists for some, or all, of their primary care needs. Pediatricians and family practitioners are primary healthcare practitioners for many children.

Reflection What do you look for in a healthcare practitioner?

Nurse practitioners, certified nurse midwives, and physician assistants are trained to deliver many aspects of primary care. Physician assistants must practice in partnership with doctors. Nurse practitioners and certified nurse midwives can work independently in some states, but not others. Some people may choose an acupuncturist, chiropractor, or naturopath for their health maintenance and consult with the medical doctor when hospitalization or special tests are needed.

There are minimum requirements to look for in any practitioner (Exhibit 17–5). Is the primary healthcare practitioner listening with full attention and not distracted with

---

EXHIBIT 17–5 CHARACTERISTICS TO LOOK FOR IN A PRIMARY HEALTH CARE PRACTITIONER

Look for someone who:

- Listens to you
- Explains things clearly
- Encourages you to ask questions
- Treats you with respect
- Understands the language that you are most comfortable speaking (or has someone in the office who does)
- Takes steps to help you prevent illness
- Is rated or certified to give quality care
- Has the training and experience that meets your needs
- Has privileges at the hospital of your choice
- Participates in your health plan, unless you choose to pay out of pocket

---

other things going on? Does the practitioner answer questions without impatience? When a client calls the office with a concern, does the staff respond, or do they refer it to the practitioner? Does the practitioner return calls? Does the entire staff treat clients with respect? Does the receptionist or billing person answer all questions and assist in a courteous way if help is needed?

KEY POINT

Staff is an extension of the primary healthcare practitioner and their attitude and actions often reflect those of their boss.

What role does prevention have in the plan for health care? Does the practitioner offer advice about a healthful diet, exercise, adequate sleep, addictive behaviors, and how to prevent minor illnesses?

Does the practitioner have additional certification and/or experience (e.g., board certified, licensed)? There are organizations that certify people in many different specialties and modalities. Is the person knowledgeable about alternative treatments or willing to listen to the search for alternative/complementary treatments? Does the practitioner have privileges at the hospital that you wish to use?

If they are already enrolled in a health plan, people's choices may be limited to doctors and healthcare practitioners who participate in the plan. If they have a choice of plans, individuals may want to first think about whom they would like to use. Then, they may be able to choose a plan that fits their preferences.

When Surgery Is Recommended

It is important for people to check their surgeons' qualifications. One way to reduce the risks associated with surgery is to choose a surgeon who has been thoroughly trained to do the procedure and has plenty of experience doing it. Surgeons can be asked about their recent record of successes and complications with a procedure. If they are more comfortable, people can discuss the topic of a surgeon's qualifications with their primary healthcare practitioner or do their own research.

People undergoing surgery will want to know that their surgeon is experienced and qualified to perform the operation. Many surgeons have taken special training and passed exams given by a national board of surgeons. People should ask if their surgeon is board certified in surgery. Some surgeons also have the letters *F.A.C.S.* after their name, which means they are Fellows of the American College of Surgeons and have passed a review by surgeons of their surgical practices. To check out qualifications, people can contact the American Board of Medical Specialists or Administrators in Medicine. (See Resources.)

From a Complementary/Alternative Modality (CAM) Practitioner

Complementary/alternative modality (CAM) covers a broad range of healing philosophies, approaches, and therapies that conventional medicine does not commonly use, or make available. People use CAM treatments in a variety of ways. Therapies may be used alone as an alternative to conventional treatment. They may also be used in addition to, or in combination with, conventional methods, in what is referred to as an *integrative approach*. Many CAM therapies are called holistic, which generally means they consider the whole person, including physical, mental, emotional, and spiritual aspects. Many are reviewed in this book. Some useful sources of information are the National Institutes of Health, National Center for Complementary and Alternative Medicine, American Holistic Nurses Association (AHNA), and Natural Healers. (See Resources.)

Most often people learn about these modalities and the therapists as referrals from friends. Today, people can go on the Internet, search for the particular modality, and find most anything they want to know. Schools often have a listing of their graduates, which can serve as a referral source. The telephone book yellow pages can be explored for alternative medicine. Primary healthcare practitioners can be good referral sources, too. Many chiropractors are knowledgeable about alternative treatments. Friends who are nurses can also be asked for ideas.

How do people know if these therapies and practitioners are appropriate for them? They can check to see if the practitioner has had training and experience. Practitioners can be asked for referrals of other clients. People should look for the same qualities as they would for any healthcare practitioner—and more. Are they holistic in their practice? Do they consider mind, body, and spirit when planning treatment? Do they explain what they are doing? Have they trained at a licensed school? Do they have certification or state licensing for what they do? It is useful for people to check the credentials of practitioners. Practitioners can be asked if their therapy has been used to treat conditions similar to the ones for which treatment is sought, if there are any side effects or cautions in using this particular therapy, and if they can they share research to support the treatment or product they use? (For more information see Chapter 21, Safe Use of Complementary Therapies.)

KEY POINT

There are many CAM therapies available for health maintenance, prevention, and treatment of illness. It is the individual's responsibility to learn about and choose the ones that are appropriate for his or her condition.

Working in partnership with their healthcare practitioners gives people the tools they need to get the quality health care they deserve. It takes work and being alert and proactive, not just accepting everything they are told. By being active participants people increase their chances of getting the best health care available.

Chapter Summary

When meeting with a healthcare practitioner, consumers have responsibilities, including preparing for the visit, informing the practitioner of medications and supplements used, other practitioners seen, and remembering instructions in detail. When diagnosed with a medical condition, consumers need to ask about the cause, symptoms, and guidelines for treatment.

Asking questions about procedures, medications, and the staff are important during a hospitalization. When facing surgery, consumers need to ask about alternatives, benefits, and risks of surgery, as well as expected pain, where the surgery will be done, and anticipated time for recovery.

A variety of questions need to be asked when considering a health insurance plan, including benefits covered, how the plan works, cost, how decisions are made, and if one's current practitioners are in the network.

When evaluating a primary healthcare practitioner, consumers should consider if the practitioner listens, explains things clearly, encourages questions, treats them with respect, speaks the same language, takes steps to prevent illness, is certified, has privileges at the hospital of their choice, and participates in their insurance plan.

By being active participants and informed consumers of their health care, people can maximize the quality of care they receive and reduce risks.

Suggested Readings

Benner, P. (2003). Enhancing Patient Advocacy and Social Ethics. *American Journal of Critical Care*, *12*(4):374–375.

Clark, C. C. (2003). *American Holistic Nurses Association Guide to Common Chronic Conditions. Self-Care Options to Complement Your Doctor's Advice*. Hoboken: John Wiley & Sons.

Ekegren, K. (2000). We Are All Advocates. *Journal of the Society of Pediatric Nursing*, *5*(2):100–102.

Fasano-Ramos, M. (2000). *Older Adult Resources*. Ventura, California: InterAge.

Ford, S., Schofield, T., and Hope, T. (2003). What Are the Ingredients for a Successful Evidence-based Patient Choice Consultation? A qualitative study. *Society of Science and Medicine*, *56*(3):589–602.

Greggs-McQuilkin, D. (2002). Nurses Have the Power to Be Advocates. *Medical Surgical Nursing*, *11*(6):265, 309.

Henderson, S. (2003). Power Imbalance Between Nurses and Patients: A Potential Inhibitor of Partnership in Care. *Journal of Clinical Nursing*, *12*(4):501–508.

Hyland, D. (2002). An Exploration of the Relationship Between Patient Autonomy and Patient Advocacy: Implications for Nursing Practice. *Nursing Ethics*, *9*(5):472–482.

Penson, R. T. (2001). Complementary, Alternative, Integrative, or Unconventional Medicine? *Oncologist*, *6*(5):463–473.

Strax, T. E. (2003). Consumer, Advocate, Provider: A Paradox Requiring a New Identity Paradigm. *Archives of Physical Medicine and Rehabilitation*, *84*(7):943–945.

Resources

American Holistic Nurses Association
800-278-2462
www.ahna.org
They have a directory of members with additional training in various modalities.

The National Library of Medicine
www.nlm.nih.gov/medlineplus/patientissues
This site has useful topics on a variety of issues effecting patients.

The National Institutes of Health
Bethesda, MD 20892
301-496-4000
www.nih.gov/niams/healthinfo/library
A place to start to find information on any medical topic, resources, research, and self-help groups.

U.S. Department of Health and Human Services
200 Independence Ave.
Washington, D.C. 20201
877-696-6775
www. healthfinder.gov
A free guide to reliable health information.

National Center for Complementary or Alternative Medicine (NCCAM)
NCCAM
P.O. Box 8218
Silver Spring, MD 20907-8218
888-644-6226
www.nccam.nih.gov
Focuses on evaluating the safety and efficacy of widely used natural products, such as herbal remedies and nutritional and food supplements; supporting pharmacological studies to determine the potential interactive effects of CAM products with standard treatment medications; and evaluating CAM practices.

Natural Healers
www.NaturalHealers.com
This site describes many complementary and alternative therapies and gives a list of schools in the United States and Canada that teach the various disciplines. Schools often have lists of graduates who are practitioners in your area.

Administrators in Medicine
www.docboard.org
Information on doctors in many states is available from state medical board directors.

American Medical Association (AMA)
AMA Chicago Headquarters
515 N. State Street
Chicago, IL 60610
312-464-5000
800-665-2882
www.ama-assn.org
"Physician Select" information is available on training, specialties, and board certification about many licensed doctors in the United States.

The American Board of Medical Specialties
800-776-2378
www.certifieddoctor.org
This site can tell you if the doctor is board certified. *Certified* means that the doctor has completed a training program in a specialty and has passed an exam (board) to assess his or her knowledge, skills, and experience to provide quality patient care in that specialty.

Agency for Healthcare Research and Quality
2101 E. Jefferson St., Suite 501
Rockville, MD 20852
301-594-6662
www.ahrq.gov
Your Guide to Choosing Quality Health Care is based on research about the information people want and need when making decisions about health plans, doctors, treatments, hospitals, and long-term care.

The National Committee for Quality Assurance (NCQA)
Health Plan Accreditation
National Committee for Quality Assurance
2000 L Street, NW, Suite 500
Washington, D.C. 20036
202-955-3500
www.ncqa.org
An accrediting agency that gives standardized, objective information about the quality of managed-care organizations, managed behavioral healthcare organizations, credentials verification organizations, and physician organizations.

Joint Commission on Accreditation of Healthcare Organizations (JCAHO)
One Renaissance Boulevard
Oakbrook Terrace, IL 60181
630-792-5000
www.jcaho.org
The Joint Commission evaluates and accredits nearly 20,000 healthcare organizations and programs in the United States. An independent, not-for-profit organization, the Joint Commission is the nation's predominant standards-setting and accrediting body in health care.

CHAPTER 18

MENOPAUSE: TIME OF THE WISE WOMAN

Objectives

This chapter should enable you to:

- Describe the three seasons of a woman's life
- Discuss how menopause is a sacred journey
- Define *menopause*
- List the three types of estrogen produced by the ovaries
- Describe what is meant by a natural hormone
- List a multistep approach to assisting women in menopausal transition years
- Describe at least six factors that can trigger hot flashes

Imagine a time long, long ago, when cycles of life were celebrated. There were ceremonies celebrating the cycles of the sun and the moon, the cycles of planting and harvesting, the cycles of seasonal change, the cycles of birth and death, marriages, and rites of passage. The cycles of our lives were honored and celebrated as necessary transitions and initiations. People knew how to stay connected to their spirit and to that which had meaning in their lives.

Reflection Do you know how to call in your spirit? Do you know how to connect to the deepest part of your soul? Do you know what your soul yearns for? Do you know what has heart and meaning for you?

Menopause is the time that helps women answer these questions. The physiological, emotional, and spiritual changes that take place, direct women's hearts, souls, and spirits. If they do not pay attention, their bodies and emotions call out to them—sometimes whispering gently, sometimes yelling to get noticed.

We must get back to remembering our roots. *Remember* means to *reconnect*, to put our members back together, to put all the pieces of ourselves back together again. Remembering our roots reminds us to reconnect to what keeps us centered and balanced in our lives. We can also reconnect to the plants that have nurtured women for centuries.

KEY POINT

Women are reminded to honor the different seasons of their lives:

The time of the maiden: of innocence, joy, playfulness, passions

The time of the mother: of unconditional loving, giving, and creativity

The time of the crone: of achieving the crowning glory of the wisdom of the elders

All of these seasons evoke celebration in honor of these transitions.

Many cultures have rites of puberty for males and females, honoring the transition into adulthood. There are trials, challenges, and initiations that evoke honor, integrity, courage, and moral character. Individuals then are welcomed into society as important and contributing members, often being given new names that honor special characteristics or individual traits. They are launched into their lives with a supportive send-off and expected to live as responsible members of the community. As their lives progress, there is another initiation when these people become elders. Respect is shown to these individuals, honoring the wisdom that they have gleaned from living life and life's experiences. The wisdom is honored and cherished, for it is passed down through generations, ensuring the future survival of the community. It is considered imperative to pass one's knowledge to others. It is not customary to keep it to oneself.

Many of the experiences that build wisdom were gathered from mistakes along the way—wisdom does not come easy. To take what life gives you and turn it into wisdom, requires courage and fortitude. "With every lesson learned, a line upon your beautiful face" (1). As with any initiation, this is not done overnight. It requires patience, endurance, and intention, and a willingness to step outside your comfort zone. The courage to forge ahead in the midst of bodily changes, can bring a new relationship with your body, that of a much deeper connection.

KEY POINT

If ever there is a time for a woman to tune into her spiritual nature, it is during menopause. If by that time she has not discovered her spiritual essence, her spirit will call upon her to start listening.

Menopause as a Sacred Journey

How does this idealistic philosophy translate into our Western culture? For the most part, gray-haired men become more distinguished with age. Gray-haired women are encouraged to dye their hair, use wrinkle-reducing creams, and hide any signs of aging whatsoever. Many women approach aging with dread, feeling like they are unappreciated and fearing they will be useless and discarded.

A more holistic approach to menopause is to view this as a sacred journey on one of life's rivers. It is an initiation into wisdom and creativity that takes time, preparedness, courage, fortitude, patience, and support. The river must be approached with respect, for you cannot predict what nature has in store for you throughout the journey. As you embark with anticipation, you do not know what will be waiting for you at the mouth of the river. You may start in peaceful waters, but may face big rapids ahead. Sometimes you get caught in the eddies and need to sit in the stillness for awhile. At times, you have to weather the storm on *terra firma*.

Because menopause is such an important and vital transition in a woman's life, it is meaningful to approach it as a time of celebration rather than a time of dread. Perhaps it is this dreaded anticipation that causes women to approach the menopausal transition with more fear and trepidation, which causes more intense symptoms. That is unknown. However, now, more than ever, women have many more options available to them so that they can embark on the menopausal journey with knowledge and many hormonal and herbal preparations that will facilitate this wondrous and sacred passage.

Taking Charge

The first thing a menopausal woman must consider is her goals. Are they to relieve symptoms, such as hot flashes, night sweats, insomnia, or vaginal dryness? Are they to have future protection against osteoporosis and heart disease? A combination? She must reflect deeply on this to make her decision. She can use her wise-woman intuition combined with true medical facts and then choose her intention. Once she decides, she needs to surround herself with a healing team. One aspect of this is finding health professionals that will support her decisions and provide information to keep her informed of new options. She needs to learn about nutritious foods to nurture her body. Keeping her body balanced with massage therapies or energy therapies could prove helpful, as could seeking a spiritual mentor. She will find it beneficial, if she's not already doing so, to exercise with a friend. She can start her own circle of women who can gather monthly to support one another. Keeping company with people who energize, not drain her, will prove to be therapeutic. With a healing team, a woman can realize that she does not have to walk this path alone.

Reflection   As you go through life passages, who will make up your healing team to offer support, guidance, and assistance?

The Energetics of Healing

Most indigenous cultures have a word in their language that means: *energy flow through the body.* The Chinese call it *chi,* the Japanese call it *ki,* in India it is called *prana.* The English language, unfortunately, lacks a word that translates into energy flow. Most other cultures are aware of the energy centers in our bodies and how to keep the energy flowing to maintain harmony and balance and to prevent disease. There are several energy systems in the body, including energy fields, energy meridians, and energy centers called *chakras.* You can learn how to look at your body in an energetic way and keep your energy centers strong. (See Healing Touch International, listed under Resources, for classes pertaining to energy healing.) Menopause is a perfect time for a woman to start observing her own energy flow and to commit to a way of life that promotes balanced energy in her body and mind. Everyone has a personal and individual energy makeup or blueprint. That is why certain things work for some people and do not work for others. The woman needs to begin looking at things energetically. She needs to learn to trust her body's inner wisdom to find medicines, herbs, and approaches that work for her individually. Finding her own balance is another example of the wise-woman way.

The Art of Mindfulness

There is a spiritual practice termed *mindfulness,* which teaches to be always present, centered, and observant in each thought that you have and in each action that you take. Mindfulness is a perfect practice during the transition of menopause. If a woman can be mindful of what is happening with each different emotion or symptom that she experiences, then she can observe the effects of different substances and situations that may trigger symptoms. When she knows what triggers a symptom, then she can modify it.

It is important for a woman to learn to be mindful of her body during this phase. She can start tuning in to her body's natural rhythms so that she will know when it needs rest, when it needs nourishing foods, when it needs quiet, when it needs play and laughter. If she believes that menopause directs her toward self-growth, then if she is mindful, she can see the connections more clearly and gain wonderful insights.

The Art of Healing

Healing is different from curing. The word *healing* means *wholeness*. Each individual has a unique energy matrix that defines wholeness. Menopause is a time for discovering and connecting to that which brings a woman closer to wholeness. Only her own inner wisdom ultimately knows what that is. During menopause, she is remembering—bringing mind, body, and spirit together to be more whole. This can be done with the use of herbs, foods, friends, exercise, quiet time, and nature. By reflecting in the quiet and the stillness, a woman will know what she needs for her own personal wholeness and healing.

KEY POINT

A new wholeness of mind, body, and spirit can be realized during menopause.

Defining Menopause

The medical definition of *menopause* is the absence of periods for 12 months in a row. Some experts define it as no periods for six months in a row, while others say if you are having menopausal symptoms unrelated to other medical pathology, then that constitutes menopause. The average age to experience menopause in the United States is age 52.

KEY POINT

Sixty million women will be experiencing the menopausal journey by the year 2020. Women's health programs that address the holistic needs of this population will need to expand.

Some blood tests can be used to confirm menopause, especially thyroid-stimulating hormone (TSH) and follicle-stimulating hormone (FSH) levels (Exhibit 18–1). It is important to rule out underlying thyroid disease by getting a TSH level, as some of the symptoms can be similar to menopause. FSH is elevated in menopause, so measuring the level can be a useful diagnostic measure.

EXHIBIT 18–1 FOLLICLE-STIMULATING HORMONE

Follicle-stimulating hormone (FSH) is produced in the pituitary gland. Through a feedback loop system, it sends a message to the ovaries each month, to stimulate ovulation. In the perimenopausal and menopausal years, there is a gradual decline in estrogen production. When the pituitary gland notices that there is less estrogen being produced in the ovaries, it produces more FSH in an effort to get the ovaries to respond by producing more estrogen. As this feedback loop continues, FSH levels start rising. A normal FSH level is under 20 mlU/ml. Many infertility specialists claim that it is difficult to conceive with FSH levels greater than 12. Some experts feel that an FSH level greater than 20, with accompanying symptoms, defines menopause. Other experts feel that a true menopausal level of FSH is more like 90 or greater, and that FSH levels between 20 and 90 are considered resistant ovary syndrome, where the woman has declining levels of estrogen, but may get a period every few months.

Saliva can be tested instead of blood to obtain hormone levels (see Aeron Life Cycles under Resources). This is equally reliable as blood tests, and less expensive, and therefore useful for people who may not have health insurance.

Estrogen

Estrogen, which is produced in the ovaries, adrenal glands, and fat cells, provides many functions. Increasingly, research reveals the many effects that estrogen has on the body. Researchers are finding more estrogen receptors in the body than were originally considered. There are estrogen receptors in the skin, the brain, the heart, the bones, the genitourinary tract, and the intestines. There are even estrogen receptors in the teeth. When estrogen levels decline in menopause, it affects all these organ systems. Through much research since the 1930s and through medical evaluation, doctors began advising estrogen replacement in the 1950s. It was believed that after menopause, estrogen replacement helped to protect against heart disease, osteoporosis, colon cancer, vaginal atrophy, and urethral and bladder atrophy. It was suggested that estrogen helped to keep skin supple, keep our teeth strong, and help our brains stay healthy, even preventing Alzheimer's disease. However, the benefits of estrogen replacement were found to be overshadowed by the risks when the results of the *Women's Health Initiative* study began to show that women who took oral estrogen with progestogen therapy showed increased risks for breast cancer, coronary heart disease, and venous thromboembolism (2).

Five times as many women die of heart disease and osteoporosis, than breast disease. Heart disease causes as many deaths each year as the next eight leading causes combined. Approximately 240,000 women die of heart attacks each year. Women are more likely to die of a first heart attack than men. The American Heart Association claims that woman's lifetime risk of heart attack is 1 in 2. (See Exhibit 18–2.)

EXHIBIT 18–2 HEART DISEASE AND WOMEN

Risks for Heart Disease

- Natural menopause occurring before age 40
- Menopause induced by surgery or illness before age 45
- Previous diagnosis of heart disease or hypertension
- Family history of heart disease especially heart attack prior to age 50
- Bulk of body fat is in upper body/waist
- Smoking
- Poor diet—low in nutrients, high fat, frequent fast foods
- Physically inactive
- No passion for life
- Inability to express anger; unresolved anger and grief
- Social isolation; limited community support

How To Strengthen Your Heart

- Exercise 3–5 times per week for 30–40 minutes
- Eat a high-nutrient diet, rich in whole grains, green leafy vegetables, low-fat protein, low sugar
- Keep your heart emotionally strong by expressing feelings
- Learn the art of forgiveness (yourself and others)
- Practice the art of the four-chambered heart
  1. Be full-hearted. Do not do anything half-heartedly.
  2. Be open-hearted. Open yourself to receiving as well as giving.
  3. Be strong-hearted. Let go of fear.
  4. Be clear-hearted. Set a clear intention.
- Herbal support:
  - Garlic
  - Onions
  - Motherwort tincture
  - Cardiovascular support tonic—hawthorne (leaf, flower, berry), motherwort, ginger, and passionflower

Twenty-eight million Americans, mostly women, have osteoporosis. Osteoporosis causes more dangerous effects than one would think. Osteoporosis leads to 1.5 million fractures each year, according to the National Osteoporosis Foundation. One out of three women older than age 50 will develop vertebral fractures. Half the women who develop a hip fracture from osteoporosis, never leave the hospital due to ensuing complications. A woman's risk of developing a hip fracture is equal to her combined risk of breast, uterine, and cervical cancer (Exhibit 18–3). The increased risk for developing osteoporosis

---

EXHIBIT 18–3   OSTEOPOROSIS: IDENTIFYING AND REDUCING RISKS

Risks for Osteoporosis:
- Surgical or abrupt menopause
- Menopause
- Strong family history of osteoporosis
- Caucasian or Asian heritage
- Small body frame/slender build
- High caffeine intake
- Smoking
- High intake of phosphates from cola drinks
- Carbonated beverages
- Frequent antacids
- Low-calcium diet
- Alcoholic beverages
- High exercise/low body fat ratio/infrequent periods as seen in athletes
- Infrequent periods
- Premature gray hair

Ways to Prevent Osteoporosis
- Regular weight-bearing exercise
- High-calcium diet (including steamed leafy greens, such as kale, dandelion, mustard greens, collards, kelp, and hijiki seaweed)
- Nourishing high-calcium and mineral teas, vinegars, herbal tinctures (including nettles, alfalfa, raspberry, oatstraw, horsetail, dandelion, and red clover)
- Soy foods
- Decreased use of alcohol, caffeine, soda pop, and antacids
- No smoking
- Care to prevent accidents and injuries
- Osteoporosis screening
- Calcium, magnesium, zinc, and vitamin D supplement

due to declining estrogen levels caused many women to consider hormonal replacement therapy, but there are safer options for women to consider. (See Exhibit 18–3.)

The ovaries produce three types of estrogen—estrone, estradiol, and estriol. Estrone (E1) was the first estrogen discovered and is very potent. This potency is attributed to many of the more intense side effects when taking it, such as breast tenderness, nausea, and headache. Estrone is possibly the estrogen most linked to an increase in breast cancer. Estradiol (E2) is the primary estrogen produced by the ovary. Estriol (E3) is the principle estrogen produced in pregnancy. It is a weak form of estrogen and has not been used much in the past, because it was more difficult to formulate a high enough dose in the laboratory. Recent research is showing that estriol may be protective against breast cancer and formulary pharmacies are making it more available now than in the past.

Options

After a woman is determined to be in menopause, or has severe menopause-related symptoms that she wants to treat, she must then decide on a regimen. If she still has an intact uterus, adding estrogen can cause a buildup of the uterine lining (or *endometrial lining*). This buildup is called *hyperplasia* and can lead to an increased risk of uterine cancer. Adding a progestin component prevents uterine hyperplasia, therefore, if a woman takes estrogen and has a uterus, it is advised that she also take a progesterone supplement. The progesterone component often causes more intolerable side effects, such as headaches, mood swings, and irritability, which causes some women to stop taking hormone supplements. Currently, there are other, more natural progestin options, with fewer side effects.

There are many types of hormone replacement options, which is good news for women. Energetically, each woman has a unique energy blueprint, therefore, regimens work differently for each woman. Using her intuition, together with sound medical advice, will allow a woman to find a regimen that works for her.

Reflection   Some women are willing to assume the increased risk for cancer and heart disease in order to obtain the benefits from hormonal replacement therapy. They claim that they're more concerned with feeling and looking their best today than with the possible risks they may face in the future. How does this coincide with your beliefs and values? What has influenced your personal beliefs and values concerning this type of view?

Natural versus Synthetic Hormones

Natural in relation to medications or hormones refers to what is identical to that which the body produces, not the source of the medication or hormone. To truly be natural, a substance would have to be extracted from the human body. When a medication is derived from a plant source, it is not naturally identical to what the human produces, although you could say it came from a natural source.

For a pharmaceutical company to obtain a patent for a drug, it cannot be human-identical (bio-identical). Therefore, a molecule in the substance must be changed to make it slightly different from what the body produces. This change in molecular structure is very minor and formulated to work almost identically to what the body would naturally produce. The patenting of a drug is what provides exclusive rights and profits to offset the cost of research and development of the drug.

When Premarin, the first synthetic estrogen, was developed, it was derived from pregnant women's urine, which is high in estrone estrogen. During the postdepression years, it became difficult to control quality in the process of obtaining the urine. For example, people other than pregnant women would submit their urine, in efforts to earn some money. This led the company to begin obtaining the urine from pregnant female horses because it was close in equivalency to human urine. The company changed the name to Premarin (*pregnant mare's urine*). In essence, Premarin is very natural, but it is mainly comprised of estrone, which is very potent and can cause many side effects. Also, the slight difference in molecular structure of synthetic hormones compared to natural, human identical hormones, may account for the minor side effects.

KEY POINT

Several years ago, private, individual pharmacies began formulating their own hormones to be human identical (bio-identical). Initially these hormones were quite expensive, but now there are many more "formulary pharmacies" and the cost has decreased to about $20–$30 per month. Insurance companies frequently pay for synthetic hormones, but not natural hormones.

The medical research that showed estrogen replacement helpful in preventing heart disease and osteoporosis was done using synthetic hormones. There is no medical research that proves that the bio-identical hormones protect the bones and heart. Menopause symptoms may go away with the human-identical hormones, but there is no assurance the bones and heart are staying healthy. Tests such as bone-density screens and treadmill tests, can evaluate the condition of the bones and heart.

Hormonal Replacement

Oral estrogens are taken daily in varying dosages, which can take a lot of juggling. It can take several weeks or more to find just the right dosage, so women need to be advised not to become discouraged or give up. It can take some time to find the right dosage for an individual, so women need to be encouraged to stay in communication with their healthcare providers, so dosages can be adjusted as needed.

There are many different types of regimens for hormone replacement. If a woman has a uterus, she must use estrogen plus a progestin. Estrogen is taken daily; the progestin component is either taken daily in a smaller dose or cyclically for 12 days each month at a higher dose. If she uses a cyclic regimen, a woman generally will have a withdrawal bleed or period each month. If she does not have a uterus, she only needs to take the estrogen component. The progestin component has been the one that usually causes the most adverse side effects such as mood swings, irritability, bloating, and headaches. The oral micronized progesterones from formulary pharmacies, and Prometrium from Solvay Pharmaceutical Co., do not seem to have as many side effects.

Examples of synthetic and natural hormones are shown in Exhibit 18–4.

EXHIBIT 18–4 EXAMPLES OF NATURAL AND SYNTHETIC HORMONAL REPLACEMENTS

Oral Estrogens
- Conjugated equine estrogen (Premarin 0.3 mg, 0.625 mg, 0.9 mg, 1.25mg, 2.5 mg daily)
- Esterified estrogen (Estratab, Menest 0.3mg, 0.625 mg, 1.25 mg, 2.5 mg)
- Estropipate (estrone) (Ogen 0.625 mg, 1.25 mg, 2.5 mg, 5.0 mg, Ortho-est 0.625 mg, 1.25 mg)
- Estradiol (Estrace 0.5 mg, 1 mg, 2 mg)

Transdermal Estrogens
Placed on skin and changed once or twice weekly. The hormone is absorbed through the skin, which bypasses the liver metabolism.
- Estradiol (Alora, Vivelle, Climara, Estraderm)

Intravaginal Ring
Inserted into vagina for 90 days then removed and replaced.
- Estradiol (Estring 2 mg)

Vaginal Creams
Generally use 1/2 applicator in vagina 2–3 times per week as needed.
- Estradiol (Estrace vaginal cream)
- Conjugated estrogen (Premarin vaginal cream)
- Estropipate (Ogen vaginal cream)
- Dinestrol (Ortho Dinestrol vaginal cream)

EXHIBIT 18-4 EXAMPLES OF NATURAL AND SYNTHETIC HORMONAL REPLACEMENTS (*continued*)

Progestins

Oral Progestins

- Medroxyprogesterone acetate (Provera, Cycrin, Amen)
- Micronized progesterone (Prometrium)
- Norethindrone Acetate (Aygestin)

Synthetic Combinations of Estrogen and Progestin

- Conjugated estrogen with Medroxyprogesterone acetate: ("Prempro" = Premarin 0.625 mg with Cycrin 2.5 mg, "Premphase" = Premarin 0.625 mg with Cycrin 5.0 mg)
- Ethinyl Estradiol (5 mcg) with Norethindrone Acetate (1 mg) daily ("Femhrt")
- Estradiol (1 mg) with Norgestimate (0.09 mg) "OrthoPrefest"

Natural (Bio-Identical) Hormones from Formulary Pharmacies

Estrogens

ORAL: Bi-est (80% Estriol, 20% Estradiol)
         Tri-est (80% Estriol, 10% Estradiol, 10% Estrone)

VAGINAL: Estriol or Estradiol cream

Progestins

- Oral-micronized progesterone 100 mg once or twice daily
- Prometrium 100 or 200 mg at bedtime (Peanut oil base—do not use if allergic to peanuts)

Multistep Approach

A six-step approach can prove helpful to women in the menopausal transition years:

1. Herbs

2. High-mineral, herbal vinegar extracts

3. Increase in soy intake

4. Physical exercise

5. Essential oils and aromatherapy

6. Breathing techniques, meditation, journaling, self-care techniques

Herbs

The wise-woman approach focuses on a nourishing and nurturing approach. The phase of menopause can be used by a woman to become more in tune with her body, her surroundings, and her attitude on how she wants to live the next phase of her life. The focus is on finding a balance in her life that supports health, vitality, harmony, and joy. Menopause is seen as a celebration. The work of childbearing and child rearing is approaching its close, lending time for joyful expression of a woman's true essence. As her children are growing and becoming adults, a woman can direct her energies to things that support her own continued growth.

> **KEY POINT**
>
> Menopause can move a woman toward more outward expression in the world, and at the same time, toward becoming more introspective.

The herbal approach allows a woman to rediscover the ways of nourishing, nurturing, and replenishing her body and spirit. It can be very gratifying for a woman to begin to learn about these wondrous plants that have been growing alongside us for centuries. Herbs can be important allies for her as she takes time to observe the plants, smell their fragrances, sit with them to discover their medicine, bask in the beauty of their colors and textures. She will find certain plants that call to her and that resonate with her own energy vibration. These will be her healing herbs. Classes on herbs and herbal medicine can help one to become more knowledgeable so that herbs can be used wisely.

There are several herbs that have been shown to be effective in controlling symptoms associated with menopause. Among these are chastetree berries, black cohosh, and licorice root (if a person has high blood pressure licorice root should not be used). Nourishing and balancing teas made of alfalfa, nettles, oatstraw, horsetail, rosehips, red clover, and licorice root can increase a sense of well-being in menopausal women. (See Resources for sources of herbal preparations.) These herbs are high in minerals and calcium for nourishing, toning, and balancing. They provide minerals to keep bones strong, and nourish the liver and adrenal glands.

Drinking a cup of tea containing these herbs in the afternoon seems to balance the blood sugar and helps give an energy boost. It can be suggested that the woman make a big pot of several quarts and keep a week's supply in the refrigerator. These teas can be consumed hot or cold, and stevia or succanat can be added to sweeten. It can be put in a thermos to carry throughout the day, using it as a reminder to nurture and nourish oneself. The Resource list at the end of this chapter offers information on making these teas.

Tea making can be used as a ritual for the menopausal woman. She can choose a beautiful teapot and mug that reflects her unique personality. As she drinks the tea she can pay attention to the color, the aroma, the flavor, and the temperature, visualizing that it is nourishing all the organs of her body as she drinks it, bringing her vitality and health.

High-Mineral Vinegar Extracts

Some women find that vinegar-based mixtures, containing mineral-rich herbs like red raspberry leaf, nettles, dandelion, and red clover are beneficial. These are high in calcium and other minerals, and help tone the liver and kidneys. The vinegar helps absorb the minerals better, especially the calcium. (Some of these preparations are available from companies that make herbal formulas, such as those listed under Resources.)

Soy Foods

The soybean contains the isoflavones, genistein, and diazein, which are plant estrogens (phytoestrogens) containing weak estrogenic activity. Isoflavones are found in many plants and legumes, such as lentils, chickpeas, cashews, and others, but highly concentrated in soybeans. Women often have to experiment with soy. Some people do not digest soy very well or have soy intolerances, so individuals must identify their responses. If a woman is able to tolerate soy, it can be another ally to provide estrogenic support. The role of soy in preventing osteoporosis is being studied. Soy intake can be increased by eating tofu, tempeh, soy milk, and fresh or roasted soybeans.

Women from Asian cultures who have a high daily soy intake, seem to have fewer menopausal symptoms than American women.

Physical Exercise

Do not underestimate the importance of exercise. Frequent physical exercise is imperative to moving through this transition with ease and health. Because people are no longer working in the fields, hauling wood and water, or being active as part of a day's work, physical exercise is needed to maintain hormonal balance and produce endorphins that help with well-being.

A woman should find some kind of movement that she enjoys and commit to moving at least four times a week, for at least 30–40 minutes. It takes three weeks at least to feel the effects of beginning to exercise again. It will not work to binge exercise. A woman should not go more than 72 hours without moving. It is useful for a woman to find the kind of movement that she enjoys, such as dancing, gardening, walking, or swimming. Yoga and T'ai Chi are excellent. Almost all community recreation centers have adult exercise classes, including water classes if there is a pool. There are lots of hiking or cycling clubs that offer all types of activities. Walking is free and easy. The woman can take mindful meditation walks where she will notice all of her surroundings and how they are changing with the seasons. This is a good way to smell the flowers and de-stress.

Reflection Do you engage in some kind of movement for at least 30–40 minutes, 4–5 times a week? If not, what prevents you from doing so and what can you do to change this?

A woman will notice immense differences in how she feels if she keeps her commitment to exercise. If she does not enjoy any type of physical activity, she could find benefit in joining a movement class that interests her from a community education center and commit to it for at least six weeks. Often, she will end up liking it, even if she didn't think she would. Exercising with a buddy can help. Of course, any weight-bearing exercise will be of additional value in helping to keep bones strong, but, initially, the woman should be advised to start with something that interests her. To prevent osteoporosis, a weight-bearing exercise program must be added to the program.

Essential Oils

There are many different essential oils that work very well to help emotional well-being. The woman should find ones that seem to call to her and experiment with ones that suit her best. Lavender is always good for calming. She can place it on her pillow to help her sleep, or put a few drops on her forehead or temples to help ease tension. It is nice to place lavender drops in the bath, too.

Clary sage is another good oil during menopause (consider the name—the *sage-ing* of the wise woman!). Orange, jasmine, and ylang ylang can evoke beauty and creativity and can also be uplifting. For more information on the use of essential oils please see Chapter 23.

Breathing Techniques, Meditation, Journaling, Self-care

Another important step is for the woman to add a disciplined, self-care program that helps her stay centered, focused, and de-stressed. Learning how to switch to deep, abdominal breathing instead of shallow chest breathing, helps oxygenate the body to give her more energy. (A technique for belly breathing is described in Chapter 4.)

Meditation techniques are good life tools that will be invaluable throughout the rest of an individual's life. There are simple meditation techniques that can be done in an instant, and yet energize for hours. Meditation can be simply looking at a sunset or a flower, or washing the dishes in a mindful manner—it doesn't necessarily have to be a formal meditation practice. There are many books and classes to help in developing techniques that work for each lifestyle. (See the section on the art of self-care later in this chapter.)

Managing Specific Symptoms

Using a multistep approach as the basic foundation, a woman can add specific herbal remedies and other measures to manage individual symptoms. Some specific suggestions are provided below:

Hot Flashes:

Several herbs could prove useful for hot flashes:

Black cohosh: normalizes estrogen levels

Motherwort: good women's herb, cools flashes, relaxes nervous tension

Chickweed: cooling, mild diuretic; helps with water retention

Sage: cooling to hot emotions (especially anger); cools night sweats

Hops: calms; promotes relaxation

American ginseng: helps nervous system; strengthens adrenal glands; de-stresses

These can be used singularly, or a woman can create combinations of her own. A cool flash formula tincture containing these herbs is available commercially (3).

Night Sweats:

Some of the triggers for night sweats include stress, sugar, alcohol, lack of exercise, and spicy foods. Reducing these can improve night sweats.

Remifemin is a standardized black cohosh extract in tablet form that can prove helpful. It is long-acting and can last well through the night. (A note about black cohosh: It is in danger of being overharvested and poached. People need to be mindful and knowledgeable about the products purchased and make pertinent inquiries as to the source of the companies' herbs.)

Some of the herbs used for insomnia can prove useful, also (see discussion below).

Insomnia:

The woman should identify potential triggers to insomnia, which include caffeine, alcohol, sugar, Nutrasweet or aspartame, lack of exercise, emotional stress, and worry. Some women have reported problems with insomnia if they have any sugar or caffeine after 3:00 P.M. (especially ice cream, candy, or sweet desserts).

Singularly or in combination the following herbs can help relax the nervous system, while being safe, gentle, and without morning grogginess:

Valerian root: sedating effects

Hops: relieves tension, anxiety, restlessness

Skullcap: decreases nervous tension and anxiety; relaxes muscles

Passionflower: sedates; antispasmodic

Journaling is a good tool for insomnia. It is helpful for a woman to journal what she did during the day, what her thoughts and feelings were, any frustrations or joys, etc. Journaling is a good daily practice for self-nurturing. (See Exhibit 18–5). There are several good books listed in the bibliography to offer some good journaling techniques, and it could be useful to take a class on journaling, also.

Don't forget that daily physical exercise is important in promoting good sleep patterns.

EXHIBIT 18–5 FREE ASSOCIATION WRITING: GUIDELINES TO OFFER WOMEN

Thirty minutes before bedtime, take your herbal sleep tincture and then sit down with a pen, paper, and a timer. Set the timer for five minutes. Then begin writing all of the things on your mind. Write down words or phrases of what you are thinking. Think of all the things you did that day and all the things you have to do tomorrow or later in the week. Free associate all the words that come to you. For instance, you may think that tomorrow you have a meeting where you need to bring a potluck item. That reminds you that you need to go to the grocery store, which reminds you that you should buy a card for your friend who is in the hospital while you are in the store. That reminds you that you should call your friend's mother to see how she is doing and if she needs any help. You also remember that you have to find your notes from the last meeting, etc. Keep writing all the things you think of until the timer goes off. Ideally, you should be done writing at least 30 seconds before the timer goes off and that you have to think really hard of what other things are on your mind to write about. If you are still writing furiously when the timer goes off, then extend the timer to 7, 8, or even 10 minutes. This exercise helps clear your mind of extraneous thoughts and worries, which in turn helps your mind relax. This relaxation helps prevent the mind chatter that sometimes makes it difficult to fall asleep, or that awakens you in the night.

Calming essential oils and hot baths help relax nervous tension and anxiety. Suggest that the woman try lavender, geranium, ylang ylang, and clary sage as essential oils to place externally on her skin, on pillows or sheets, or in bathwater.

The spiritual state could affect a woman's sleep patterns. She should ask herself questions such as: What is my spiritual connection? How do I create mindfulness and centeredness? How do I nurture myself? She should be encouraged to be open to asking some hard questions. Insomnia may not only be an adjustment to hormonal and physical changes, but also a signal that her spirit is calling out to her. When she does not listen to the stillness and misses her spirit calling, her spirit may awaken her at night to get her attention.

Decreased Libido:

During menopause, the fluctuating hormone levels can cause changes in libido. Some women experience an increased sex drive, while others experience a decrease. When women are under stress, libido is one of the first things affected. In our fast-paced society, and with all the many things women do in a day, making love is sometimes the last thing on their minds.

There are herbs that will enhance libido, and some women report good results with hormonal therapies as well. However, other factors need to be examined. In a quiet and reflective state, the woman can ask her body's inner wisdom to speak its truth. She needs to be willing to hear the truth and answer some tough questions. Is she truly in a relationship that supports her as the person she truly is? Does the love she gives out, return to her in the way she desires? Is she around people that love, support, and energize her, or does she feel drained by them? Does she get the companionship that she desires? Does she receive the communication from her partner that she wishes for? Is she too fatigued; does her body need a deep rest?

High stress can cause the adrenal glands to work overtime. This leaves a person feeling depleted, with no extra energy for expressing sexuality. There are herbs that help strengthen the adrenal glands (e.g., American ginseng), which in turn may increase libido. However, herbs do not take the place of rest, sleep, and stress-reduction strategies, that offer the adrenal glands a chance to recover.

Reflection   What do you notice about the way your energy and stress levels affect your libido?

Vaginal Dryness:

Vaginal dryness can be attributed to the decreased estrogen affects on vaginal and vulvar tissue. The vulvar and vaginal tissue becomes thinner and atrophies. This can cause irritation and discomfort, painful intercourse, and contribute to urinary incontinence.

This can be treated by oral hormone replacement and/or prescription estrogen cream that is applied to the vulvar and vaginal tissue. The estrogen cream is available as a synthetic hormone or as a bio-identical hormone.

The herbal options include creams and salves that are soothing and healing to vaginal tissue and mucus membranes, and moisture-enhancing teas and tinctures. Salves can be made from marshmallow root, calendula blossom, and licorice root. It is common to find a calendula-comfrey cream or gel in health food stores. These herbs help promote nourished, well-lubricated, and supple vaginal and urethral tissues. These salves can be used daily at first and then weekly—as often as needed to provide relief.

Triggers to Hot Flashes

You have probably already heard the expression, "It's not a hot flash, it's a power surge." This comes from the energy principle that hot flashes signify a rewiring of our nervous system towards intuition. Some energy theorists believe that hot flashes are an actual energy release. It may be a release of toxins or a type of cleansing and clearing. If a woman notices that hot flashes usually occur after an exposure to an intense substance, then this theory makes sense.

KEY POINT

It is interesting to note, that in the United States, approximately 60 to 70 percent of women experience hot flashes. In other countries, there is much less reported experience of hot flashes: 30 percent in Canada, 17 percent in Navajo women, 9 percent in Japan, and 0 percent in Mayan women. It is not certain whether the hot flashes are not reported, or whether they are actually not experienced or not deemed uncomfortable. Many indigenous cultures, such as the Mayan, do not have a word in their language that translates into *hot flash*.

Declining estrogen levels cause vasomotor symptoms, such as hot flashes, but there may be other triggers. If a woman tunes in to her body and identifies these triggers, sometimes she can modify her experience of hot flashes. It is good for her to keenly observe and keep a diary of her symptoms to identify her own personal triggers. Common triggers to hot flashes are:

Sugar   The effects that sugar and refined carbohydrates have on causing hot flashes and PMS, such as symptoms of mood swings, headaches, fatigue and low energy, anxiety and restlessness, insomnia, and breast tenderness cannot be emphasized enough. If a woman became a Sherlock Holmes for a few weeks, and analyzed her sugar intake and her body's response, chances are she would notice a connection. One way to identify this is to eliminate all sugar and wheat for three weeks, and then gradually add them back in, in moderate amounts. This can be an extremely difficult undertaking for many people. It takes a lot of preparation, but the rewards at the end are worth it. People who have done this often notice an unbelievable increase in energy, as if a cloud or veil has lifted. They have increased mental clarity and alertness. There also tends to be some weight loss, which is a benefit that many would welcome!

Sometimes a little sugar or wheat products, especially ingested in the afternoon or later, can cause night sweats and insomnia. It is very common to experience hot flashes and night sweats after a special evening going out to dinner, where a woman may have a little wine, pasta, dessert, or richer foods that she may not normally eat.

Spicy or hot foods   Some spicy foods, such as curry, hot peppers, or cayenne can trigger hot flashes or night sweats. The woman needs to observe her own personal response to hot, spicy foods.

Alcohol   Although a glass of wine or beer may be relaxing and calming, alcohol breaks down into sugars and also can be a trigger for hot flashes. The woman's personal response to alcohol needs to be observed.

Aspartame or Nutrasweet   It is important to read labels, as these chemical sugar substitutes can be found in more products than realized and can worsen menopausal symptoms.

Stress   Stressors are different in everyone. Identify your own stressors and pay attention to them. Are they signaling that you need to honor your wise-woman ways and your intuition? Are they signaling you to be more gentle with yourself, or more nurturing? Often times, it's the frequent little things that cause the most stress, not the big disasters. Reflect on the hot flash you just had. Was there a message in it for you?

Chronic Sleep Deprivation   New studies are showing that Americans are chronically sleep-deprived. Adults actually need about eight hours of sleep each night, especially in our fast-paced society. Lack of sleep places extra stress on the adrenal glands that are already depleted during menopause. This is also a paradox, because during menopause, women are awakened at night due to hot flashes or night sweats, and their sleep is disrupted often. Therefore, it is difficult to obtain a restful night's sleep. Keeping a consistent sleep schedule by going to sleep and awakening at the same times each day, together with some herbs that help promote sleep, will sometimes help establish a better sleep pattern.

Anxiety and Worry   It is difficult to let go of worries and trust and go with the flow. If a woman has a worry, she can either take action to relieve it, or let it go. She must consider if it is worth worrying about. A woman can allow a hot flash to help her keep in tune with what worries are important to her. For example, if a woman is worried about a medical symptom, she must recognize that action is needed and get it evaluated. In anxiety-producing situations, deep-breathing techniques can help her to get through, as can learning techniques to help her stay centered, calm, and detached from the outcome.

Anger   The relative increase in testosterone in relation to the declining levels of estrogen, can cause more aggression or assertiveness, which can make a woman feel out of control. Women say they become quick to anger and they do not like that feeling. Some women say that after they have reflected on the situation they realized that their anger may have been legitimate, but that it was out of proportion, and they wish they could have controlled it better. A woman may benefit by asking herself: *Is this anger so intense because I have been silent for too long, and now cannot hold it in any longer? Do I really need something to help me temper this anger, so I can be more balanced and not so out of control?* Often, when women begin a nourishing self-care program, including herbs or hormones, the anger and ensuing hot flashes diminish.

The Art of Self-Care

Woman's nature is to give and they tend to give a lot. Therefore, it is imperative that women also learn how to receive. The more you give, the more it is necessary to receive also, for then you can be replenished to give again. This is the true art of recycling.

Reflection The more you give, the more you need to receive, in order to pass the giving around the circle. Does what you give balance with what you receive?

When someone offers something to us, it is a gift to them for us to receive it. This may need to be reinforced to women as they are encouraged to receive as part of their own nurturing. Women who have been other-oriented for most of their lives may find it hard to receive and care for self. They may be receptive if it is put in the perspective that they can help others much more if they are energized and not depleted.

Each individual must develop her own self-care model that energizes and supports her, and then make a disciplined commitment to integrate it into her daily life. Some suggestions that can be offered to women are presented in Exhibit 18–6.

EXHIBIT 18–6 SELF-CARE HINTS TO NOURISH AND ENERGIZE YOU

- Give gratitude to your body every day. While you are taking a shower, allow the water to flow over every body part, mindfully acknowledging how it serves you, and be grateful that this day you are healthy.
- Scan your body energetically and notice areas of tension or discomfort that may need your nurturing attention.
- Embrace humor. Add levity every day. Smile and laugh often.
- Have music in your life in some way.
- Allow your creativity to flow: Sing a song, bake a cake, or paint a picture. Start by doing easy and simple things first.
- Search to find your passion and allow it to unfold.
- Find a connection to your spiritual essence, whatever that may be.
- Allow quiet time often (for reflection and basking in the stillness). Discover how much quiet time you need and honor that. Create a healing space in your home or outdoors where you can go to be quiet.
- Spend time with nature, mindfully drinking in your surroundings to nurture and replenish you.
- Create rituals to mark the passing of time or the special events in your life.
- Share a connectedness with others. Surround yourself with friends that are loving, supportive, stimulating, and energizing.

The Celebration

It is important to honor the transitions in life and mark one's changing seasons with ritual. A woman can create her own ritual or ceremony to acknowledge and celebrate the wise-woman she has become. She can invite a small circle of women, or include special family, friends, and children, give gratitude, sing a song, light candles, share stories, and give blessings. A shared feast can follow the ceremony. A woman can use her own inner wisdom, intuition, and creativity to make her ceremony a special one.

Indigenous cultures look at life in a circle. We are all equal because we are all equidistant from the center or the source. We all travel the circle through the seasons of our lives and we all pass in each other's footsteps at some point on the wheel. We must remember that we do not travel the circle alone. We are all connected, all related. Women need to reach out to each other, knowing that they all share the energy of

---

EXHIBIT 18–6 SELF-CARE HINTS TO NOURISH AND ENERGIZE YOURSELF *(continued)*

- Learn to care without rescuing or enabling.

- Honor your own body rhythms for rest, work, and play. Practice self-acceptance.

- Be open to possibilities and be willing to step outside your comfort zone to try new things or new attitudes. A trusted friend can help lend clarity if you are unsure.

- Be open to receiving and be willing to ask for help. Human nature causes you to want to give and help others. There are people around you that want to reach out and all they need is to be asked. Your gift back to them is allowing yourself to receive from them.

- Check in. If someone or something fires up your emotions negatively sit with it and ask yourself, is the problem the issue or is it the way I am reacting to the issue?

- Be open to looking at your own issues and past patterns, and be willing to make changes that may move you towards a higher level of awareness and communication. Menopause is a time to claim your power and sometimes stand your ground over things that you have tolerated for way too long. However, remember that being in power is walking the path of the heart.

---

their heart connections. When they have times of doubt or despair, they can call on the energy of the worldwide circle of women that will uplift their spirits and give them hope. When they have moments of joy and bliss, they should send it out to others. At midlife, women can learn to walk the path of the heart, using the gifts of the wise woman: compassion, understanding, and unconditional love.

Chapter Summary

Menopause is defined as the absence of menstruation for 12 consecutive months. This is a significant event for women, not only because of the physiological challenges that are present, but because it happens at a time when they can take stock of many aspects of their life. From this standpoint, menopause is viewed as a sacred journey into wisdom and creativity.

A multistep approach is useful for women as they face the menopause transition. Useful strategies include the use of herbs, high-mineral, herbal vinegar extracts, soy, essential oils, and exercise and self-care techniques. Women should try to identify triggers for hot flashes, which could include sugar, spicy foods, alcohol, artificial sweeteners, stress, chronic sleep deprivation, anxiety, and anger. Individualized plans are essential to address each woman's unique needs.

Menopause can be used as a time to launch new self-care behaviors that allow women to nurture themselves and receive from others. New experiences and opportunities are possible.

References

1. Saliers, E. (1997). "Get Out the Map" in: Indigo Girls *Shaming of the Sun* (CD), EMI Virgin Songs, Inc.

2. Writing Group for the Women's Health Initiative Investigators. (2002). Risks and Benefits of Estrogen Plus Progestin in Healthy Postmenopausal Women: Principal Results from the Women's Health Initiative Randomized Controlled Trial. *Journal of the American Medical Association,* 288:321–333.

3. Developed by Shelley Torgove, Clinical Herbalist, *Apothecary Tinctura.* 1275 Madison St. Denver, CO, 303-399-1175, 800-220-5838.

Suggested Readings

Adams, K. (1999). *The Write Way to Wellness—A Workbook for Healing and Change,* New York: Warner Books.

Anderson, S. and Hopkins, R. (1992). *The Feminine Face of God.* New York: Bantam Books.

Andrews, L. (1993). *Woman at the Edge of Two Worlds. The Spiritual Journey Through Menopause.* New York: HarperCollins.

Bolen, J. S. (1995). *Crossing to Avalon: A Woman's Midlife Pilgrimage.* San Francisco: HarperCollins.

Borysenko, J. (1996). *A Woman's Book of Life. The Biology, Psychology, and Spirituality of the Feminine Life Cycle.* New York: Riverhead Books.

Crawford, A McQ. (1996). *The Herbal Menopause Book.* Freedom, CA: The Crossing Press.

Ivker, R. (1997). *Thriving.* New York: Crown Publishing Co.

Klaiber, E. L. (2001). *Hormones and the Mind. A Woman's Guide to Enhancing Mood, Memory, and Sexual Vitality.* New York: HarperCollins.

Lee, J. (1996). *What Your Doctor May Not Tell You About Menopause.* Sebastopol, CA: BLL Publishing.

Linn, D. (1997). *Quest: A Guide for Creating Your Own Vision Quest.* New York: Ballantine Books.

Mehl-Madrona, L. (1997). *Coyote Medicine.* Santa Fe: Bear and Co.

Mortimer, J. E. (2002). Hormone replacement therapy and beyond. *Geriatrics, 57* (6):25–32.

Myss, C. (1997). *Anatomy of the Spirit. Seven Stages of Power and Healing.* New York: Harmony Books.

North American Menopause Society. (2003). Amended Report from the NAMS Advisory Panel on Postmenopausal Hormone Therapy. *Menopause: The Journal of the North American Menopause Society, 10*(1):6–12.

Northrup, C. (2001). *The Wisdom of Menopause. Creating Physical and Emotional Health and Healing During the Change.* New York: Bantam Books.

Northrup, C. (1998). *Women's Bodies, Women's Wisdom: Creating Physical and Emotional Health and Healing.* New York: Bantam Books.

Quinn, J. (1999). *I Am a Woman Finding Her Voice: Celebrating the Extraordinary Blessings of Being a Woman.* New York: Eagle Brook, an Imprint of William Morrow and Co., Inc.

Soule, D. (1995). *The Roots of Healing. A Woman's Book of Herbs.* Secaucus: Carol Publishing Group.

Thoule, S. P. (1998). *A Woman's Book of Soul. Meditations for Courage, Confidence and Spirit.* York Beach, ME: Conari Press.

Weed, S. (1996). *Breast Cancer? Breast Health.* Woodstock, NY: Ash Tree Publishing.

Resources

Bio-identical (Natural) Hormones
To find a pharmacy in your area contact: International Academy of Compounding Pharmacies
800-631-7900

Energy Healing
Healing Touch International
12477 W. Cedar Dr., Suite 206
Lakewood, Colorado 80228
303-989-0581

Organizations
American Menopause Foundation
350 Fifth Ave, #2822
New York, New York 10118
212-714-2398

HERS Foundation (Hysterectomy Education Resources and Service)
422 Bryn Mawr Ave.
Bala Cynwyd, PA 19004
215-667-7757

Menstrual Health Foundation
104 Petaluma St.
Sebastopol, CA 95472
707-829-3154

The North American Menopause Society
c/o Department of Obstetrics and Gynecology
University Hospitals of Cleveland
11100 Euclid Avenue
Cleveland, OH 44106

Saliva Hormone Testing
Aeron Life Cycles
1933 Davis St., #310
San Leandro, CA 94457
800-631-7900

CHAPTER 19

ADDICTION: DISEASES OF FEAR, SHAME, AND GUILT

Objectives

This chapter should enable you to:

- Describe what is meant by an addiction
- List at least five types of addictions
- Discuss at least five significant areas that can be affected by addictions
- Describe at least three characteristics of addicts
- Describe four measures that can aid in healing the body of the addict

Addictions are among the most common diseases in the United States. An estimated 20 percent of our population lives with the pain of being addicted to something. Each person who is an addict affects about 10 other people who experience pain, stress, fear, shame, and guilt just as the addict does.

Clearly addictions of all sorts are major problems in our society. The magnitude of alcohol addiction is seen in the statement of William C. Menninger, MD, who said, "If alcoholism were a communicable disease a national emergency would be declared" (1). We have lived to see that epidemic with a myriad of related abuse problems across the United States. Other addictions, such as gambling or exercise, appear more subtle, but cause many of the same problems.

Scenarios of Addictions

The following are scenarios of a variety of addictions:

- They must gamble no matter what the costs. Loss of home, "maxed out" credit cards, risky loans, and threats on their lives do not stop them.
- They are driven to the next new sexual conquest in spite of the risk of HIV and AIDS, hepatitis, loss of their marriages and children.
- They must eat and vomit even though they weigh 90 pounds and have painful dental problems from stomach acid damaging their teeth when they vomit. Additionally, they just got out of the hospital because of cardiac problems and electrolyte imbalances in their blood.
- They must eat the whole container of food (usually not vegetables, but ice cream, cookies, chips, etc.). It happens in secret especially if their weight is more than 250 pounds.
- They need the cocaine to complete some important work task, but they cannot get the sustained high anymore. Their heart hurts while their nose runs and bleeds.
- They drive drunk for the seventh time since their last DUI and lose their drivers' licenses.
- Their best friends died in an automobile accident last year after they used a lot of drugs and marijuana. They continue to grow their own pot.
- They worked 90 hours again this week and missed their youngest child's birthday. They have to get that promotion.
- The collection of newspapers and important magazines are a fire hazard. The cats (37 of them) cause waste that is a health hazard. Things are getting moldy and smelling. The addict is getting sick. The Department of Health threatens to condemn the home.
- They must run another 15 miles today even though they have not had periods for more than 12 months. It does not matter that it is 10 P.M. If they hurry, they can do it before midnight.

These scenarios depict some extreme late-stage addictive behaviors. Before people get to this stage, a nonjudgmental health risk appraisal with hopeful feedback can start the healing process.

Reflection   Was there anyone in your family who had an addiction? How did that impact that person and the rest of the family? How did the family address this issue with the person?

Definition of Addictions

Addictions are behaviors people do repeatedly that result in problems in one or more major areas of their lives. All addictions are the result of attempts to relieve or control feelings of anxiety, vulnerability, and anger. They are related to problems with impulse control and self-esteem. The repetitious behaviors that constitute an addiction include misuse, overuse, and abuse of alcohol, food, work, sex, shopping, smoking, money, power, relationships, exercise, drugs (prescription, nonprescription, and "street" drugs), and collections of "stuff" (papers, memorabilia, guns, etc.). You probably could add a few more to the list of things that are used addictively to escape facing a feeling.

KEY POINT
_____

Significant areas that potentially are affected by addictions include:

- Physical and mental health (e.g., accidents, depression, etc.)
- Spirituality: loss of hope, belief, and peace; isolation from supports; anger at God, creator, supreme being
- Relationships: family, mate (partner), parents, children, and friends
- Work: poor performance; overachievement; poor working relationships; attendance problems; workaholism
- Legal: litigation, DUI, violence, stealing, tax evasion, sexually acting out
- Financial: loss of income/savings; living in guilt, fear, and shame over spending

Prognosis for Addicts and Their Families

The prognosis may look bleak and appalling, but it is not. Early identification, education, and intervention can lead to prevention of part or all of the problems noted above. Intermediate and late interventions can reduce the severest symptoms of the addiction-related diseases and problems. Later in this chapter, assessment and intervention will be addressed. These techniques help reduce the inevitable destruction. So the prognosis can be excellent when specific steps are followed and there is support for all who are directly involved.

Who Are Addicts?

At the very least, 1 out of every 10 people suffers with some type of addiction. Addicts are represented in all strata of society. Everyone is at risk. Addicts are presidents, teenagers, generals, nuns, homeless individuals, grandmothers, rabbis, doctors, nurses, accountants, "skid row" people, pilots, school dropouts, valedictorians, and beauty queens. The types of people who become addicts are not determined by social status, income, education, ethnicity, sex, or any other demographic characteristic.

Are addicts bad people? No, although they sometimes do very bad things. Most addicts do not know why they repeat actions that keep hurting themselves and others. At first, many do not really think they have a problem. They believe they can cut back on their behaviors whenever they desire. They repeatedly try to stop the addiction, and often succeed in exercising some control although the problem remains. As the behavior begins to bother others they may make promises to stop, however, there comes a point when they cannot control the outcomes of their addictive behaviors. They do not know how to break the pattern (2).

Next, addicts may feel fear, shame, and guilt. They want to stop, but the urges are out of their control. Some may not want to stop because they cannot conceive living without the habit that they believe allows them to function. If they muster a super human effort and manage to stop acting out the addiction, they suffer severe anxiety and pain. With drugs, alcohol, gambling, and food addictions there can be tremendous physical pain, as well as anxiety and emotional devastation.

KEY POINT

Withdrawal symptoms from some addictions can include insomnia, headaches, extreme irritability, anxiety, upset stomach, sweating, and chills.

Lastly, addicts lose all hope, suffer guilt, lie in their shame, and hide themselves in constant fear (beginning paranoia). Prison, chronic illnesses, financial ruin, suicide attempts, and death are frequently the final results of untreated addictions.

Addicts cannot imagine life without the escape and feelings of relief that their addiction gives them. Most of the addicts have a need to escape from some emotion that is not at a conscious level.

Persons who have loved ones who are addicts suffer many feelings, too. Families, friends, and the addicts themselves need compassion, love, support, and information to recover their lives. It is possible. People need to know they are not alone, and there is hope. Addicts are not bad, worthless, and hopeless. No matter what society tells us, the fact is that addicts are sick people (3). Since 1957 the American Medical Association recognized alcoholism as a disease. The Diagnostic and Statistical Manual IV (DSM IV), a guide for identifying mental illnesses and their characteristics, lists various addictions as diseases (4). These listings are helpful because they acknowledge many addictions as treatable conditions.

Commonalties Among Addictions

There are similarities among many addictions. Most addicts contributed significantly to the development of their problems, which can cause society to have limited sympathy for them. However, just as many people with heart disease have contributed to the development of their illnesses because of lifestyle choices they have made. People who stray from the special diets they follow knowing they are putting their lives in jeopardy contribute to their medical problems just as much as persons who abuse alcohol and drugs. Yet, society considers people with traditional medical diagnoses as legitimately needing help and care despite their responsibility for causing their problems. There is less support and sensitivity for those who are addicted.

> **KEY POINT**
>
> Addicts deserve reasonable help and support just as any person with a disease. They are sick people who need help and healing desperately. People in their lives also need healing because loving and living with an addict makes people close to them hurt and sick, too.

Help, Hope, Healing, and Health

How can you help addicts and yourself if you have relationships with them? There are risk factors and risk patterns associated with the development of addictions. Identification of those patterns and the persons at risk is ideal. You can use a health risk appraisal questionnaire such as the Efinger Addictions Risk Survey (EARS) to identify persons at risk. See Exhibit 19–1. Please feel free to make copies for future use.

The EARS asks questions that are nonoffensive to most people. The survey includes topics that are common experiences and assigns a score to the degree the experience affects the person. It does not appear as invasive or judgmental like many other surveys and screening tests. For example, the traditional alcohol surveys ask questions about alcohol use that are likely to cause an alcoholic to deny or outright lie. In typical nursing and health assessments, the questions evoke an underestimation of drinking, smoking, and sexual behaviors. These surveys encourage the addicts to lie to health professionals and to feel guilt and fear.

People should not be made to feel guilty about their addictions; it is the only way they know how to cope with life. With a risk assessment of behaviors and thought patterns, they can be helped to identify the patterns of behaving and thinking that are leading them to addictions that are hurting, damaging, and eventually going to destroy their

---

EXHIBIT 19–1 EFINGER ADDICTIONS RISK SURVEY (EARS)

1. Various stresses and losses occur at all stages of our lives. Please check Column A if any of these losses or stresses occurred or are occurring in your life. Please check Column B if the item checked in Column A still causes you emotional pain.

Column A	Stresses, Losses, and Feelings	Column B
Yes, I had or have this stress/loss.	*Check the left column if you have or had these stresses or losses. Check the right column if it still causes you pain.*	*Yes. Still causes me some pain.*
	Feelings of shyness as a child.	
	Felt other children were favored.	
	Frequent illnesses as a child.	
	Feelings of aggression.	
	Addicted mate.	
	More than two panic or anxiety attacks.	
	Few friends I can count on for help.	
	Bothered or worried about addicted parent.	
	Can't count on spiritual advisor; minister, priest, rabbi, or other.	
	When I need help, I'm uncomfortable asking for it.	
	Insomnia.	
	Death of a pet.	
	Guilt in some areas of life: religion, sexual activities, parenting.	
Total:	Add column A and B.	Total:

Total of Columns A and B _____

Indicator:	Early risk	10–13
	Intermediate risk	14–19
	Late risk	20–23
	Probable addictions	24–26

EXHIBIT 19-1 EFINGER ADDICTIONS RISK SURVEY (EARS) *(continued)*

2. When you have leisure time, how often do you have these feelings or reactions? Please check the box in the column that applies to you. Answer the questions as you would in a normal week. For example, do not respond as you would when you are on vacation.

Feelings or Reactions to your leisure time	1 Never	2 Almost Never	3 Sometimes	4 Often	5 Most of the time
Tired					
Do not want to exercise					
Bored					
Anxious or uptight					
Want to shop					
Want to gamble					
Want to make love					
Want to have a drink					
Lonely					
Column Totals:					
Multiply by:	× 1	× 2	× 3	× 4	× 5
TOTALS					

Total of:

Col. 1 _____

Col. 2 _____

Col. 3 _____

Col. 4 _____

Col. 5 _____   Add the totals of the five columns:

Total of 5 columns _____

Addiction indicators:　Early risk　　　　24–27

　　　　　　　　　　　Intermediate risk　28–34

　　　　　　　　　　　Late or high risk　35–39

　　　　　　　　　　　Probable addiction　40–45

EXHIBIT 19–1   EFINGER ADDICTIONS RISK SURVEY (EARS) *(continued)*

Please check the column that most applies to the frequency you have these feelings or perform the following behaviors.

Behavior or feelings you may experience	Almost always	Frequently	Sometimes	Almost never
3. How often do you wear a seat belt?	1	2	3	4
4. How often do you feel overwhelmed?	4	3	2	1
5. How often do you feel the need for some help to change a low or sad mood?	4	3	2	1
6. How often do you do a creative activity?	1	2	3	4
7. How often do you worry about your family or being alone?	4	3	2	1
8. How often do you worry about your past?	4	3	2	1
9. How often do you worry about criticism by others?	4	3	2	1
10. How often do you feel guilty about some behavior?	4	3	2	1
11. How often are you annoyed by criticism of what you do?	4	3	2	1
12. How often do you feel grief over a loss or death of someone?	4	3	2	1
13. How often do you wish you could tell your parents, mate, or family what they've done to hurt you?	4	3	2	1

Add the numbers in the boxes you checked.

EXHIBIT 19–1 EFINGER ADDICTIONS RISK SURVEY (EARS) *(continued)*				
Behavior or feelings you may experience	Almost always	Frequently	Sometimes	Almost never
Enter the totals from the previous page in the appropriate columns.				
14. How often are you fearful about the results of something you've done?	4	3	2	1
15. How often have you had legal problems?	4	3	2	1
16. How often do you feel compelled to do something you really wish you didn't do?	4	3	2	1
17. How often are you lonely?	4	3	2	1
18. How often have you had a problem enjoying sexual activity?	4	3	2	1
19. How often do you feel compelled to control your anger or resentments?	4	3	2	1
20. How often are you concerned about your job performance or other responsibilities?	4	3	2	1

Totals of the numbers in the boxes you checked.
Add each of the columns' totals   _____

_____

_____

_____

TOTAL   _____

Addiction indicators:	Early risk	40–45
	Intermediate risk	46–54
	Late or high risk	55–64
	Probable addiction	65–80

lives. They can be shown new patterns of living, behaving, and thinking that will help them to live more comfortably with less anger, victimization, and fear. They can be given hope that they can live happier and more serene, courageous lives without their addictions and avoidance of feelings. The new patterns can be applied to dealing with all addictions because they all have some common sources of feelings that result in the damaging behaviors. It is clear that the early addictive behaviors are often effective in coping with anxiety, anger, and other uncomfortable events. The intermediate addictive behaviors can have both effective and painful, damaging results. The late behaviors have ineffective results. There is no relief at this stage for addicts. They are obsessed prisoners of their addictions.

Recognizing these stages of early, intermediate, and late addictive behaviors provides hope that help can be given at earlier stages. Earlier help and hope leads to quicker healing.

Denial

Denial is a strong barrier to seeking help, hope, and healing. Denial exists for the addict, as well as for the loved ones because of the fear, shame, and guilt associated with every addiction. Gentleness, acceptance, promotion of self-esteem, and recognition of pain when communicating with an addict helps to reduce denial. When family members or healers provide compassion to an addict, they enhance treatment effectiveness and provide an opening to reduce denial.

KEY POINT

The addict's denial must be confronted.

The need for denial causes an addict to try to manipulate others. Open compassionate confrontations and interventions are necessary in helping the addict consider beginning any type of healing and recovery process. Confronting and risking the anger of the addict may save his or her life. At times it is hard for family and traditional healers to be compassionate. Many stereotypes exist that influence feelings toward someone who has caused turmoil and pain to self and others by his or her addictions.

At this stage, a noncaring attitude directed toward the addict by family and friends is common. Some parents may wish their drug-addicted child were dead. Some people, who have lost a child to addiction or an accident, grieve and start their own addictions to sexual activities, excessive shopping, work, controlling another child, religion, and secret things that they often feel too ashamed to share.

Efinger Addictions Risk Survey (EARS)

EARS is a health risk appraisal survey for addictions. It can help identify those at risk for addictions at an early stage of their disease (Exhibit 19–1). When the risks are identified, there can be interventions, education, motivation, and reduction of the horrendous costs of addictions to the persons, their families, and society. Risk identification provides information about where the problems may be. It gives a focus for the most effective counseling, education, and support interventions to reduce the progression of the risks to addictions. It appears that if the major areas of pain, fear, shame, and guilt vulnerability can be addressed first and ameliorated, addicts may be more amenable to change, to attending therapy, and to be motivated to work on their problems.

Discussion of Risk Scores

The EARS scores are divided into early, intermediate, late, and probable addiction risk scores. There is flexibility in the scoring. The scores serve as a general framework to assess addictions risk.

Early Risk Indicators   Early risk indicators are events or predictors that occur in childhood or adolescence that reflect behaviors and attitude characteristic of persons who later became addicts. Feelings of shyness as a child are one of the earliest indicators. This could be reflected through low self-esteem or other uneasy feelings when dealing with people. Some of these children have been abused and are fearful and insecure. They often have experienced a nonsupportive environment at home or school. Frequent illnesses experienced by a child set a pattern of thinking that medications or drugs can fix everything. The child may feel different from classmates and friends, and they become isolated and lonely. A lack of coping skills to deal with loss can be reflected through unresolved death of a pet. In fact, any of the responses in Question 1 that are checked as still causing pain are risk indicators. The more items that still cause pain, the greater the risk.

Question three, regarding almost never wearing seat belts is an early risk indicator. Perhaps it reflects the rebellion a potential addict feels toward society. This could also indicate lack of self-care or a subtle self-destructive attitude. It also represents an effort to be in control of how rules are applied in the addicts' lives. Research supports this behavior as an early risk. The number of close relatives who have a serious addiction problem should be analyzed, also. The genetic component of addictions and depression are major early warning risks.

Intermediate Risk Indicators   Intermediate risk indicators are predictors that occur in childhood, adolescence, and early adulthood that reflect behaviors and attitudes that are characteristic of persons who later became addicts. Being very reluctant to ask for help, rarely asking for help, and having few people to count on are intermediate risk indicators. Not viewing leisure time positively is a precursor to serious risk.

KEY POINT

Addicts often feel anxious or uptight, frequently bored, tired, lazy, and lonely when faced with leisure time. The need to avoid the quiet time alone reflects their discomfort with inner feelings and thoughts.

Feelings of isolation are a common experience. Persistent guilt, insomnia, panic attacks, and not feeling spiritually connected are serious patterns of intermediate risks. Unresolved pain related to the loss or death of a person is not an unusual experience when people receive no help with grieving. However, when this feeling is added to the other patterns of feelings and behaviors, the person is at risk.

Late Risk Indicators   Late risk indicators are predictors and stresses that affect healthy functioning of the person's spiritual, mental, physical, and economic life. All of the risk indicators already mentioned can be found to a greater degree in the late risk indicators. When questions 4, 7, 8, 9, and 10 to 20 are primarily marked "almost always," late risk for addiction is strongly present. The degree of risk is related to the higher scores. For example, when there is a lack of any creative activity, and the "almost never" column is marked, the risk score increases.

Driving while under the influence of drugs or alcohol is a serious late risk that leads to legal problems. That behavior and other problems in legal, financial, work, or intimate relations are patterns that approach the strongest late risk indicator category.

Probable Diagnosis of an Addiction   The scores for many of the risk indicators listed previously will be higher when there is a probable diagnosis of an addiction. In addition, there may be arrests, serious illnesses, admissions to the hospital (greater than two related to the addiction), and suicidal feelings. These require immediate attention by their healthcare providers and family members (2).

Treatment Modalities and an Essential Paradigm Shift

The medical model of addictions management has not had a successful record of arresting and healing these diseases. A paradigm (worldview) shift toward a holistic approach is essential to access the healing tools and energy to begin effective treatment and healing. We only need a small window of hope to access a spiritual connection to the vast energy of love, compassion, and acceptance to start the healing for the addict and those involved.

Medications, therapy, supervision, and support groups, such as the anonymous groups for narcotics (NA), alcoholics (AA), gamblers (GA), overeaters (OA), etc. have a role in holistic healing, but treatment methods must go beyond those common resources. Holistic treatment addresses the mind, body, and spirit.

Holistic Approach to Healing Using Feedback on Risk Factors

The areas of risk identified by the EARS can be individually addressed using a holistic approach. Most of the stresses and fears (work, relationships, etc.) can be decreased through use of imagery and progressive relaxation.

All transitions and changes are stressful. Planning relaxing activities for the period of time between the completion of employment activities and the start of home responsibilities can reduce stress. This is a time when people feel anxious and addictive thoughts strongly enter their minds. Simple strategies, such as clarification of job description and responsibilities, can reduce work-related stress. Reducing interruptions at work and home when involved in tasks requiring concentration can decrease irritability and stress.

Anxiety (panic) attacks are instant triggers for addictions. The thoughts with the emotional and bodily responses during an anxiety attack feel life threatening. Seeking help is essential.

A strategy that can help control an anxiety attack is to slow down breathing, look up, focus on an object, and repeat, "These feelings are terrifying, but they are not dangerous. I will not be harmed." This action seems very simple, yet it works to get people through the panic. A thought, even a prayer, can interrupt the body's responses.

Support groups for losses, illnesses, and painful life events can be healing experiences for many people. Addicts feel acceptance and hope with the knowledge that they are not alone as they experience the group support. Sometimes the groups may be spiritual or religious in orientation.

Coping skills, assertiveness, conflict resolution, and crisis management techniques increase the comfort of daily living. With these capabilities people can interrupt the cycle of victimization and vulnerability leading to addictions.

The identified risk factors lead to specific treatment strategies. The education, interventions, and treatments include integration of mind, body, and spirit healing (5).

Healing the Mind

Addictions create alterations in optimal brain chemistry. Abnormal neurotransmitters (chemicals that help send impulses through the nerves) of the brain can cause and perpetuate addictions. Healing the mind is essential to permanently heal addictions and restore normal brain chemistry.

KEY POINT

A neurotransmitter can be thought of as a brain messenger.

A diet rich in vitamins, amino acids (proteins), essential fatty acids, and minerals needs to be integrated into daily living. Some food supplements help the brain manufacture chemicals like the neurotransmitter norepinephrine that boosts energy and mood; examples of these supplements include:

- Glutamine has been successfully used to reduce alcohol cravings in early recovery.
- Tyrosine is an important building block for norepinephrine.
- Tryptophan; a precursor for serotonin. Foods high in tryptophan are popcorn, turkey, chicken, and dairy products.
- Serotonin, another neurotransmitter, that creates a calm, relaxed state and promotes sleep. Absence of sufficient serotonin is a trigger for addictions.

Hypoglycemia (low blood sugar) can cause depression, anxiety, panic attacks, and mood swings leading to increased addictions. Another neurotransmitter, histamine, regulates mood and energy. High levels of histamine cause the mind to race and lead to obsessive–compulsive thoughts and behaviors. Methionine, an amino acid, reduces the impact of histamine on the brain.

The mind has habits of thought that are responses to physical imbalances. Blocked energy (*chi* or *qi* or *life energy*) causes imbalances in the brain. The blockages occur throughout the body and affect the mind in harmful ways. Disturbances in brain chemistry can be reduced by helping the person to alter negative thoughts through therapy, prayer, meditation, and other modalities. Next, the body must be integrated into the holistic approach to healing (6, 7).

Healing the Body

The body has many systems that affect all other aspects of healing. In turn, the body is affected by the mind, spirit, and the energies within and without. Touch and movement have key roles in healing addictions.

Massage

Touch is a gesture of support. When someone touches, respects, and cares for an addict's body, the addict is aided to reconnect physically and center emotionally, important healing steps because avoiding problems and dissociating from the body are common among addicts. The person is more connected to his or her body and able to discuss and come to terms with their addiction.

Massage has a powerful impact on the body, releasing endorphins, substances that have a mood-enhancing effect. Self massage of hands and ears help reduce cravings. The ear has pressure points that stimulate the body's natural pain relievers.

Full body massage releases tension and blocked energy. Loosening the tight muscles sends the body messages to cut down on the production of stress hormones. Massage also moves lymphatic fluid through the body. This movement of fluid assists in the body's natural cleansing processes and enhances immune response. Acupressure can help people deal with stress, depression, anger, and the issues underlying their addictions.

Hatha Yoga

Hatha yoga simulates the parasympathetic nervous system and removes tension from all major muscle groups. Yoga helps the addict to become more physically aware, leading to greater mental self-awareness. Eventually, as peaceful body responses are developed, the addict becomes sensitive to how his or her behavior can change. The person experiences the ability to feel better without their addictions. The connection between mind and body heals in an integrated way.

Acupuncture

The use of acupuncture reduces cravings and unblocks energy (*chi* or *qi*). The body feels better and there is a release of the healing neurotransmitters. It restores harmony in the body. These results are related to the skill of the practitioner.

Other Body-Healing Therapies

Dance therapy, shiatsu, Ta'i Chi Ch'uan, reflexology, aromatherapy, chiropracty, acupuncture, qigong, therapeutic touch, and healing touch are major complementary therapies. Some other treatments include homeopathy, hypnotherapy, herbals, biofeedback, and music therapy (8, 9, 10). (See Chapter 21, Safe Use of Complementary Therapies, for additional alternative therapies that could prove useful.)

Healing the Spirit

Spiritual healing encompasses the removal of grudges, negative views of self, and compassion for self and others. Forgiveness, making amends, and acceptance of self and others promotes spiritual love and healing. These practices also remove the fear, shame, and guilt that are characteristic of addictions.

KEY POINT

Addicts need support and a spiritual awakening to acknowledge that total healing is possible for them.

Healing the spirit is a wonderful experience for addicts. Addicts have lost focus and are unaware of their own identities and purposes. They become disconnected from the purpose of their creative energy, their inherent goodness, and ability to love and be loved (11). With support and guidance through the process, addicts may experience relief from their compulsions in a brief time frame. The willingness to heal opens the channels for healing to occur. The process is a personal empowering journey. From its deepest perspective, an unresolved longing causes addictions. This awareness is a message that opens the heart and soul of an addict to see that addicts have lost their way. All addictions have a common source. If only the obvious addiction is addressed, the cause will remain and there is the risk that when one addiction pattern starts to diminish, another will start to take over. This happens because the sources of the addictions have not been identified, addressed, and healed. The new addiction's role is the same as the old addiction's role. Therefore, if patterns of behavior and the needs for the patterns are identified; then intervention, education, support, and prevention can be implemented.

Reflection   In For Whom the Bell Tolls, *Ernest Hemingway stated that "We become stronger at our broken places." How have you seen this occur in your own life?*

Chapter Summary

Addictions are behaviors people do repeatedly that result in problems in one or more areas of their lives. People can be addicted to gambling, drugs, alcohol, sex, eating, work, collecting, or exercise. Health, spiritual, relationship, work, legal, and financial problems can result from addictions. Addicts may not believe they have a problem, feel shame, live in fear, experience guilt, and lose hope. The body of the addict can be healed using measures such as a good diet, supplements, massage, yoga, acupuncture, and other body-healing therapies. Forgiveness, making amends, and acceptance of self and others are important aspects of healing the spirit of the person who has an addiction.

References

1. Federation of American Hospitals. (1981). Alcoholism and the Increasing Role of the Hospital. *Federation of American Hospitals Review.* 14:4.

2. Efinger, J. (1984). *The Development of a Health Risk Appraisal Instrument for Alcoholism.* University of Pennsylvania (Dissertation).

3. Bailey, J. (1990). *The Serenity Principle.* New York: Harper & Row.

4. American Psychiatric Association. (1994). *Diagnostic and Statistical Manual of Mental Disorders.* 4th ed. Washington, DC: American Psychiatric Association.

5. Schaub, B. and Schaub, M. (1997). *Healing Addictions.* New York: Delmar.

6. Kabat-Zinn, J. (1995). *Wherever You Go There You Are.* New York: Hyperion.

7. Katherine, A. (1998). *Boundaries: Where You End and I Begin.* Center City, MN: Hazelden.

8. Apostolides, M. and Yunker, T. (1996). How to Quit the Holistic Way. *Psychology Today,* 29(5):34.

9. Dossey, B. M. (1997). *Core Curriculum for Holistic Nursing.* Gathersburg, MD: Aspen.

10. Woodham, A. and Peters, D. (1997). *Encyclopedia of Healing Therapies.* NY: Dorling.

11. Myss, C. (1997). *Energy Anatomy.* Audiotapes. Sounds True.

Suggested Readings

Beattie, M. (2001). *Codependent No More and Beyond Codependency.* New York: MJF Books.

Burns, L. (1999). *An Investigation of Risk Indicators for Substance Abuse Among Nurses.* Philadelphia: University of Pennsylvania.

Carnes, P. (2001). *Out of the Shadows: Understanding Sexual Addiction.* 3rd ed. Center City, MN: Hazelden.

Claude-Pierre, P. (1997). *The Secret Language of Eating Disorders: The Revolutionary New Approach to Understanding and Curing Anorexia and Bulimia.* New York: Times Books.

Dossey, L. (1998). *Be Careful What You Pray For—You Just Might Get It: What We Can Do About the Unintentional Effects of Our Thought, Prayers, and Wishes.* San Francisco: HarperSanFrancisco.

Dreher, D. (1998). *The Tao of Womanhood: Ten Lessons for Power and Peace.* New York: William Morrow.

Durham, M. (2003). *Painkillers and Tranquilizers*. Chicago: Heinemann Library.

Hausenblas, H. and Fallon, E. (2002). Relationship among body image, exercise behavior, and exercise dependence symptoms. *International Journal of Eating Disorders*, 32(2):179–185.

Kushner, H. (1997). *How Good Do We Have To Be? A New Understanding of Guilt and Forgiveness*. Boston: Little, Brown and Co.

Lee, S.G. (2000). *Light in the Darkness: A Guide to Recovery from Addiction: A Physician Talks Openly About His Own Addiction to Sex*. Newport News, VA: Five Star Publications.

Rich, P. (2000). *Clinician's Guide to the Healing Journey Through Addiction*. New York: Wiley.

Schwartz, J. and Beyette, B. (1996). *Brain Lock: Free Yourself from Obsessive-Compulsive Behavior: A Four-Step Self-Treatment Method to Change Your Brain Chemistry*. NY: HarperCollins.

Stewart, G. (2000). *Teen Alcoholics*. San Diego: Lucent Books.

Summers, M. and Hollander, E. (1999). *Everything In Its Place: My Trials and Triumphs with Obsessive Compulsive Disorder*. New York: Jeremy P. Tarcher/Putnam.

West, M. (2000). *An Investigation of Pattern Manifestations in Substance Abuse-Impaired Nurses*. Chester, PA: Widener University.

West, M. (2002). Early risk indicators of substance abuse among nurses. *Journal of Nursing Scholarship*, 34(2):187–193.

Wright, J. (2003). *There Must Be More to This: Finding More Life, Love, and Meaning by Overcoming Your Soft Addictions*. New York: Broadway Books.

Internet Resources

http://pathfinder.com/thrive

Search engine: *http://infoseek.go.com*

Mental health, addictions, and specific Web sites.

CHAPTER 20

SYMPTOMS AND CHAKRAS

Objectives

This chapter should enable you to:

- Describe the characteristics and purposes of chakras
- List the names and locations of the seven main chakras of the body
- Describe a symptom of imbalance or dysfunction for each of the seven chakras

Chakras

The word *chakra* is a Sanskrit word for spinning vortices, or wheels, of energy. Many ancient systems of belief have this understanding of energy in and around the body with entry points located at distinct places along the body. The chakras are like the input valves for the body to receive nourishing energy from the universe around it and output valves to help release or transfer energy. The energy received is transformed into useable energy for the body. However, the chakras also extend outward to affect everything and everyone. It is thought to be vital to the health of all aspects of the body—physical, emotional, mental, and spiritual—that the chakras be open, flowing, and healthy.

From a physical standpoint, the energy received through the chakras affect the hormones, the organ systems, and the cellular functions of the body. Each chakra has been associated with a particular nerve plexus (group of nerve endings) or endocrine system (organs of the body that secrete necessary hormones for health and well-being). The chakras

335

receive energy from outside the body and transform it internally to stimulate some form of hormonal-gland response or nervous system response, which in turn affects the entire body (1).

There seems to be a general acceptance of the existence of seven main chakras of the body (Figure 20–1). The crown chakra and the root chakra are the only two without a corresponding pair. The five central chakras exist on the front of the body and the back of the body. The main channel of energy exists from the top of the head, or crown, to the base of the spine. All chakras meet in this channel and connect with each other through nadi. *Nadi* are fine threads of energy that help connect the pairs of chakras to the main channel of energy through the body and to each other. In this way, all the chakras are connected together and can affect each other.

Figure 20–1: The Chakras

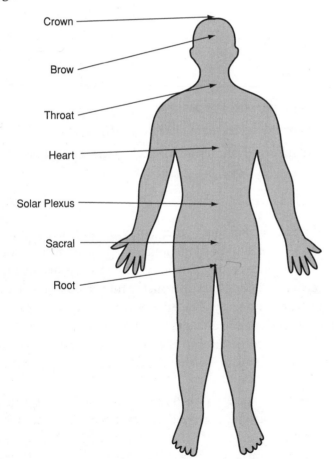

The chakras are vortices of energy that receive nourishing energy from the universe and send out energy from the body. They have distinct names, often described for the area of the body over which they reside.

The first, or *root chakra,* comes downward from the base of the spine. The second, or *sacral chakra,* is a pair of chakras located just below the umbilicus (belly button) on the front and lower back portion of the body. The third, or *solar plexus chakra,* is a pair of chakras located where the ribs form a "v" on the front of the body and the middle of the back on the body. The fourth, or *heart chakra,* is a pair of chakras located between the breasts and between the shoulder blades. The fifth, or *throat chakra,* is a pair of chakras located at the point of the Adam's apple in the neck and the curve of the neck on the back of the body. The sixth, or *brow chakra,* is a pair of chakras located in the middle of the forehead on the face and directly behind on the back of the head. The seventh, or *crown chakra,* is a single chakra located on the top of the head. These seven make up the chakras of the physical body. Some believe there are more chakras that affect the nonphysical portion of our existence (2).

The Root Chakra

In the yogic tradition, the root chakra is called *muladhara,* or the manifestation of life energy. The center relates to the lower portion of the body—hips, legs, and feet—and to the functions of movement and elimination. The normal desire to move and dance are reflections of a healthy root chakra (3).

In addition to the physical aspect, this chakra relates to feeling secure in the world, feeling grounded to the earth, and the will to survive. It deals with the sense of joy and vitality. The root chakra governs the adrenal glands, which are responsible for secreting hormones that, in frightening situations, help one to be more alert and escape danger if necessary. If the chakra is not balanced or unhealthy from prolonged stress, problems such as high blood pressure and anxiety can be seen (4). One often feels a sense of lacking presence, of not being here, or low on physical energy. In persons with HIV/AIDS and cancer, this chakra is often severely damaged or nonfunctioning.

Energy can be seen through color and heard through sound. The vibrational energy of the root chakra is associated with the color red (the slowest vibration on the color spectrum) and the sound of bumble bees (5). It can also be related to the first sound "Do" in the scale "Do-Ray-Me-Fa-So-La-Ti-Do."

The Sacral Chakra

This chakra is known as the *svadhisthana chakra* in yogic tradition and is related to the life force and vital body energy. The reproductive organs and the lower abdomen are affected by this chakra, especially the gonads (endocrine organs of sexuality and reproduction). Nutrients and the absorption of fluids through the intestine are also related to this chakra. The color vibration that relates to this chakra is orange and the sound is the one of a flute or the sound "Ray" (6).

Psychologically, this chakra deals with feelings and emotions. It also relates to the expression of sexuality and desires, pleasures, and feelings about reproduction (7). Relationships will occur easily and fall into place when the sacral chakra works properly.

> **KEY POINT**
>
> Creativity or the desire to create another human being or other things is greatly affected by the sacral chakra.

When imbalanced or nonfunctioning, the sacral chakra will cause problems with emotions, feelings of sexuality, or ability to reproduce or create. If energy is deficient to this chakra, one may feel a lack of emotions or flat. There may be a tendency to avoid emotions altogether. Some may have problems feeling passion about anything or anyone. If the chakra is overactive, one may experience mood swings or be very emotional (8). Another possibility is the need for constant pleasurable stimulation. Chemical addictions often occur when this chakra is not functioning appropriately (9). Addiction to drugs and alcohol help hide and deaden the emotional and physical pain of our feelings about ourselves while giving us temporary and distorted feelings of pleasure.

The Solar Plexus

The third chakra, or solar plexus, is also known as the *manipura* and is associated with one's own power, strength, and ego identity. It also centers around the issues of the will to think, control, exert authority, display aggression, and warmth, as well as the physical components of digestion and metabolism (10). With this chakra intact, one has the ability to start things and see them through to completion. The color associated with this chakra is lemon yellow and the sound is of the stringed instruments, such as the violin, or the sound "Me" (11).

Physically, imbalances or malfunctioning of this chakra can lead to obesity (being overweight), diabetes (elevated blood sugar), hypoglycemia (low blood sugar), heartburn, gallbladder problems (stones or infection), and stomach ulcers. Most of us have felt the "pit in the stomach" when someone verbally or physically attacks us. In fact, one may feel nauseous or even vomit. Our stomach "gets into knots" when we get nervous or fearful, and things are out of our control.

Emotionally, one feels timid or dominating when there is an imbalance. There can be feelings of anger and rage that sit within this chakra. Some persons who are passive-aggressive (act disinterested, but are really angry inside) have imbalances in this chakra. Lack of self-worth or a hidden sense of shame is often found within this chakra. A healthy outlet is one of assertiveness, or being able to state your needs and feelings freely and clearly while respecting others and yourself (12).

The Heart Chakra

This chakra, in the Indian tradition, is called the *anahata* and is the center of love. It has the qualities of loving self and others, harmony, compassion, openness, giving, peace, and grace (13). The heart chakra is called the transformation center, because at the heart level one begins to deal with his or her spiritual side. Whereas, the first three chakras dealt with the physical, emotional, and mental components of the self, the heart center speaks to the soul. It is through this chakra we experience the feeling of unconditional love or the deep love for others (14). This love is of a pure or spiritual kind of caring. The heart chakra is felt open when one cries tears of happiness or joy, or in those instances where the heart strings are pulled. The color associated with the heart is emerald green and the sound is of bells or "Fa."

The heart, circulation, and respiratory systems are related to this center on the physical plane. Imbalances can be seen through physical problems, such as heart disease, high blood pressure, poor circulation, angina (chest pain), asthma, emphysema, bronchitis, or pneumonia. Without a properly functioning heart and lungs, life is not possible and death will result.

Psychologically, imbalances in the heart can leave one feeling self-hatred or lacking self-esteem. One may avoid interpersonal relationships for fear of being hurt or unloved. Some choose isolation to avoid this pain. Others may have suffered from neglect, abandonment, or abuse (15). Grief weighs heavy on the heart and, if left unresolved, can create many problems. Some choose to give their hearts away, leaving very little for themselves, therefore feeling very empty and lonely.

Forgiveness is not necessarily letting others off the hook, but releasing the anger and hurt you experienced from the action. Forgiveness of the self is one of the hardest things to do because we tend not to feel worthy of it. By showing compassion to ourselves, we are able to better show compassion to others. Forgiveness and the release of old grudges helps the heart energy to expand.

Reflection Is there anything that you have done for which you are unable to forgive yourself? What prevents you from offering or receiving this forgiveness from yourself?

The Throat Chakra

The center of creative energy, the throat chakra is also called the *vishuddha*. It deals with issues surrounding communication and expression. By using the voice, one is able to create sounds of speech or song to express oneself. This connection to others by sound allows you to reveal who you are. The throat chakra relates to the neck, esophagus, throat, mouth, and ears (16). The sound of wind blowing through trees or the note "So" is associated with this chakra. It resonates to the vibration color of turquoise or light blue. Some describe it as an electric blue.

Physically, a healthy throat chakra is one revealing a clear voice that communicates thoughts, feelings, and ideas concisely. If the chakra is unbalanced, one may speak softly or with a hoarseness. Having a "frog in the throat" or "choking" on words are descriptions of the free flow of speech being impeded. Other symptoms of imbalance are knots in the neck muscles, tight throats, and clenched jaws (17).

Emotionally, people need to express themselves and their talents, knowledge, and ideas. Hindering this expression may reflect a poor self-esteem or identify family patterns that suppressed the individual's need to create or communicate. Grief can become locked here when emotions are not released through words or tears. Anger and stress can inflame the temporomandibular joint (in front of the ears) with teeth gnashing and grinding at night.

One way of opening this chakra is through sound—speaking, singing, chanting, or toning. By opening your mouth and emitting sound, the vibration clears the throat and it becomes stronger. Additionally, the throat chakra is the communicator from the heart to the soul. It allows us to "sing to our heart's content" and allow music to "soothe the soul." It lets us speak from our heart and make sounds reflecting our emotions. Silence can be used to actively listen to others or the surroundings. By actively listening, one can learn to communicate more effectively by hearing exactly what the other is saying (18).

The Brow Chakra

This chakra, known as the *ajna center*, is also called the third eye. It is associated with the pituitary gland, which controls most of the hormonal functions of the body (19). The brow chakra relates to memory, dreams, intuition, imagination, visualization, insight, and psychic perception. This chakra is all about seeing, within and without (20). The color associated with the brow chakra is deep indigo blue or deep purple. The sound of "La" or waves crashing on the beach help with this center.

KEY POINT

Physically, the brow chakra relates to the eyes, brain, nose, and head. Any imbalance will result in problems with these organs.

Sinusitis, headaches, and poor vision may be seen as imbalances in this chakra. From an emotional standpoint, the brow chakra deals with compassion of putting oneself in another's shoes, being sensitive to the needs of others, and a sense of humor (21). Mentally, recognizing patterns helps people predict that which will occur next in addition to providing insight into their behaviors. Remembering recent events, long-term events, and even past lives is encoded within this chakra. Stored images that can be seen like a movie in one's head allow one to view the same scenario again or re-play it, making changes to produce a different outcome. Dreams are another mental component of the brow chakra, whether they be daydreams or those occurring in sleep. The symbology of dreams provides a great deal of insight to feelings, thoughts, and desires (22).

Imbalances with the brow chakra may be seen with hallucinations, delusions, night-mares, and misguided thinking (23). Some people may be insensitive to others' needs either deliberately or simply by not having observed them. These are the people who just don't seem to take the hint for whatever you are trying to tell them. Others are not able to see what is in front of them; they are blinded by inaccurate thinking.

The Crown Chakra

The seventh chakra or crown chakra is called the *sahasrara* center in yogic tradi-tion. It is often called the spiritual center or center of connection to the oneness of the universe. The crown chakra relates to the divinity of self and our connection to a higher source however one defines it. The crown chakra also relates to intelligence, thought, consciousness, and information. An alignment to a Higher Power is seen through this center. It is associated with the color white or lavender and the sound "om" or "Ti." The pineal gland is an endocrine gland that is not well understood. Its purpose is to deal with the body's rhythms and timing (24).

KEY POINT

The crown chakra is the one with the highest energy vibration of the physical body.

There does not seem to be much dysfunction with this center on the physical level. Some people with imbalances may experience a sense of disconnection, a "holier-than-thou" thinking, or rigid belief system of thinking. These people can be described as hav-ing their heads in the clouds or being spacey (25). Those with psychiatric disorders or drug abuse will often have distortions or irregularities with their crown charkas.

The crown chakra is the center of our connection to the oneness of the universe. It allows people to define who they are in relation to the universe and to experience their higher selves as whole. It is where they connect to the higher power and experience the oneness with all of creation in peace and grace.

Putting It All Together

An understanding of what the various chakras represent and symptoms associated with their imbalances can provide important information as to the status of the mind, body, and spirit. It can be helpful for people to consider if certain physical symptoms that they experience on a regular basis are related to emotions that are blocking a chakra. For example, problems with weight control or chronic upset stomach could be associated with feeling a sense of low self-worth or unexpressed anger. Learning to be assertive in expressing feelings in a healthy manner could improve the physical symptoms. Meditating and thinking of the color associated with the specific chakra that is expressing itself as imbalanced could prove useful. Also, healers who work with the energy fields, such as healing touch practitioners, can assist in balancing the chakras.

Chapter Summary

Chakra is a Sanskrit word for spinning vortices of energy. Chakras transform energy from the universe into useable energy for the body. In turn, chakras send out energy from the body to the universe. The seven main chakras of the body are the crown, brow, throat, heart, solar plexus, sacral, and root. The names often refer to the area of the body over which they reside. Specific symptoms can be manifested when there is imbalance or dysfunction of a chakra. Changing thought patterns, working with an energy therapist, and using specific sounds and meditating on colors associated with the chakra are some of the ways that chakras can be balanced and symptoms improved.

References

1. Gerber, R. (1996). *Vibrational Medicine: New Choices for Healing Ourselves.* Santa Fe: Bear & Company, p. 131.

2. Ibid., p. 128.

3. Hover-Kramer, D. (1996). *Healing Touch: A Resource for Health Care Professionals.* Albany, New York: Delmar Publishers, p. 62.

4. Ibid., p. 62.

5. Ibid., p. 62.

6. Ibid., p. 63.

7. Judith, A. and Vega, S. (1993). *The Sevenfold Journey: Reclaiming Mind, Body, and Spirit Through the Chakras.* Freedom, CA: Crossing Press, p. 87.

8. Ibid., p. 89.

9. Hover-Kramer, p. 63.

10. Judith and Vega, p. 128.

11. Hover-Kramer, p. 63.

12. Judith and Vega, p. 131.

13. Ibid., p. 162.

14. Hover-Kramer, pp. 64–65.

15. Judith and Vega, p. 165.

16. Hover-Kramer, p. 65.

17. Judith and Vega, p. 205.

18. Ibid., pp. 211–212.

19. Hover-Kramer, p. 66.

20. Judith, et al., pp. 225–228.

21. Hover-Kramer, pp. 66–67.

22. Judith, et al., pp. 226–228.

23. Ibid, p. 229.

24. Hover-Kramer, p. 67.

25. Judith and Vega, p. 261.

Suggested Readings

Buhlman, W. (1999). *Chakra Technique and the Vibrational Technique.* Chatsworth, CA: Spiritual Adventures.

Lee, I. (2002). *Healing Chakra. Light to Awaken My Soul.* Mesa, AZ: Healing Society, Inc.

Pond, D. (1999). *Chakras for Beginners. A Guide to Balancing Your Chakra Energy.* St. Paul, MN: Llewellyn Publications.

Wauters, A. (2002). *The Book of Chakras. Discover the Hidden Forces within You.* Haupauge, NY: Barrons Educational Series.

Wauters, A. (1997). *Chakras and Their Archetypes: Uniting Energy Awareness and Spiritual Growth.* Berkeley, CA: Crossing Press.

CHAPTER 21

SAFE USE OF COMPLEMENTARY THERAPIES

Objectives

This chapter should enable you to:

- List three factors that have stimulated Americans' interest in complementary therapies
- Discuss at least three philosophical differences between holistic and conventional approaches
- Describe the role of self-awareness in health and healing
- List at least five questions that should be asked to guide the decision to use a complementary therapy
- Describe the five major categories of complementary therapies
- Describe the alternative systems of medical practice of traditional Chinese medicine, acupuncture, homeopathy, Ayurvedic medicine, and naturopathy
- Describe the manual healing methods of chiropractic, craniosacral therapy, energy medicine/healing, massage therapy, Trager approach, Feldenkrais method, and Alexander therapy

- Describe the mind–body therapies of meditation/relaxation, biofeedback, guided imagery, hypnotherapy, yoga, and T'ai Chi
- Give an example of a pharmacologic and biologic treatment
- Describe herbal medicine

Complementary therapies have been used for a long time throughout the world, however, it has been primarily since the 1990s that interest has soared in the United States. It was during that decade that the landmark study by David Eisenberg and his colleagues, published in the prestigious *New England Journal of Medicine*, revealed that one-third of Americans were using alternative therapies—a figure that grew to 40 percent (1). By the turn of the century, Americans were spending over $27 billion annually for complementary and alternative therapies, most of which was out of pocket. To say this caught the medical community's attention would be an understatement!

There are many factors that have contributed to the growing use of complementary therapies. The interest in preventive health has stimulated individuals to explore practices and products that they can use independently, and many complementary therapies, such as meditation and dietary modifications, fit the bill. Growing reports of adverse drug reactions and other complications from conventional medical care have led people to explore natural means to manage illness. The personalized attention provided by practitioners of complementary therapies offers people a superior experience to the abbreviated and often impersonal office visits and hospital stays. Further, research proving the benefits of complementary therapies is growing by the day.

The heightened attention to complementary therapies also has created much confusion regarding the safety of using many of these therapies. Questions emerge, such as: Why and when is it appropriate to use these therapies? Are these therapies consistent with my health beliefs? How do I choose a practitioner or a therapy? And, above all, are these therapies right for me?

Mystery and what seems to be a strange language surround many complementary treatments. Even the terminology used to describe these types of therapies is confusing. These therapies were first called (and continue to be called) *alternative* therapies. This term does not fit for many because it creates an either-or choice situation. Because it is felt by many that these therapies can be used in conjunction with western medical treatments, the word *complementary* conveyed a clearer meaning. Clarifying even more the joint use of several methods of treatment at the same time, use of the term *integrative* has evolved.

KEY POINT

The evolution of terms used in describing complementary therapies is most evident in the changed name of the division of the National Institutes of Health that investigates and researches these types of practices and products. First established as the Office of Alternative Therapies, in 1998, it was upgraded to the National Center for Complementary and Alternative Medicine. Along with the name change has been an increase in its annual budget. This means there are more monies available for the ongoing research of these therapies.

Terms such as *holistic* and *natural* are frequently used to describe complementary therapies. *Allopathic* is another word that describes western conventional medicine. Some feel that using the term *traditional medicine* to describe today's practice of medicine is incorrect. It is felt by many that *traditional* indicates the use of a treatment since the beginning of time and, therefore, *conventional* better describes the present use of western medical treatments.

History

Many complementary therapies originated from ancient and non-western healing traditions, many of which have their roots in spiritually based healthcare systems. These systems use such measures as prayer, meditation, drumming, storytelling, and mythology to help people in their search for wholeness by allowing them to experience sacred moments in their lives. Spirituality is not in itself religion, but underlies and enhances all world religions. It is also seen as a drive to become a complete, balanced person and is believed by many to be related to intuition, creativity, and motivation (2). Most ancient and non-western cultures express healing as being in balance and harmony.

Holistic Health Beliefs

There are many components to a holistic health belief that are assumed. Today the term *holistic* is being used freely and yet many of the basic concepts that underlie its true meaning are not understood or fully embraced by those using it. The most basic of these concepts is the concept of wholeness. Many ancient healing traditions have as a belief that wellness exists when there is balance of the physical, emotional, mental, and spiritual components of our being. Your physical body has an innate physical tendency to work toward equilibrium or homeostasis. It has a built-in potential to maintain physical health or optimal function of all body systems and a complex natural ability to repair itself and overcome illness. In the quest for balance emotionally, you strive to feel and express your entire range of human emotions freely and appropriately. Mentally, you seek a sense of self-worth, accomplishment, and positive self-identity. Spiritually, you seek a connectedness to others and to a higher or divine source. This balanced state is seen as wellness in a holistic approach to health care. Illness is considered an imbalance of these components.

Holistic health is the balance among your physical, emotional, mental, and spiritual components.

Healing is seen as an ongoing, lifelong process and when viewed in a positive manner, is seen as a continual journey of self-discovery. All healing is self-healing and conventional (western) medical treatments and complementary treatments help by creating an environment that supports your personal perceived needs in your attempt to balance the components of your beingness. Yet, there are some philosophical differences between the holistic and conventional (western) medical approaches:

- The holistic approach to healing seeks the root of the problem (the cause of the imbalance) and tries to re-establish a balance of mind, body, and spirit, while conventional medical approaches are more disease oriented and seek more to remove or block signs and symptoms of physical illness.

- In western medical approaches people have been conditioned to turn over the responsibility of healing to the healthcare provider. However, participation in one's own healing process is a requirement of a holistic approach to health care. In the holistic approach to health care self-responsibility is a key component. Being a passive recipient or expecting others to fix it is not part of the holistic caring process. This belief in seeking balance or healing is carried out in partnership. The person and the caring provider each have responsibilities. Learning how to partner is a very important concept that conventional medicine, until now, has not strongly emphasized.

- Another element of the holistic approach to health care is the requirement of self-care. The caring and nurturing of all aspects of one's self supports a healthier balance and results in more productivity and a fuller participation in the life experience.

- A holistic orientation to health recognizes the interconnectedness of the mind, body, and spirit. If any aspect of yourself is not attended to and nurtured it cannot function to its capacity and has a detrimental effect on the other components of your health. Imbalances are identified and addressed before they become disease processes.

Self-awareness then becomes paramount in this dance or movement between balance and imbalance of our mind, body, and spirit. This self-awareness is supported and/or learned through many of the complementary therapies. Many of the therapies can precipitate an awareness of emotions as well as a physical awareness. It may have been the physical complaint that directs a person to seek the therapy, but the awareness of an emotional component may surface in the process. Knowing this is of importance when seeking complementary therapies. This is also why these therapies are referred to as holistic: they involve all aspects of the person. Recognition and choosing to act upon this self-awareness is part of the personal healing process.

Reflection How do you react when you experience headaches, indigestion, and other symptoms? Do you quickly try to eliminate them with medications, or do you first take time to understand the underlying causes so that you can prevent them in the future?

Acute and Chronic Illness

Pharmacological and technological advancements have equipped conventional medicine to handle acute conditions effectively and efficiently. Heart attacks can be halted, shattered bones mended, and infections eliminated. Unfortunately, as medical technology has increased, the caring components of medical care seem to have shrunk. Hospital stays and office visits are shorter; healthcare providers seldom have ample time to learn about the whole person, or to teach and empower the person for self-care. For these reasons, conventional medicine is less successful at managing chronic conditions than at treating acute illnesses.

KEY POINT

Less than 25 percent of the healthcare dollar in the U.S. today is spent on prevention and acute care; the balance is spent on the management of chronic conditions.

Persons with chronic conditions are increasingly integrating complementary therapies into their medical care. They find that complementary practitioners invest more time in getting to understand their clients, encourage an active provider–client partnership, empower clients for self-care, promote healthy lifestyle practices, and tend to see the whole person rather than merely treat the symptoms (3).

Self-Awareness: Body Wisdom

The journey toward self-awareness like anything else begins with the first step, and a beginning point is physical body awareness. Physical body awareness appears to be a foreign concept in western society today as most people have been taught to deny, ignore, or push through early signs the body may express. Self-awareness is a major developmental pearl that provides key information that influences choices in making informed decisions when choosing a therapy that is most appropriate and/or safe at any given point in time.

> ### KEY POINT
>
> Self-awareness enables one to make informed decisions.

As body awareness develops, awareness of feelings and thoughts follows. This knowledge and understanding leads to inward focusing. Inward focus and awareness protects and guides in many ways. Most of us have been directly taught by our parents, teachers, and others how to get around our weaknesses and imbalances. We tend to ignore body messages until they scream so loudly that we finally are incapacitated and forced to stop and take notice.

Befriending and listening to the body is a lifelong process that continues to be refined as more attention is paid to it. Paying attention leads to learning the body's wisdom versus overriding it. Learning how to recognize this wisdom increases personal knowledge and with this knowledge comes personal power. Power to be more in control of knowing the best choice to help the body regain or move toward balanced health.

Self-awareness feeds into self-responsibility in a more holistic approach to maintaining wellness. Rather than following the pattern of expecting others to provide information of what is best, self-awareness provides the ingredient of self-involvement in illness prevention. This journey of exploration and self-discovery can be fascinating and removes the image of the body as foreign territory. This voyage begins with small steps and requires notation of results obtained. This tuning into the body, instead of tuning out, allows the body to be worked with in a cooperative way.

Self-awareness better equips a person in making an initial choice of which complementary therapy to experience and provides information after receiving the therapy. Paying attention to the physical, mental, and emotional responses after receiving a treatment is invaluable in making future treatment decisions. Were the reasons for choosing a particular therapy satisfied? In what way? How long? What new information was obtained about the body and the mind? This information allows for the choice to continue an old pattern of ignoring the messages received, or paying attention, learning, and deciding to make new informed choices.

> ### KEY POINT
>
> Paying attention to their physical, mental, and emotional responses helps people to determine what is best for their health rather than relying on the decisions of others.

The continued evolution of this self-awareness can become very powerful and self-empowering. Becoming more involved allows for greater participation in decision making in healthcare or wellness choices. This gentler, friendlier approach to body–mind maintenance allows for less fault finding with the body, less rushing ahead without will power, and less blindness to personal weaknesses. Self-awareness and self-acceptance are major components that propel a person on the journey toward a more balanced mind, body, and spirit and establish a more personal feeling of control of life in general.

Selecting a Therapy

Deciding to use a complementary/alternative therapy requires much consideration and forethought. In order to be safe and appropriate many questions need to be asked.

KEY POINT

If a person desires to use complementary/alternative therapies (CAT), he or she must be committed to being an active participant in regaining and/or maintaining health.

A major consideration is how to work effectively with a primary healthcare provider. Is conventional medical care required to monitor a particular medical condition? If so, developing a partnership with the conventional healthcare provider is crucial. Cooperation by the provider and the person seeking CAT is essential. For proper assessment of CAT effects, if combining conventional medicine and CAT, the conventional healthcare provider needs to be informed. Clear baseline assessment information of current symptoms or concerns is needed. The person must be prepared to keep a diary of information to assist in evaluating CAT results. Decisions need to be made regarding the safety of combined therapies or the impact of postponing conventional medical care while using CAT. Agreements need to be reached regarding follow-up visits with the western medical care provider, if necessary, during or after receiving CAT. Some suggestions for using CAT safely are listed in Exhibit 21–1.

Choosing a Practitioner

Deciding which therapy to receive is part of the process, but deciding which provider will deliver that therapy requires just as much serious thought and investigation. There are some important steps in selecting a treatment specialist.

First, people need to be urged to take their time. They should gather names of practitioners by contacting professional organizations, ask for recommendations from people they

---

EXHIBIT 21–1 SUGGESTIONS FOR SAFELY USING COMPLEMENTARY AND ALTERNATIVE THERAPIES (CAT)

- Know your reason for choosing CAT. Is it out of frustration with experiences of western conventional medicine? Increasing awareness of other cultures' approaches to health and illness? A desire for wellness or to explore a wholeness approach to health? Friends' positive experiences that have aroused your curiosity?

- Use CAT under the supervision of a qualified doctor if you have a serious medical illness

- Understand and establish your goals in using CAT

- Beware of mixing and matching conventional and complementary/alternative (CAT) therapies on your own

- Do your homework and gather information; don't rely merely on testimonies of persons who have used a therapy

- Avoid the more is better fallacy

- If something sounds too good to be true it generally is

- Keep an open mind and use the best of conventional medicine and CAT

- Ask questions of practitioners before selecting their therapy, such as:
  - What is it?
  - How does it work?
  - What health conditions respond best to this CAT?
  - When is it best to use it /not use it?
  - What should I expect?
  - What are the possible harmful effects?
  - What is the cost and length of a session?
  - How long must I use the therapy/receive treatment?
  - What information and resources are available to help me learn about this CAT?
  - Do you need to be licensed or certified to practice this CAT? If so, are you?
  - What professional organizations can be contacted to get information about practitioners of this CAT?

respect, and check local directories. Once a few practitioners are identified, they can be called and asked questions regarding education, experience, and credentials/certification. Some therapies require degrees, while others require training with specific criteria. People need to beware of any pressure or claims about cures. A brochure can be requested, as can the names of some of the practitioners' clients who can be contacted for references. State licensing boards can provide information about standards that practitioners need to meet.

The information collected needs to be reviewed. People need to assess their own comfort level with the qualifications (educational background/licensing/certification), or lack of, and the practitioner's manners in interacting with them. They may want a consultation visit. During this visit, they should be clear about their goals, review the goals with the practitioner, discuss organizing a treatment plan, and inquire about side effects and/or adverse reactions. Also, people need to remember to budget their time and expenses appropriately to attain their goals.

After an initial session, re-evaluating is helpful. People need to understand that it is their decision to continue the sessions or not: They are in charge. They should consider the practitioner's professionalism, willingness to answer questions, ability to listen, understanding of concerns, and their overall feelings of ease with this provider. People need to trust their judgment and confidence in the practitioner's skills and degree of healing relationship established.

Reflection   Have you ever received care from a healthcare practitioner who did not treat you with respect or listen to your concerns? How did this influence your ability to feel in charge of your care? How can you avoid behaving in the same manner when you care for others?

Common Complementary and Alternative Therapies

Now that the basic information influencing choices of approaches has been discussed, it is time to take a closer look at some specific choices. There are a variety of ways of categorizing CAT therapies. Some common categories and alternative and complementary approaches will be discussed are:

- Alternative systems of medical practice, including traditional chinese medicine, acupuncture, homeopathy, ayurvedic, naturopathy
- Manual healing therapies, including chiropractic, osteopathy/craniosacral therapy, energy therapy/energy medicine, bodywork therapy, such as massage therapy, movement therapy (Trager approach, Feldenkrais method, and Alexander therapy)
- Mind–body therapies, including meditation/relaxation, biofeedback, guided imagery, hypnotherapy, yoga, T'ai Chi

- Pharmacologic/biologic treatments, including aromatherapy, vitamins, minerals, other supplements
- Botanical medicine/herbal medicine

Some therapies overlap into several categories. For example, T'ai Chi and yoga fit under both movement and mind–body therapies.

Alternative Systems of Medical Practice

Traditional Chinese Medicine

What It Is   A complex and sophisticated ancient system of health rooted in Chinese culture that has been passed down from generation to generation. Traditional Chinese medicine (TCM) approaches the person as a whole, sees mind, body, and spirit as inter-related elements that are intertwined with nature and the universe. It embraces many theories, methods, and approaches, and emphasizes prevention. Some of the basic principles inherent in TCM are listed in Exhibit 21–2.

How It Works   Diagnostic approaches are based on identifying patterns of disharmony or imbalance and consist of

Examination or assessment of the voice, pulse, and respiration

Observation of overall appearance, eyes, skin, and tongue

Questioning about functions of the whole person (both physical and emotional)

The patterns determined by this investigative process are the basis upon which the treatment plan is made. Treatments then are focused on restoring or maintaining harmony and balance of the chi's flow.

EXHIBIT 21–2 BASIC PRINCIPLES INHERENT IN TRADITIONAL CHINESE MEDICINE

- Qi (chi) believed to be the vital life force or invisible flow of energy that circulates through specific pathways in plants, animals, and people called *meridians*, which are necessary to maintain life
- Yin and yang, which is the interaction of opposing forces and seen as complementary aspects
- Five phases theory of fire, earth, metal, water, and wood
- Five seasons of summer, autumn, winter, spring, and late summer
- View of mind, body, and spirit as the three vital treasures

---

Various therapies may be prescribed to treat patterns of disharmony. Some of these therapies are diet; herbal remedies; massage; acupuncture, or insertion of very fine needles at specific points on the body to stimulate and balance energy flow; acupressure, which is the application of finger pressure over specific points to also stimulate the flow of chi; moxibustion, or the burning of a special herb (mugwort) over acupuncture points in order to stimulate the energy flow through the energy channels; qigong (pronounced *chee–gong*), involving low-impact stretches, abdominal breathing, meditation, and visualization and/or possibly T'ai Chi (pronounced *tie–chee*), which is a form of movement meditation designed to unite body and mind, improve muscle tone, and encourage relaxation. Individualized plans determine the number of sessions prescribed for any of these forms of treatment.

Acupuncture

What It Is   As already mentioned, acupuncture is one of the treatment methods used in traditional Chinese medicine. Acupuncture is used to unblock the pathways (meridians or channels) at specific juncture points through which the chi or life force flows. The theory is that disease or illness results from the blockage or obstructions of the pathways, therefore clearing the blockages allows the chi to run freely through the meridians and restores health.

Archeologists have traced the use of acupuncture as far back as the Stone Age. Americans began to take note in 1972, after President Richard Nixon visited China. It was during that trip that a news reporter developed an appendicitis and used acupuncture for his emergency appendectomy. He wrote of this event and stimulated much interest and many visits by western physicians to observe the use of acupuncture in China. The National Institute of Health has demonstrated the effectiveness of acupuncture for pain management following dental surgery, and for controlling nausea and vomiting in pregnancy, after chemotherapy, and post surgery.

How It Works   It has been determined that acupuncture stimulates physical responses, such as changing brain activity, blood chemistry, endocrine functions, blood pressure, heart rate, and immune system response. More specifically medical research has shown that acupuncture can regulate blood cell counts, trigger endorphin production, and control blood pressure.

Acupuncture needles are sometimes inserted and removed immediately, and at other times they are allowed to remain in place for a period of time. Sensations described as rushing, warmth, or tingling are experienced. As the immune system is stimulated, a sense of well-being is experienced. Acupuncture is used both to maintain health and to treat illness or pain.

What It Helps   The World Health Organization has described more than 100 different health conditions that acupuncture can treat. Much positive research has supported the use of acupuncture in the treatment of alcohol and drug addiction.

Words of Wisdom: Cautions   Many sources tell us that one of the biggest advantages of the use of acupuncture is the lack of harmful side effects. A feeling of lightheadedness or euphoria after a treatment has been reported, which is stabilized by a few minutes of rest.

Homeopathy

What It Is   *Homeopathy* is a system of medical practice that is based on the principle that "like cures like." It is a therapeutic system that assists self-healing by giving small doses of remedies prepared from plant, animal, and mineral substances. This system uses diluted (the more diluted the better) portions or remedies to cure symptoms of disease. The remedies encourage the body to eliminate symptoms by encouraging the symptoms to run their course instead of suppressing them. Symptoms are considered signals as the body works to restore natural balance. During this process of self-healing the immune system is stimulated, healing is accelerated, and the body is strengthened.

Dr. Samuel Hahnemann (1755–1843), a German physician, is known as the father of homeopathy. He became familiar with the ancient "Law of Similars," which states that a substance that would cause illness or a set of uncomfortable symptoms when taken in large amounts by a healthy person, could accelerate healing if taken in minuscule amounts by a sick person.

In the 1830s homeopathy was used in most of Europe, Russia, Latin America, and the United States. It appealed to the well educated and affluent—including the British Royal Family. In 1880 homeopathic medical colleges were in most major cities and by 1900 homeopaths were recognized as legitimate physicians. After the Civil War medicine changed and by 1914 the American Medical Association controlled the standard for medical education and rejected homeopathy. By 1970 homeopaths became almost nonexistent. However, interest in natural remedies and concern over the growing incidence of adverse drug reactions has stirred a new interest in homeopathy.

How It Works   Remedies of healing compounds are made through a process of *serial dilution*. One single drop of a plant substance is mixed with 100 drops of water and shaken. This mixture is called C. One drop of that solution is then mixed with another 100 drops and shaken. This is repeated and the number of repetitions indicates the number placed before the C. For instance, the process repeated 30 times would be called a *30C dilution*. During this process each dilution actually becomes higher in potency.

KEY POINT
_____

The more dilute a homeopathic remedy is, the higher its potency.

It is not clearly understood how homeopathic remedies work but there are a number of theories. One theory is the *hologram theory*—meaning no matter how many dilutions occur a complete essence of the substance remains. Another theory is that the "water has memory"—meaning the original substance leaves an imprint of itself on the water molecules.

Homeopaths believe everyone expresses illness and heals in unique ways. This differs greatly from conventional western medicine, which lumps symptoms into categories and believes that everyone with the same disease can be treated in the same way.

Diagnostic methods in homeopathy work toward obtaining a composite picture of a person, taking into consideration the physical, emotional, and mental aspects. A person is encouraged to tell his or her story while the homeopath observes many things, including dress, posture, tone of voice, and rate of speech. Homeopathic practitioners refer clients to conventional medical physicians for drugs and surgery when appropriate. The focus is on how a person is expressing a particular problem or condition so an individualized plan can be made for treatment. Homeopathic practitioners will determine the remedy that can most closely mimic the sick person's pattern of symptoms.

There are two types of homeopathic approaches for treatment: classical and nonclassical. A *classical* homeopath will prescribe a single remedy for a specific problem after determining a symptom picture and matching it to an individual's constitution. The *nonclassical* approach would be trying to match a symptom to a remedy without having the detailed individualized information about the person with the symptom(s).

What It Helps   Homeopathic remedies benefit arthritis, pain, anxiety, muscular aches and pains, asthma, sinusitis, allergies, headaches, acute infection, skin disorders, circulatory disorders, infant and childhood illnesses, digestive problems, pregnant and lactating women, endocrine imbalances, and cardiovascular problems.

Words of Wisdom: Cautions   There could be the potential for using remedies to treat serious conditions instead of seeking appropriate conventional care. This is especially true if someone is trying to self-treat an illness.

Because symptoms can get worse before they get better, it may be hard to determine if a remedy is working or if a side effect requiring immediate western medical attention is occurring.

Because dosages are different from conventional western medicines it would be better to seek the advice of a qualified homeopath rather than using an over-the-counter remedy.

Homeopathy can be used for minor acute care, but it is best to become informed by seeking a group study program instead of trying over-the-counter remedies or reading related literature.

Ayurvedic Medicine

What It Is   *Ayurveda* is a sophisticated ancient healing system derived from Hindu and Indian culture, and practiced in India for 4,000 years. It is a way of life, a philosophy of living, which supports the belief in the interconnectedness of mind, body, and spirit and of the individual to the environment. It teaches and emphasizes individual responsibility in becoming an active participant in maintaining healthy body systems. The focus is on prevention and regaining good health.

KEY POINT

Ayurveda means *science of life*. In sanskrit *Ayur* means *life* and *Veda* means *knowledge*.

Ayurveda views individuals as composed of five elements: earth, water, fire, air, and space. Ayurvedic philosophy holds that there are three basic operating principles or *doshas* that govern the function of health. It is believed that a person is born with a particular *dosha* (body type) or combination of doshas and that the basic constitution is expressed through this body type. There is also a belief that the mind has a powerful influence on the body, therefore a major role for a person is to become aware of the positive and negative thought patterns that support or destroy health.

How It Works   By assessing an individual's physical and emotional makeup, food and environmental preferences, and lifestyle a particular dosha or body type is determined. Knowing the specific elements that make up this dosha along with basic patterns, 24-hour cycles, seasons, and stages of life associated with each of the doshas, a particular health plan is developed.

Some diagnostic methods used are detailed history-taking through questioning (family, interpersonal relationships, and job situation), pulse diagnosis, tongue diagnosis, and other observational skills (eyes, nails, and urine).

A treatment plan's goal is to help a person arrive at a lifestyle that results in a balance of body and mind for optimum health. Treatment suggestions may include a combination of:

- Nutritional suggestions, including the six tastes that are important to include in every meal (sweet, sour, salty, pungent, bitter, and astringent)
- Herbs (which are classified according to the six tastes)
- Exercise (specific for each dosha/body type)
- Breathing exercises (called *pranayama*)
- Meditation exercises (to help develop moment-to-moment awareness and cleansing of the body)
- Massage (marma therapy)
- Aromatherapy (to help balance body functions, emotions, and memories)

- Music (certain tones or rhythms to be used at certain times of the day)
- Purification technique called *panchakarma* (that includes five procedures or therapies to be experienced over the course of one week)

What It Helps   In addition to being appropriate for a wide range of physical and emotional illnesses, Ayurveda benefits anyone who is interested in optimum health.

Words of Wisdom: Cautions   Physical side effects are rare, although there may be occasional side effects from certain Ayurvedic herbs. It is always best to seek advice from a practitioner who is experienced or who has been educated in the Ayurvedic principles.

Naturopathy

What It Is   Naturopathic medicine grew out of the nineteenth century medical system, and was given its name by Dr. John Scheel in 1895, and was formalized by Benedict Lust in 1902. It was popular in the early 1900s, but with the development of antibiotics and vaccines in the 1940s and 1950s that popularity declined. It wasn't until the 1970s that interest was renewed.

Naturopathy is a way of life, viewing health as more than the absence of disease. It looks at symptoms as signs of the body eliminating toxins and believes that a person should be treated as a whole, looking at physical, psychological, emotional, and genetic factors. A naturopath's emphasis is on finding and treating the cause (not just symptoms), self-responsibility, education, health maintenance, and disease prevention. The basic belief is that the body has the ability to heal itself and an innate ability to maintain health, so any treatment focuses on a combination of natural healing methods that strengthen the body's natural abilities. Techniques and approaches are used that do no harm and support and restore harmony within the body.

A practice is generally built around two or more therapeutic approaches such as traditional Chinese medicine or acupuncture; clinical nutrition; counseling; dietary and lifestyle modifications; exercise; herbal medicine; homeopathy; hydrotherapy; or osteopathy.

Training for a doctor of naturopathic medicine (ND) varies from a four-year graduate level education within a naturopathic medical college to training from a correspondence school.

How It Works   As the primary role of a naturopath is as an educator, recommendations and encouragement for self-responsibility for health are offered and the person must make a commitment to change. The first visit involves a medical history with detailed assessment of lifestyle habits, diet, occupation, family dynamics, emotional, environmental, and genetic influences. Diagnostic procedures, such as laboratory testing and X-rays may be used and if specialized care, surgery, or hospitalization is warranted referral is made to other healthcare professionals as appropriate. Naturopaths prefer the least invasive intervention and do not do emergency care, although some may practice natural childbirth. Naturopaths pay attention to a person's individuality and susceptibility to disease.

What It Helps   There is unlimited potential for most health conditions to respond to this type of approach.

Words of Wisdom: Cautions   Natural therapies are less likely to cause complications, but choose the practitioner that knows his or her limitations with any of the approaches practiced.

Manual Healing Methods

Chiropractic

What It Is   History tells us that the use of manipulation as a healing technique was used as early as 2700 B.C. by the Chinese. The Greeks (in 1500 B.C.) and Hippocrates (460 B.C.) also used spinal manipulation to cure dysfunctions of the body.

Daniel Palmer founded chiropractic in the Midwest in 1895 and it is now the fourth largest health profession in the United States. Palmer believed that all body functions were regulated by the nervous system and that because nerves originate in the spine, any displacement of vertebrae could disrupt nerve transmission, (which he called *subluxation*). He hypothesized that almost all disease is caused by vertebral misalignment, therefore spine manipulation could treat all disease. Today the theory has changed to what is being called intervertebral motion dysfunction. The key factor in this theory involves the loss of mobility of facet joints in the spine.

KEY POINT

Chiropractors believe that a strong agile and aligned spine is the key to good health.

How It Works   The spine is made up of 24 bones called vertebrae with discs of cartilage cushioning between each vertebra. The spinal cord runs through the middle of the vertebrae with many nerves branching off through channels in the vertebrae. Chiropractors believe that injury or poor posture can result in pressure on the spinal cord from misaligned vertebrae and that this can lead to illness and painful movement.

The chiropractor identifies and corrects the misalignments through manipulation, which are called adjustments. Muscle work is also incorporated as muscles attach and support the spine. Manipulation and muscle work can be done by hand and/or assisted by special treatment tables, application of heat or cold, or ultrasound. Some chiropractic physicians also advise about nutrition and exercise. The first visit includes a detailed medical history and examination of the spine. Sometimes X-rays of the spine are also obtained. The findings are reviewed by the chiropractor and a plan is established with a suggested number of follow-up treatments.

What It Helps   Chiropractic is useful for lower-back syndromes, muscle spasms, mid-back conditions, sports-related injuries, neck syndromes, whiplash and accident-related injuries, headaches, arthritic conditions, carpal tunnel syndrome, shoulder conditions, and sciatica.

Words of Wisdom: Cautions   With a conscientious, professionally trained chiropractor there are few side effects, however, some soreness may be experienced for a few days after a spinal adjustment and occasionally symptoms may get worse. Manipulations are contraindicated in persons with osteoporosis and advanced degenerative joint disease as these might be worsened by spinal adjustment.

Craniosacral Therapy

What It Is   The basic belief of craniosacral therapy (CST) is that an unimpeded cerebrospinal fluid flow is the key to optimum health. Craniosacral therapy was developed in the early 1900s and is an offshoot of osteopathy and chiropractic.

William Sutherland, an osteopathic physician, developed craniosacral therapy, which at that time was called cranial osteopathy. He believed that the bones of the skull were movable and that they move rhythmically in response to production of cerebrospinal fluid in the ventricles of the brain. This belief contradicts the teachings of anatomy in western medicine, which holds the bones of the skull fuse together at two years of age and are no longer movable after this point in the physical development of the body.

Craniosacral therapists also believe that by realigning the bones of the skull, free circulation of the cerebrospinal fluid is restored, and strains and stresses of the meninges (that surround the brain and spinal cord) are removed, which allows the entire body to return to good health. William Sutherland researched his theory over 20 years and documented physical and emotional reactions to compression on the cranial bones.

Craniosacral therapy was further advanced by John Upledger who performed scientific studies at Michigan State University from 1975–1983. His findings validated craniosacral therapy's capability to help evaluate and treat dysfunction and pain. The Upledger Institute in Palm Beach Gardens, Florida trains practitioners in this discipline.

How It Works   Trained practitioners palpate the craniosacral rhythm by placing their hands on the cranium (skull) and sensing imbalances. This approach is painless as the practitioner uses gentle touch (less than the weight of a nickel) to sense the imbalances in the rhythm and stabilize it. Recipients report a release of tension and a state of deep relaxation and peace. Practitioners work in a quiet setting and use no needles, oils, or mechanical devices. They take a medical history, observe, and question about any symptoms. As with other alternative therapies, a person may experience a brief period of worsening symptoms following treatment (usually for only 24–48 hours) as the body adapts to the changes that occurred during the session.

What It Helps   Anxiety, headaches, central nervous system disorders, neck and back pain, chronic ear infections, chronic fatigue, motor coordination difficulties, facial pain, temporomandibular joint (TMJ) dysfunction, and sinusitis.

Words of Wisdom: Caution   As with any integrative therapy, use with the exclusion of western medical advice is not recommended.

Energy Medicine/Healing

What It Is   Energy medicine and energy healing are called *hands-on healing* and *hand-mediated biofield therapies*. Energy field theory (biofield theory) is based on quantum physics law. These laws recognize matter as energy and hold that all living things generate vibrational fields. Validation of the existence of human energy fields is beginning to emerge through research studies.

KEY POINT

In energy healing, subtle energy is seen as the core of life and the central force in healing.

Therapeutic Touch (TT) is one of these techniques and was developed by Dolores Krieger, a nursing professor at New York University, and Dora Kunz, a healer from Canada, in the 1970s. The concept of universal life force is central to these forms of therapy—like *qi* (called *chee*) is in traditional Chinese medicine and acupuncture. Two other therapies that use hands to alter energy fields and assist in the healing process are Healing Touch and Reiki. Healing Touch was developed for healthcare professionals by Janet Mentgen, a nurse from Denver, Colorado, and includes a varied collection of energy techniques. Reiki is an ancient Buddhist practice that was rediscovered by Dr. Usui, a Japanese physician, through ancient Tibetan texts. A Japanese-American woman who studied with Dr. Usui later introduced Reiki in the United States.

These modern interpretations of ancient practices should not be confused with faith healing as they are not practiced within a religious context. The goal of this form of healing is to accelerate the personal-healing process at all levels of mind, body, and spirit. These forms of treatment are not meant for diagnosing nor are they to replace conventional medicine or surgery.

Each technique has a process that is learned through training, reading, and practice. Therapeutic Touch can be learned through short courses. Healing Touch is learned through various levels of training over a period of two-to-three years and criteria must be met for certification as a practitioner. Reiki is learned from a Reiki Master and includes two degrees that can be learned in weekend courses. The Master degree takes longer study and a mentorship.

KEY POINT

Although conventional scientific medicine has no evidence to support the existence of human energy fields, many of the diagnostic instruments used for diagnosis and treatment of disease are energy-medicine devices. Examples of these devices that measure electromagnetic frequencies are: electrocardiogram (ECG), electroencephalogram (EEG), electromyogram (EMG), ultrasound (US), and magnetic resonance imaging (MRI). It is these electromagnetic frequencies or energy fields that skilled energy healers/practitioners literally feel and work with to create repatterning.

How It Works   These therapies are based on the belief that health exists when there is an abundance of energy flowing without obstruction throughout a person and between the person and his or her environment. Energy therapists help individuals create an environment that supports this self-healing. This is in essence what happens when a person interacts in a caring relationship. Healing may occur on the physical, emotional, mental, or spiritual levels as this process works with the whole person.

Practitioners center themselves in preparation for a treatment session so they are consciously present for the client. Their focus is completely on the person receiving the treatment without any preoccupation or thought process in any other direction. Practitioners assess the energy field, clear and balance it through hand movements and/or direct energy in a specific region of the body. The end result expressed by most people after receiving a session of energy healing is extremely deep relaxation. Reiki involves a similar process and helps restore balance to a person's energy field.

What It Helps   Research supports the use of energy healing to relieve pain, anxiety, stress, and tension, and to accelerate wound healing and to help maintain health and a feeling of well-being. There are unlimited uses for these therapies when provided by a trained practitioner.

Words of Wisdom: Caution   Always be concerned about claims of curing, and know the credentials of the practitioner offering the treatment.

Massage Therapy

What It Is   Massage is the third most common form of alternative treatment in the United States after relaxation techniques and chiropractic. It consists of the therapeutic practice of kneading or manipulating soft tissue and muscles with the intent of increasing health and well-being and assisting the body in healing.

There are many different types of massage, such as lymphatic massage, sports massage, Swedish massage, shiatsu massage, myofascial release, trigger point massage, thai massage, and infant massage. A form of deep tissue massage that is known as structural integration is called *rolfing*. This system works deeply into muscle tissue and fascia to stretch and release patterns of tension and rigidity and to return the body to a state of correct alignment.

How It Works   Besides stretching and loosening muscle and connective tissue, massage also:

- Improves blood flow and the flow of lymph throughout the body
- Speeds the metabolism of waste products
- Promotes the circulation of oxygen and nutrients to cells and tissue
- Stimulates the release of endorphins and serotonin in the brain and nervous system.

KEY POINT

Massage can be seen as a form of communication from the therapist that brings comfort, gentleness, connection, trust, and peace.

What It Helps   Massage is good for health maintenance as well as an adjunct to healing. Many conditions may benefit from massage, such as chronic pain, fluid retention, circulatory problems, fatigue, muscle tension and spasms, anxiety and stress, muscle strain or sprain, and insomnia.

Words of Wisdom: Caution   There are a few contraindications that will be screened by the therapist when taking a medical history at the first visit. This is a reason for choosing a well-trained and qualified massage therapist. Ask for credentials.

Bodywork—Movement Therapy

The Trager Approach
What It Is   In the 1920s, a physician, Milton Trager, developed a method of passive gentle movements with traction and rotation of extremities to help reeducate muscles and joints. Through this method muscle tightness is relieved without pain and the end result is a sense of freedom, flexibility, and lightness.

How It Works   Through smooth joint movements and gentle rhythmic rocking of body parts, communication is made with the nerves that control muscle movement to release and reorganize old patterns of tension, pain, and muscle restriction. A session lasts 60-to-90 minutes, and after a session, instructions are given for a series of simple movements (called *mentastics*) to help maintain the results of the treatment. Deep relaxation of mind and body is also promoted during these movements.

What It Helps   Chronic pain, severe disability, muscle spasms, fibromyalgia, temporomandibular pain (TMJ), headaches, plus many other neuromuscular disorders.

Words of Wisdom: Caution   With a trained practitioner there are no harmful side effects.

Feldenkrais Method

What It Is   Feldenkrais teaches a person how to alter the way the body is held and moved. It is a gentle method of bodywork that involves movement. Moshe Feldenkrais developed this method after suffering a knee injury. He studied and combined principles of anatomy, physiology, biomechanics, and psychology and integrated this knowledge with his own awareness of proper movement.

How It Works   By developing awareness of body movement patterns and changing them through specific exercises, flexibility, coordination, and range of motion improve. Through instruction a teacher guides a person through a series of movements, such as bending, walking, and reaching. These movements can help reduce stress and pain and improve self-image. It is believed these movements access the central nervous system. There are two types of sessions: (1) a set of movement lessons learned with a group called *awareness through movement* and (2) individual hands-on sessions called *functional integration*. The results benefit mind and emotion, as well as the physical body.

KEY POINT

Feldenkrais teaches a person to be aware of the way the body moves and to use proper movement.

What It Helps   Strokes, arthritis, bursitis, back pain, spinal cord injury, cerebral palsy, multiple sclerosis, digestive difficulties, respiratory difficulties, musculoskeletal difficulties, and concentration problems.

Words of Wisdom: Caution   There are no known side effects or unsafe conditions when provided by a trained practitioner.

The Alexander Therapy

What It Is   Alexander therapy is an educational process that identifies poor posture habits and teaches conscious control of movements that underlie better body mechanics. Frederick Mathias Alexander, an Australian actor who lost his voice while performing, developed this therapy. Discouraged by only temporary relief from medical treatments he began studying how posture affected his voice. After nine years of study and perfecting his technique he began to train others.

How It Works   Alexander therapy teaches simple exercises to improve balance, posture, and coordination. It is done with gentle hands-on guidance and verbal instruction. It results in release of excess tension in the body, lengthens the spine, and creates greater flexibility in movement.

What It Helps   Many conditions that result from poor posture can be greatly helped. This technique is taught in many drama and music universities throughout the world.

Words of Wisdom: Caution   Safe therapy when performed by a credentialed therapist.

Mind-Body Therapies

Meditation/Relaxation

What It Is   Relaxation involves practices that shut down the fight and flight response of the body and settles the mind. Meditation is an ancient art of focused attention and is a practice to help the body reach a relaxed state. Relaxation has been found to reduce stress, which leads to many physical and mental health benefits. Herbert Benson, MD, from Harvard, researched meditation and documented its many benefits is his book titled *The Relaxation Response* (4).

KEY POINT

Some of the benefits of reduced stress include decreased heart rate, breathing rate, blood pressure, and brainwaves; improved mood; increased awareness and spiritual calm.

How It Works   Two forms of meditation are *concentrative meditation* and *mindfulness meditation*. The former involves focusing on a sound, an image, or one's own breathing. By doing this process a person reaches a state of calm and deepens attention and awareness. The latter form of meditation brings full awareness in the present moment. Mindfulness meditation teaches one to not allow outside distraction to interrupt focus on the present moment. This helps a person to slow down, become more relaxed, and have more insight into what is occurring in the immediate moment.

What It Helps   Unlimited usage for physical symptoms, anxiety reduction, increased energy level, and increased sense of well-being.

Words of Wisdom: Caution   Occasionally negative emotions or thoughts can surface indicating a need for referral for further professional consultation.

Biofeedback

What It Is   *Biofeedback* is a process of learned control of physical responses of the body. Through this therapy a person develops a deeper awareness and voluntary control over physical processes.

With biofeedback, a person learns to use thought processes to control bodily processes.

How It Works   Through the use of instruments a person is trained to relax and monitor changes through certain feedback devices. Meditation, relaxation, and visualization techniques are taught and these techniques ultimately teach psychological control over physical processes.

What It Helps   Tension headaches, chronic pain, anxiety, asthma, and high blood pressure.

Guided Imagery

What It Is   Guided imagery is a mind–body technique that helps a person use imagination to relieve symptoms, heal disease, or promote relaxation. It is based on the belief that the mind and body are interconnected and work together in the healing process.

How It Works   A person can use guided imagery alone or be led by a practitioner. Sessions can last 10-to-30 minutes. Different imaging is used as a person is guided through the process. A quiet place is needed, free from distractions. Numerous studies have demonstrated physiologic and biochemical changes.

What It Helps   Almost any medical situation can benefit from guided imagery, especially if problem solving, relaxation, decision making, or symptom relief is useful. It is used frequently to prepare for surgery and to speed recovery after surgery. It can be used to enhance the immune system, reduce stress, and to induce a sense of well-being.

Words of Wisdom: Caution   This is a harmless healing technique. This technique may reduce the need for medications, but medications should not be adjusted or stopped without first checking with a primary healthcare professional.

Hypnotherapy

What It Is   *Hypnotherapy* is a state of focused concentration or relaxation that is guided by a therapist. In this state a person is open to suggestion.

Hypnosis dates back to ancient China and Egypt and was even included as part of surgical procedures. In the eighteenth century Franz Mesmer, an Austrian physician, was known for a process of inducing trance states in people and is credited with introducing hypnotism into medicine. The term *mesmerize* was used to describe his process.

A surgeon, James Braid, developed the technique further in the mid-nineteenth century and used it for pain control and as anesthesia in surgery. But because over the years Vaudeville performers, magicians, and others exploited it, hypnosis became associated with superstition, quackery, and evil. It wasn't until 1958, when Milton

Erickson, an American psychotherapist, demonstrated how psychosomatic symptoms could be resolved with hypnotherapy that the American Medical Association finally accepted hypnotherapy.

How It Works   In a trance state, a state between sleep and waking, which is called an *alpha state*, a person is very relaxed. It is like awakening in the morning and not being fully conscious or fully connected with the surroundings. In this state a person is very receptive to suggestions from a therapist. Everyone is unique in his or her receptivity to entering into a guided trance state. No one can enter this state by force and in this state there is full awareness of everything that is happening. In this hypnotic state past events can be more easily remembered and trauma and anxiety around such events can be resolved. When this happens past events no longer affect present behavior negatively.

What It Helps   Hypnotherapy is a therapeutic tool that can be very helpful in managing many situations, including fears, anxiety, chronic pain, addictions, poor self-control, low self-esteem, and behavioral problems.

Words of Wisdom: Caution   Situations that interfere with hypnotherapy are extreme fear, religious objections, skepticism, inability to trust the therapist, and inability to relax. Hypnotherapy is not suitable when there are serious psychiatric conditions.

Yoga

What It Is   Yoga uses stretching, breathing, body postures, and relaxation/meditation to restore and promote good mental and physical health. It has been practiced in India for thousands of years and, although it was introduced in the United States in the 1890s, it didn't become popular until the 1960s. The goal of yoga is to create balance between movement and stillness, which is said to be the state of a healthy body. Postures require little movement, but require mental concentration. Originally yoga was developed as part of a spiritual belief system, but our western culture primarily uses it as a health practice for improved flexibility, strength, relaxation, and physical fitness.

KEY POINT

Yoga consists of breathing exercises, various stretching postures, and meditation.

How It Works   There are many styles of yoga and most are performed in a class. Yoga consists of breathing exercises and various postures or poses (*asnas*) that promote stretching and toning. There are beginning, intermediate, and advanced stages of practices within the various styles of yoga. Each posture has specific benefits and each session usually ends with some form of a relaxation exercise or meditation. People have been known to practice yoga well into their 80s.

What It Helps   Headaches, asthma, back pain, sciatica, insomnia, balance, coordination circulation, concentration, flexibility, endurance, physical strength, range of motion, and immunity.

Words of Wisdom: Caution   Certain positions can cause muscle injury if the body is forced into those positions. Knowing personal limitations and consistent practice are important keys to obtaining the most benefit from yoga.

T'ai Chi

What It Is   *T'ai Chi* is a discipline that has been practiced in China for centuries. It is a form of slow-moving exercise that assists in uniting the mind–body connection. It is a martial art form that has been described as *meditation in motion*. It combines physical movement, breathing, and meditation to bring about relaxation and a feeling of well-being. There are various styles of T'ai Chi and some involve up to 108 different movements and postures. Much concentration and discipline is required and it takes time to learn the proper motion and coordination. People of all ages and physical capabilities can practice the art form, and it develops endurance, and flexibility, decreases fatigue, and improves overall physical health.

How It Works   The Chinese believe T'ai Chi helps to increase the flow of *qi* (*chi* or *universal life force*) circulating throughout the body. The movements are learned in rhythmic coordinated patterns that slowly flow from one series of movements into another. Focus is placed on breath and the body's motion, which in turn rejuvenates, stretches, strengthens, releases tension, opens points, and calms and quiets the mind at the same time. The slow turning, twisting, and stretching allows every part of the body to be exercised without strain.

What It Helps   High blood pressure, nervous disorders, immune system, balance, stress-related disorders, circulation, panic attacks, concentration, insomnia, muscle tone, dizziness, internal organs, fibromyalgia, and spine and back problems.

Words of Wisdom   Few problems if done within individual limitations.

Pharmacologic and Biologic Treatments

Aromatherapy

What It Is   *Aromatherapy*, an offshoot of herbal medicine, is the therapeutic inhalation or application of essential oils distilled from plants. It is a pharmacologic treatment because the chemicals found in the essential oils are absorbed by the body and result in specific effects. The benefits are either physical or mental/emotional or both.

How It Works   Essential oils stimulate the release of neurotransmitters in the brain. The sense of smell connects with the part of the brain that controls the autonomic (involuntary) nervous system. The resulting effects are calming, pain reducing, stimulating, sedating, or euphoric. These oils can also be applied to the skin through the use of carrier oils or lotions. Many have antibacterial, antiviral, antifungal, and anti-inflammatory and antiseptic properties. Oils placed on the skin are absorbed and enter the circulatory system and intercellular fluid. Inhaled oil attaches to oxygen molecules and circulate throughout the body. These oils are able to penetrate cell walls and transport oxygen and nutrients to the cell. (See Chapter 23 on Aromatherapy for more information.)

KEY POINT

Essential oils are very potent and are obtained through steam-distillation of various parts of plants (leaves, flowers, blossoms, fruits, bark, gum, bulbs) and grasses.

What It Helps   Anxiety, headaches, depression, arthritis, fatigue, bronchitis, pain, bruises, sinusitis, colic, nausea, hormonal imbalance, indigestion, muscle strain, skin conditions, and many other conditions/symptoms.

Words of Wisdom: Caution   There are many cautions with these very powerful essential oils.

- Use oils according to direction
- Use only diluted oils—use in a carrier oil or lotion
- Test for allergic reactions
- Know what you are using
- Use oils only from reputable companies
- Store oils in a cool place
- Keep away from children
- Never apply oils to eyes
- Some oils should never be taken internally (eucalyptus, hyssop, mugwort leaf, thuja, pennyroyal, sage or wormwood)

Herbal Medicine

What It Is   Besides a way to accent flavor in foods, herbs and plants have been used by many cultures to treat illness for thousands of years. Herbal medicine is also called *botanical medicine* or *phytotherapy* (*phyto* means *plant*). Herbs are used as prevention, as well as for treating illnesses. Many drugs are derived from plants; however, most of the ingredients in today's drugs are chemicals. Medicinal uses of herbs and plants come from different parts of a plant. Some examples are leaves, flowers, stems, seeds, berries, bark, fruit, and root depending on the plant and its specific use.

Herbal medicine is used as the main form of healing in about 80 percent of the world.

Conventional medicine's approach to using plants is to pinpoint the active ingredient in the plant, and extract it rather than use the whole plant. It is believed by many herbalists and other traditional healing systems (such as traditional Chinese medicine and Ayurvedic medicine) that isolating and using a specific ingredient may reduce the healing power of the plant and also possibly remove the built-in buffers that protect against side effects. This is based on the belief that active ingredients in plants work together synergistically. This means that the action of two or more plant ingredients working together produces an effect that can't be produced with the individual extracted ingredient alone.

Herbs are prepared in many different forms: teas, infusions, decoctions, tinctures, extracts, tablets, capsules, injections, oils, creams, and ointments.

How It Works   Herbs have classifications according to their effects on a person just like western drugs. Classifications are, such as adaptogenic, antihelmintic, anti-inflammatory, antimicrobial, antispasmodic, astringent, bitters, carminative, delmucent, diuretic, expectorant, hepatic, hypotensive, laxative, nervine, stimulant, and tonic. It is important to work with a knowledgeable practitioner in order to have guidance in selection both from the standpoint of the proper herb for the proper condition and also in selecting the right purity and potency of the herb. It is very important to use herbal preparations from a source that uses standardized dosages to guarantee the correct amount of herb in each batch produced. It is important to have guidance for the length of usage of an herb and whether it is being used as a tonic (prevention) or as a treatment.

Much research is being carried out presently that is allowing for a greater understanding of safe usage, especially in combination with western medications. The information is changing almost daily. (For more information, see Chapter 22 on Herbal Remedies.)

What It Helps   Herbs are helpful for a wide range of illnesses frequently treated by western medicines, however, knowing how to use them safely alone or in combination requires monitoring by a knowledgeable person. Herbs provide vitamins and nutrients that enhance wellness, so they are very effective as preventative agents.

If an informed practitioner is not available for guidance then a reliable resource that provides detailed information and safety measures is a must.

Words of Wisdom: Caution   Infants, children, and pregnant women or women attempting pregnancy need special cautions and need to always seek supervision of any herbal usage. Likewise, anyone with chronic or serious illness or anyone using western medications needs to inform and seek the guidance of a knowledgeable healthcare professional. Taking responsibility for becoming informed about herbs helps with the safe use of herbal preparations, however, seeking the advice of a professional herbalist is the greatest safety.

Remembering to inform your healthcare provider when seeking medical care is also of prime importance, especially if any western medicine is prescribed. This will help prevent any side effects from any potential drug–herbal interactions that could occur due to incompatibility.

Today there are many options available in the quest to maintain or regain health and wellness. Being prepared to make appropriate individual choices regarding these options requires considerable thought and a thorough investigation. This investigation leads to an understanding of the concepts of wholeness (the inseparableness of mind/body/spirit) and insights into personal health beliefs. This investigation also leads to greater knowledge of self-awareness, self-responsibility, and self-nurturance and provides a clearer vision of personal needs and more personal power in developing a partnership with the healthcare provider.

A broader view of health allows for the realization that optimum health is a lifelong journey rather than an ultimate state of being. The goal of this journey is the maintenance of balance between health and illness. The attempt at maintaining this balance is thwarted with many challenges and choices. What is the extent of your personal knowledge of your health and wellness status? Is there a need to consult with a conventional medical healthcare provider if you choose to integrate a complementary therapy in your journey? What do you know about the origin, today's use, and safety of a specific non-western medical therapy? Is it safe to combine the use of conventional and complementary healthcare therapies? Is the practitioner of choice knowledgeable and appropriately educated and trained? Will there be communication between your providers if necessary? In directing your own health care, these are but a few of the questions that need to be addressed. Selection of an appropriate complementary therapy requires much consideration and the information provided here is offered as beginning guidance and assistance along the journey of self-discovery and balanced health.

Chapter Summary

Americans have shown a growing interest in complementary therapies due to their interest in preventive health, concern about adverse drug reactions, and personalized care offered by complementary practitioners. Although new to many Americans, many complementary therapies originated from ancient and non-western healing traditions that have been used in other parts of the world for centuries.

Holistic care is not the same as complementary or alternative therapies. Holistic care implies a balance and harmony among mind, body, and spirit. It assumes that individuals take an active role in achieving maximum wellness. Although people can use complementary or alternative therapies as part of holistic care, the use of these therapies does not guarantee holism.

The five major categories of complementary therapies are: alternative systems of medical practice, manual healing therapies, mind–body therapies, pharmacologic/biologic treatments, and botanical/herbal medicine.

Complementary therapies need to be used wisely. To use complementary therapies safely, people need to gather information to base decisions on facts, establish goals, and keep an open mind. They need to ask questions before using a complementary therapy, such as what conditions respond best to it, how does it work, what should be expected, how long must it be used, and what are the harmful effects?

References

1. Eisenberg, D. (1998). Advising Patients Who Seek Alternative Medical Therapies. *The Integrated Medical Consult, 1*(1):4–5.

2. Fontaine, K. L. (2000). *Healing Practices: Alternative Therapies for Nursing.* Upper Saddle River, New Jersey: Prentice Hall.

3. Eliopoulos, C. (1999). *Integrating Conventional and Alternative Therapies: Holistic Care for Chronic Conditions.* St. Louis: Mosby, Inc.

4. Benson, H. (1975). *The Relaxation Response.* New York: Morrow.

Suggested Readings

Carlson, L. K. (2002). Reimbursement of Complementary and Alternative Medicine by Managed Care and Insurance Providers. *Alternative Therapies in Health and Medicine, 8*(1):38–49.

Cerrato, P. L. (2001). Complementary Therapies Update. *RN, 61*(6):549–552.

Chopra, D. (1991). *Perfect Health, The Complete Mind/Body Guide.* New York: Harmony Books.

Credit, L. P., Hartunion, S. G., and Nowak, M. J. (1998). *Your Guide to Complementary Medicine.* Garden City Park, New York: Avery Publishing Group.

Decker, G. (1999). *An Introduction to Complementary and Alternative Therapies.* Pittsburgh: Oncology Nursing Press, Inc.

Dillard, J. and Ziporyn, T. (1998). *Alternative Medicine for Dummies.* New York: IDG Books Worldwide, Inc.

Earthlink, Inc. (2000). *Alternative Healthcare: Is It the Right Alternative for You?* Blink. June/July, p. 27.

Eisenberg, D. M. (1997). Advising Patients Who Seek Alternative Medical Therapies. *Annals of Internal Medicine, 127*(1):61–69.

Eisenberg, D., et al. (1993). Unconventional Medicine in the US: Prevalence, Costs and Patterns of Use. *New England Journal of Medicine, 328*(4):246–252.

Huebscher, R. and Shuler, P. A. (2003). *Natural, Alternative, and Complementary Health Care Practices.* St. Louis: Mosby.

Kirskey, K. M., Goodroad, B. K., Kemppainen, J. K., et al. (2002). Complementary Therapy Use in Persons with HIV/AIDS. *Journal of Holistic Nursing, 20*(3):250–263.

Knaster, M. (1996). *Discovering the Body's Wisdom.* New York: Bantam Books.

Marcus, C. L. (1999). Alternative Medicine: The AMA Reviews Scientific Medicine. *Clinician Reviews, 9*(2):87–90.

Krohn, J. and Taylor, F. A. (2002). *Finding the Right Treatment. Modern and Alternative Medicine: A Comprehensive Reference Guide That Will Help You Get the Best of Both Worlds.* Point Roberts, WA: Hartley & Marks Publishers.

McCaleb, R. S., Leigh E., and Morien, K. (2000). *The Encyclopedia of Popular Herbs: Your Complete Guide to the Leading Medicinal Plants.* Roseville, CA: Prima Publishing.

McGovern, K., Lockhart, A., Malay, P., et al. eds. (2003). *Nurse's Handbook of Alternative and Complementary Therapies,* 2nd ed. Philadelphia: Lippincott Williams & Wilkins.

Morrison, J. (1995). *The Book of Ayurveda: A Holistic Approach to Health and Longevity.* New York: Fireside.

Olshansky, E. (2000). *Integrated Women's Health: Holistic Approaches for Comprehensive Care.* Gaithersburg, Maryland: Aspen Publications.

Skinner, S. E. (2001). *An Introduction to Homeopathic Medicine in Primary Care.* Gaithersburg, MD: Aspen Publishers, Inc.

Smith, D. W., Arnstein, P., Rosa, K. C., and Wells-Felderman, C. (2002). Effects of Integrating Therapeutic Touch into a Cognitive Behavioral Pain Treatment Program. *Journal of Holistic Nursing, 20*(4):367–387.

Stephenson, N. L. N. and Dalton, J. (2003). Using Reflexology for Pain Management. *Journal of Holistic Nursing, 21*(2):179–191.

Trivieri, L. and Anderson, J. W., eds. (2002). *Alternative Medicine: The Definitive Guide*, 2nd ed. Berkeley, CA: Celestial Arts.

Weil, A. (1999). *Self-Healing*. Watertown, MA: Thorne Communications, Inc.

Williams, G. (1999). *The Future of 21st Century Health: Getting the Right Care*. Harvard Business School Consumer-Driven Health Care Conference.

Wisneski, L. (1999). *The Integrative Medical Consult*. Integrative Medicine Communications. Newton, MA.

Resources

Alternative Systems of Medical Practice

Acupuncture

Acupuncture and Oriental Medicine Alliance
6405 43rd Avenue Ct., NW, Suite B
Greg Harbor, WA 98335
253-851-6896
www.AOMalliance.org

American Academy of Medical Acupuncture
4929 Wilshire Blvd, Suite 428
Los Angeles, CA 90036
800-721-2177
www.medicalacupuncture.org

American Association of Acupuncture and Oriental Medicine
5530 Wisconsin Avenue, Suite 1210
Chevy Chase, MD 20815
888-500-7999
www.aaom.org

Ayurvedic Medicine

Ayurvedic Institute
11311 Menaul NE, Suite A
Albuquerque, NM 87112
505-291-9698
www.ayurveda.com

Homeopathy
  National Center For Homeopathy
  801 N. Fairfax Street, Suite 306
  Alexandria, VA 22314
  703-548-7790
  www.homeopathic.org

  North American Society of Homeopathy
  1122 E. Pike Street, Suite 1122
  Seattle, WA 98122
  206-720-7000
  www.homeopathy.org

Naturopathy
  American Association of Naturopathic Physicians
  3201 New Mexico Avenue NW, Suite 350
  Washington, DC 20016
  866-538-2267
  www.naturopathic.org

Bodywork—Movement Therapy

The Alexander Therapy
  American Society for the Alexander Technique
  PO Box 60008
  Florence, MA 01062
  800-473-0620
  www.alexandertech.com

The Feldenkrais Method
  Feldenkrais Guild of North America
  3611 SW Hood Avenue, Suite 100
  Portland, OR 97239
  800-775-2118
  www.feldenkrais.com

The Trager Approach
  Trager International
  24800 Chagrin Blvd., Suite 205
  Beachwood, OH 44122
  216-896-9383
  www.trager.com

Manual Healing Methods

Chiropractic
American Chiropractic Association
1701 Clarendon Blvd.
Arlington, VA 22209
800-637-6244
www.amerchiro.org

Federation of Chiropractic Licensing Boards
901 54th Avenue, Suite 101
Greely, CO 80634
970-356-3500
www.fclb.org

World Chiropractic Alliance
2950 N. Dobson, Suite 1
Chandler, AZ 85224
800-347-1011
www.worldchiropracticalliance.org

Craniosacral Therapy
Upledger Institute
11211 Prosperity Farms Road
Palm Beach Garden, FL 33410
561-622-4706
www.upledger.com

Energy Medicine/Healing
American Holistic Nurses Association
P.O. Box 2130
Flagstaff, AZ 86003
800-278-2462
www.ahna.org

Colorado Center for Healing Touch
12477 W. Cedar Drive, Suite 206
Lakewood, CO 80228
303-989-0581
www.healingtouch.net

Nurse Healers Professional Associates
3760 South Highland Drive, Suite 429
Salt Lake City, Utah 84106
801-273-3390
www.therapeutic-touch.org

International Society for the Study of Subtle Energies and Energy Medicine
11005 Ralston Road, Suite 100D
Arvada, CO 80004
303-278-2228
www.issseem.org

Reiki Training International
P.O. Box 2765
Indianapolis, IN 46206
800-506-1144

International Center for Reiki Training
21421 Hilltop St., Suite 28
Southfield, MI 48034
800-332-8112
www.reiki.org

Massage Therapy
American Massage Therapy Association
820 Davis Street, Suite 100
Evanston, IL 60201
847-864-0123
www.amtamassage.org

Associated Bodywork and Massage Professionals
800-458-2267
www.abmp.com

Massage Bodywork Resource Center
www.massageresource.com

Mind-Body Therapies
Biofeedback
Association of Applied Psychophysiology and Biofeedback and
Biofeedback Certification Institute
10200 West 44th Avenue, Suite 304

Wheat Ridge, CO 80033-2840
800-477-8892
www.aapb.org

Guided Imagery
Academy for Guided Imagery
30765 Pacific Coast Highway, Suite 369
Malibu, CA 90265
800-726-2070
www.interactiveimagery.com

Nurse Certificate Program in Imagery
Beyond Ordinary Nursing
PO Box 8177
Foster City, CA 94404
www.imageryrn.com

Hypnotherapy
American Board of Hypnotherapy
2002 E. McFadden Avenue, Suite 100
Santa Ana, CA 92705
800-872-9996
www.hypnosis.com

American Society of Clinical Hypnosis
140 N. Bloomingdale Road
Bloomingdale, IL 60108
630-980-4740
www.asch.net

Society for Clinical Hypnosis
128-A Kings Park Drive
Liverpool, NY 13090
315-652-7299
www.hypnosis-research.org

Meditation/Relaxation
American Meditation Institute
60 Garner Road
Averill Park, NY 12018
518-674-8714
www.americanmeditation.org

The Stress Reduction Clinic
Department of Medicine
University of Massachusetts Medical Center
45 Lake Avenue North
Worcester, MA 01655
508-856-1616
www.umassmed.edu/behavmed/clinical.cfm

The Center for Mind-Body Medicine
5225 Connecticut Avenue, NW, Suite 414
Washington, DC 20015
202-966-7338
www.cmbm.org

Tai Chi

Classic Tai Chi
Synerchi Publishing
PO Box 165
Penfield, NY 14526
www.classictaichi.com

Yoga

American Yoga Association
PO Box 19986
Sarasota, FL 34236
800-226-5859
www.americanyogaassociation.org

Yoga Alliance
122 W. Lancaster Avenue, Suite 204
Reading, PA 19607
877-964-2255
www.yogaalliance.org

Yoga Science Research Foundation
1228 Daisy Lane
East Lansing, MI 48823
517-351-3056
www.yogasite.com

Pharmacologic and Biologic Treatments

Aromatherapy

Institute of Aromatherapy
Aromatherapy Consultant Program
3108 Route 10 West
Denville, NJ 07834
973-989-1999
www.instituteofaromatherapy.com

National Association for Holistic Aromatherapy (NAHA)
4509 Interlake Avenue North, Suite 233
Seattle, WA 98103
206-547-2164
www.naha.org

The Institute of Integrative Aromatherapy
P.O. Box 18
Issaquah, WA 98027
877-363-3422
425-557-0805 (Office and Fax)
www.Aroma-RN.com

Herbal Medicine

Herb Research Foundation
4140 15th Street
Boulder, CO 80304
800-748-2617
303-449-2265
www.herbs.org

American Botanical Council
6200 Manor Road
Austin, TX 78723
512-926-2345
www.herbalgram.org

American Herbalist Guild
1931 Gaddis Road
Canton, OH 30115
770-751-6021
www.americanherbalistsguild.com

CHAPTER 22

HERBAL REMEDIES

Objectives

This chapter should enable you to:

- Define *phytochemical*
- Discuss the actions of a tonic, an adaptogen, and an immune stimulant
- List at least eight forms in which an herb can be used
- Describe three precautions to observe when wildcrafting herbs
- Discuss precautions when using herbs with children
- Describe the common use and cautions of at least five popular herbs

Advances in medical technology have given us antibiotics, laser surgery, and organ transplants that have changed the face of health care. However, this mushrooming of technology has come at a cost, including new risks and the insidious belief that health-care professionals and technology are the sources of health and healing.

We have not always looked to technology for solutions to health problems. There was a time when our ancestors were very aware of and connected to the healing power of nature. It was a natural part of human existence. Unfortunately, much of this information has been lost or ignored. Throughout the last century, in our quest for modern technology, we thought that we might be able to improve on nature.

But a change is taking place in which we are rediscovering that one needs to venture no further than the kitchen spice cabinet, backyard garden, or nearest woods to discover the abundance of herbs that can be readily used to influence human health and well-being. Indeed, we are literally surrounded by a bounty of medicinally charged leaves, flowers, seeds, barks, and roots. We are learning of the healing power of nature. Common garden weeds, such as St. John's Wort, and garden perennials, such as echinacea, are offering natural ways to improve health and treat illnesses. Many benefits can be found in developing a relationship with plants.

Employing the use of herbs from a holistic perspective is the best way to maximize their healing potential. This means using herbs in a way that addresses the whole person—mind/body/spirit—within the dynamic environment as opposed to just trying to control, suppress, or alleviate symptoms. It is important to incorporate the appropriate herbs into a larger effort of care that includes other lifestyle decisions and factors, such as nutrition, exercise, and stress reduction (much of which has been addressed in other chapters of this book).

KEY POINT

Rather than control specific symptoms, herbal therapy, when used holistically, considers the needs of the whole person mind, body, and spirit.

Historical Uses of Herbs and Folklore

Let's take a quick look at where herbs have fit into the history of medicine. In the United States, an untold amount of information from millennia of cultural plant medicine use by indigenous people has been lost in just a few generations (Exhibit 22–1). Fortunately, other countries and cultures have, to varying degrees, protected centuries of experiential data and records of plant use and effectiveness.

What remains quite valid about our history with plants is the fact that we have co-evolved with them through the ages, creating a very special and unique relationship. Plants contain most of the substances that are vital to our health, but not only in the form of vitamins, minerals, and enzymes. They also contain hormones and compounds that stimulate our body to produce chemical messengers known as neurotransmitters that are responsible for major communication systems within our bodies. There is a myriad of materials known as *phytochemicals* (plant chemicals) and science seems to be uncovering, on a daily basis, new active ingredients and information regarding our health con-

EXHIBIT 22–1   WISDOM OF THE ANCIENTS

One particularly interesting remnant of an ancient system of herbal use is referred to as *the Doctrine of Signatures*. This system suggested that the physical characteristics of the plant indicated its function or action. In other words, the color, shape, or appearance of the plant signified how it could be used. For example, a plant with a thick yellow root would indicate use for liver problems or red stems for blood conditions. This explanation is an over simplification of a very intricate, insightful system of which too little information has survived to make it relevant or safe for use today. However, it is evidence of the tremendous depth of understanding and relationship people the world over once had with their environment.

nections with plants. These phytochemicals occur in plants in mind-boggling numbers and combinations. They exist in delicate balances, buffering, strengthening each other, and creating synergy within the plants.

KEY POINT

Synergy is the combined and/or cooperative action of individual parts that allows the total effect to be greater than the sum of their individual effects.

Phytochemicals are stored by the plants in concert with the sun, soil, air, and water and they exist as a product and service of the plants' own healthy growth, function, and reproduction. Because of our co-evolution they also occur in forms that our bodies can, for the most part, readily digest, assimilate, and utilize for maintaining vital and healthy function. Yes, there is still a lot of research to be done, but while science continues to unravel the mysteries we can begin to reacquaint ourselves with and take advantage of the wealth of knowledge handed down to us by our ancestors. Today, 80 percent of the world's population still relies on plants as part of their primary health care. This percentage is not just a reflection of less-developed countries, it includes those with advanced concepts of health care such as Germany and China where the systems recognize the undeniable benefits of integrating both modern conventional technology and traditional wisdom. (The scope of this subject extends far beyond what can be addressed in this chapter. For those interested in learning more about the history of herbal medicine, please refer to the Suggested Reading list at the end of the chapter.)

Reflection   What has been your attitude about the medicinal use of plants? Have you believed herbal medicine to be quaint folklore or legitimate therapy that just hasn't yet been proven in the laboratory? How does this influence your use of these products?

Phytochemicals' Actions on the Body

Now that we know that individual plants contain hundreds, maybe thousands, of different phytochemicals in varying combinations it is important to also develop a sense of how they work in our bodies and how those actions differ from synthetic pharmaceuticals. Foremost, the very reason most of our modern drugs came to be was to provide a particular action: To do one thing and do it with authority. This is generally achieved through potent blocking, suppressing, and overriding mechanisms in the body. As a result, we have many very powerful and effective drugs at our disposal. However, along with their power comes a ponderous incidence of side effects even when properly taken. Recently published research documents complications from properly prescribed and used pharmaceuticals as the fourth leading cause of death in this country. Herbs, on the other hand, with their warehouse of constituents, often do a variety of things at once on different levels (Exhibit 22–2); they support, strengthen, and balance our systems.

Herbs provide as important a role in helping to maintain good health as they do treating the symptoms and underlying causes of disease. In addition, many herbalists feel the range of influence on specific situations can be increased by combining a number of herbs and creating a formula or compound. The goal is to address different body tissues, thereby strengthening the overall effect of the remedy. For example, someone with PMS could use a formula that may include dandelion leaf to relieve symptoms of fluid retention, black cohosh to ease cramping, and chaste tree to help rebalance hormones and alleviate anxiety. So, depending on how deep a relationship you would like, becoming familiar with some of the known plant phytochemicals and their actions would give you an added advantage in choosing the herbs that would be most effective in a given situation and avoid possible side effects or conflicts with other herbs or treatments.

Getting Started

In getting started it is important to familiarize yourself with the different forms in which herbs are available and their advantages and disadvantages. From the holistic

---

EXHIBIT 22–2   ACTIONS OF HERBS

Tonic: an action nourishing to tissues or organ systems, such as with hawthorn for the heart

Adaptogen: the action of helping regain normal function in the presence of stress such as Siberian ginseng

Immune stimulant: stimulating the immune system to recognize and mount a fight against an illness inducing invaders, such as with echinacea

perspective the form of herb is just as important a consideration as the type of herb. If it's a tea and the person doesn't "do teas," it's not of much use. Most of us are used to taking our medicines in the form of a pill, but this is not the only way, nor is it always the best or most effective method. Remember that a pill is a form that must first be digested before the medicine it contains can be absorbed, assimilated, and utilized. This is a process that is often compromised when someone is dealing with an illness. Teas and tinctures are in liquid form, so they are more readily available to the body to absorb. Also, there is a whole science involving the solubility of phytochemicals in different solutions, some releasing their properties more readily in alcohol, others in water.

KEY POINT

Herbal remedies can be used in many forms, such as extracts, teas, infusions, decoctions, tinctures, capsules, compresses, poultices, liniments, salves, or ointments.

Most herbal remedies at some point in their creation, unless you just eat them fresh or dried in an unaltered state, involve an extraction process. Extracts are made by separating the active constituents (phytochemicals) from the inactive ones (which may include sugars, starch, etc.) with the use of a solvent. This concentrates the active ingredients, which can then be kept as fluid (known as a liquid extract) or condensed and dried into a powder (referred to as powdered extract, which can then be put into capsules or made into tablets). A more potent form of the herb is created by these processes and is generally more effective for dealing with health imbalances than simply eating fresh or raw dried herbs.

Tea is a liquid extract, with water being the solvent. This a great way to get your daily medicine, particularly tonic herbs, that nourish the body's various tissues and systems, especially when taken over a period of weeks or months—it also doesn't seem much like medicine. A cup of tea is a thoughtful thing to do for yourself or someone else, providing you the opportunity to add your own caring intention to the preparation. Relatively speaking, it is often the least expensive way to take your medicine.

There are two methods of tea making: infusion and decoction. An *infusion* is a gentle form of preparation designed to preserve the valuable nutrients and essential oils and is used to prepare the more delicate parts of plants—leaves, flowers, and fresh berries. Generally speaking, the herbs are placed in a covered container and steeped in freshly boiled water for 10–30 minutes. The proportions used will vary depending if the herbs are fresh or dried, usually 1 teaspoon dried or 2 teaspoons fresh to 1 cup of water, or 1 ounce of dried herb (roughly 2 ounces of fresh) to 1 quart of water. The second method, *decoction*, is used for harder parts of the plant (roots, bark, and seeds), which are gently simmered for 15 minutes to an hour. There are some wonderful books that extol the virtues of medicinal teas that include tried and true recipes to make it easy. Supplies are readily available at most health food stores, in ready to steep bags or as loose bulk herbs to custom blend to your needs and desires. For those interested, there is little that can be more gratifying than growing, picking, and using some herbs of your own and it is fairly easy. But, teas may not be for everyone. They do take time and space, can be cumbersome to travel with, and may not appeal to some taste buds, although most herbalists will tell you that the tasting of the herb can be a very important part of the healing relationship. Additionally, there are some phytochemicals that are not water soluble, (meaning that they are not accessible to water extraction).

There are health situations when forms other than teas are more appropriate. In these cases other liquid extracts can be used such as tinctures, which will vary depending on the solvent used—generally alcohol, vinegar, or glycerin. Again, these preparations are made by the active ingredients literally being pulled out of the plant into the solution, the solvent then acts as a preservative. Of the three types of solvents, food grade alcohol is most often used as it is the strongest and provides the longest shelf life, up to three years or longer. However, regardless of the type of solvent used, all tinctures are easy to carry and are readily absorbed by the body's digestive process. Some people object to the taste of alcohol tinctures (even though most can be concealed in juice or tea) and there are situations when even small amounts of alcohol are undesirable. The extracts made with glycerin are nonalcoholic and sweet tasting (so, child-friendly), but are considerably weaker in potency than the alcohol extracts. Likewise, vinegar extracts are not as potent as alcohol tinctures and not readily available commercially; but there are those who feel that vinegar, especially apple-cider vinegar, adds healing properties of its own. When using tinctures follow specific manufacturers' recommendations for dosage.

Capsules may contain crushed, dried herbs or the more concentrated powdered extract. The size of the capsule will determine the dose of the unaltered dried herb, with the standard "double 00" capsules holding 500 mg. If the contents are powdered extract the strength will be higher. This is one compelling reason why it is so important to develop the habit of reading labels, so you know as clearly as possible what exactly you are getting. (See Table 22–1.)

External forms of herbal medicines also are extremely effective and with many possible variations in form and content, they can be useful in a wide array of situations. For example, an infusion or decoction of echinacea or goldenseal can be used as a gargle to ease the inflammation of a sore throat. A compress is made by soaking a soft cloth in a warm or cool tea made with the appropriate herb and applied to an injury, sore, or wound to speed healing. A poultice is similar, but the herb itself is applied to the skin. This could be as quick and simple as crushing a fresh plantain leaf and pressing it to a bug bite or sting to bring relief, or as specific as mixing a combination of herbs, say garlic, mustard, and onions, wrapping them in gauze and securing them over the

TABLE 22–1 POINTS TO CONSIDER IN REGARD TO STANDARDIZED EXTRACTS AND WHOLE PLANT PRODUCTS

Standardized Extract	Whole Plant Products
• Highly purified standard amount of specific constituents	• Can confirm active constituents present at a certain level
• Nonsynthetic powerful medicine	• Does not interfere with the natural synergistic balance of nature's intent
• Some herbs have organ-specific activities and indications	• Promotes traditional or holistic approach; prevention and nutrition
• Insures proper identification of plants	• Some variations in concentration of components depending on growing conditions
• Promotes more allopathic approach of treating symptoms	• Record of thousands of years of use and efficacy
• Clinical testing and research data are available	• Less expensive than standardized extracts
• Evidence of increased incidence of side effects	• Solvents and preservatives typically include alcohol, vinegar, water, and glycerin
• May lose all other activity, but targeted effect	
• Solvents such as hexane are involved in the extraction process; solvent residues can be liver toxins	
• Takes plant constituents out of context; perpetuates the idea that we can outsmart or improve upon nature	

Note: It stands to (holistic) reason to determine what will serve the individual best in each situation. Perhaps employing standardized extract in more acute cases and relying on whole plants for the majority of health needs involving nutrition, prevention, and tonification (tonics). The important issue is having access to, and being able to use, what works best for the individual in a given scenario.

chest to break up the congestion of a cold. Herbal tea bags make a handy poultice (wet thoroughly and bandage where needed). Yet another very effective way to use a tea is as an herbal steam inhalation, breathing in the medicinal steam to lessen the inflammation, irritation, and discomfort of sinus infections or head colds. This also is a great idea to add to your routine to prevent illness as many herbs that are used this way are antiviral and antibacterial with the steam helping to keep the mucous membranes in top condition to fend off infection causing bugs.

Liniments are tinctures that are used only externally. Because the alcohol they contain is usually the isopropyl (rubbing) type, a liniment absorbs quickly on skin, carrying the medicine into the tissues. Salves and ointments are semisolid preparations designed for application to the skin using oil-base substances or beeswax with dried herbs. They are not meant to blend into the skin but to form a protective outer layer that holds the medicine in place and prolongs the time that the herbs remain moist. (Included in the Suggested Readings are books that go into great detail about making your own remedies, some providing extremely helpful illustrations of each step and pictures of commonly used herbs. In addition there is a list of suppliers for finding needed materials.)

Cultivating Herbal Wisdom

Once you have made the decision to incorporate herbal medicine as part of your holistic health approach there are some general guidelines and tips that can help make your relationship with plants rewarding and safe. Become familiar with a few herbs. A single herb can offer multiple health benefits, so you may find most of your herbal needs can be met from a few plants. Attend one of the increasingly available classes and workshops. To locate courses and events check with local health food stores, wellness centers, and universities. Also, the American Herbalists Guild and the American Botanical Council (listed in Resources) are great organizations to check with regarding educational programs.

When deciding where to buy herbs try to purchase locally and organically grown produce when possible. Become attuned to looking for sustainably harvested products (plants that are collected in an ecologically and environmentally-conscious manner). This may require a little investigation, but is well worth the effort. Search for reputable companies, particularly those with the reputation of being in the business for more reasons than just making a profit. The quality of the medicine will be enhanced by the social consciousness and good intentions of the company producing it.

Some precautions are needed when gathering your own herbs from the wild (*wildcrafting*). First, be absolutely sure that you properly identify the plant as there are many examples of different plants that resemble each other very closely, some of them being very toxic. Be aware of the potential for chemical/pesticide contamination where you pick. For instance, don't pick along busy roads where the plants are exposed to many different pollutants from auto exhaust to detergent-laden runoff. Also, know plants well enough to avoid picking them if they are endangered species. All of these precautions can be disregarded if you are in a position to grow some herbs on your own. There are some books listed at the end of this chapter to help you do that.

For best results when using herbs be consistent; take them in the recommended amounts and with the recommended frequency. If taking something long term (as a tonic) it is a good idea to omit the herb at regular intervals. For instance, five days on/two days off or one month on/one week off, the individual situation and the herb used will help determine the schedule.

When treating a specific condition avoid starting herbs that are generally promoted as good for the condition without some assessment. Consider how you feel and what may have contributed to or precipitated the situation. Do not ignore symptoms or delay seeking the most appropriate care or therapy. If you have a known problem consult with a healthcare practitioner, especially if you are taking other medications. The ideal approach in these situations is to work with an experienced professional herbalist. If you don't know of one, try contacting the American Herbalists Guild to see if there is a member in your area. In lieu of an herb-savvy healthcare professional, the safest way to proceed is with one herb at a time.

KEY POINT

Remember that the term *natural* does not necessarily mean *safe!*

You will do well to remember that herbs are medicines and need to be used appropriately and correctly. It is important to know the dosage range and understand that a higher dose doesn't necessarily mean greater effectiveness. Also in regard to safety you must consider individual allergies and sensitivities, particularly if taking an herb for the first time start with a low dose (perhaps half the recommended dose) and work up to a standard dose over a couple days.

KEY POINT

When using herbs with children particular attention must be paid to dose. A general rule of thumb is to use half the adult dose for children ages 7–12 and one quarter of the dose for children below 7 years of age. Of course, the same guidelines of safety must be applied as are considerations for the specific situation and individual child. Using herbs with infants should only be done with the guidance of a healthcare practitioner.

Be aware that there are definitely situations when the use of specific herbs is inappropriate and contraindicated (should be avoided) as they may give rise to side effects or complicate the situation. This is particularly true during pregnancy and breastfeeding. Although there seems to be information released daily regarding drug/drug and food/drug interactions. To date there is relatively little that is known about interactions between synthetic pharmaceuticals and herbs. Until more research is available, use common sense and check several reliable resources, including the practitioner who prescribed the medication. Healthcare providers need to be kept aware of all medicines, herbs, remedies, and supplements that are being taken by their patients. A growing number of pharmacists are becoming more knowledgeable about herbs and many have access to computer databases that can help alert people to possible undesirable interactions to avoid side effects. The literature shows that most problems related to using herbs arise from misuse, allergic reactions, or improper combining with pharmaceuticals, all of which can be avoided by taking the responsibility to use herbs wisely, thoughtfully, and with respect for the abundance of health that they offer.

The following pages list some of the more popular and useful herbs readily available, along with a combination of information gathered from time-tested experience and what modern science has validated. This information is by no means all encompassing, but offered as a place to begin.

Quick Review of Some Popular Herbs

Burdock *(Arctium lappa)*

FAMILY: Compositae
OTHER NAMES: Beggars buttons, cockle buttons, cocklebur, burr seed, hardock
HABITAT: Open fields, roadsides, and waste places
PARTS USED: Root and seed
COMMON USES: Blood cleanser/purifier (Alternative)
CAUTIONS: Do not take during pregnancy. May cause dermatitis in sensitive individuals.

Burdock is a large biannual plant growing up to 6-feet-tall with huge leaves, and a deep taproot, which can reach 30 feet in length. Small purple flowers appear at the top of a single stalk in late spring of the second year and mature into seed heads, which readily stick to almost anything they touch. These are also known as beggars buttons because they were once used to fasten clothing together. The concept of Velcro® is based on the sticky nature of burdock seed heads.

In Japan, the long taproot is known as *Gobo* and is used for food. Fresh, sliced, young roots can be slice and added to a stir-fry or soup to make a nutritious meal. In general, it is an important tonic herb, which is considered gentle and nourishing. Traditionally, burdock root has been used as a blood purifier because of its ability to support the body's function in elimination of waste products via the liver. Herbalists use the root as a mild diuretic (increasing fluid elimination through the kidneys) and to promote sweating during some illnesses. A decoction of the root or tincture of the seeds can be used for dry-skin disorders, such as eczema and psoriasis. Additionally, some cases of acne respond to treatment with burdock.

A root poultice or oil infusion of leaves can be applied to skin sores and leg ulcers. A compress made with a strong decoction will help treat topical fungal infections.

Black Cohosh *(Cimicifuga racemosa)*
FAMILY: Ranunculaceae
OTHER NAMES: Black snake root, fairy candles, bugbane
HABITAT: Densely shaded, deciduous woods
PARTS USED: Dried root and rhizome
COMMON USES: General anti-inflammatory, menopausal symptoms, menstrual cramps, antispasmodic, sedative
CAUTIONS: Large doses (over 2 teaspoons) may cause headache. Do not use during pregnancy or while nursing. Take with food to avoid stomach irritation with long-term use.

Black cohosh is a perennial plant, which often reaches 6 feet in height and produces a rather showy spike of white flowers in mid-summer. It is a spectacular site when the sunlight filters down though the woodland canopy and strikes individual "candles" setting them a-glow. This herb was greatly valued by Native Americans as a remedy for joint pain. It is often used as part of a formula (in combination with other herbs) to reduce inflammation of joints and soft tissues. This is an action people have found useful in easing the discomfort of some forms of arthritis, bursitis, and fibromyalgia. It is also normalizing to the female reproductive system, providing relief of uterine pain and decreasing menopausal symptoms, such as hot flashes and anxiety. Because black cohosh can reduce spasms, it can be an aid in treating whooping cough and relaxing tense muscles. Black cohosh can also be used as a tincture or a decoction.

Calendula *(Calendula officinalis)*
FAMILY: Compositae
OTHER NAMES: Pot marigold

HABITAT: Mediterranean area, however, it can be cultivated in any good garden soil.

PARTS USED: Flower petals

COMMON USES: Topically for healing skin and mucous membranes, internally for stomach ulcers, fevers, and menstrual cramps

CAUTIONS: Do not take during pregnancy.

This bright yellow member of the marigold family is native to the Mediterranean region and lacks the strong smell of its more familiar nonmedicinal cousin. Almost anyone can easily grow calendula in a sunny location.

Calendula's anti-inflammatory and wound-healing properties make it a very useful herb. As an ointment, it can be applied to bruises, cuts, and scrapes. In the form of a tincture, it is a wonderful mouth rinse for red, irritated gums, gingivitis, and pyorrhea. A tea can be used as an aid in healing mouth tissues after oral surgery, as well as treating a sore throat or mouth ulcers. Just gargle and rinse. A poultice or compress can be applied to varicose veins and bruises. A tea or glycerite tincture used topically can help with healing bedsores. Although calendula is considered a mild remedy, it is effective as a tea to sooth unpleasant conditions like stomach ulcers. Externally it can often reduce the effects of eruptions, such as measles or shingles. For day-to-day use, calendula cream makes skin feel soft and silky. In the form of a lotion it is an excellent beauty aid for cleansing and soothing the skin.

Chaste Berries *(Vitex agnus-castus)*

FAMILY: Verbenaceae

OTHER NAMES: Chaste tree, monk's pepper, hemp tree

HABITAT: Mediterranean region of Asia

PARTS USED: Fruit

COMMON USES: Female tonic, kidney tonic, and thyroid tonic

CAUTIONS: Do not take during pregnancy or while nursing. May cause *urticaria* (itching).

Vitex is a deciduous shrub growing up to 10 feet high with flower spikes made up of dense, showy clusters of pale, lilac blue flowers. In folklore, the plant was given the name of *monk's pepper* because of the alleged use of the fruit in monasteries for its ability to reduce male libido.

As a female tonic, Vitex can be used to reduce common symptoms associated with imbalances of the menstrual cycle and menopause. It is believed to work through the female pituitary gland, which is responsible for the secretion of the hormones that regulate the ovaries. Because of this mechanism of action, it is a primary herb in helping menopausal symptoms, such as hot flashes and mood swings. It may decrease water gain in women with PMS and help rebalance hormones when coming off birth control pills. It has been found effective in the treatment of certain types of ovarian cysts and has been shown to reduce some types of acne during puberty in both males and females. Vitex can be safely taken for months at a time with intermittent breaks to check if it is still needed.

Chaste tree can be used as a tea or a tincture.

Cinnamon *(Cinnamomum zeylanicum)*
FAMILY: Lauraceae
OTHER NAMES: Cassia
HABITAT: Tropical Asia
COMMON USES: Antiviral, antibacterial, analgesic (pain relieving), mild digestive disorders and intestinal cramping in children and adults, flatulence, circulatory stimulant
PARTS USED: Bark
CAUTIONS: Do not use with active stomach ulcers or during pregnancy. Some individuals may be sensitive and develop contact irritation.

Cinnamon is an evergreen with dense, leathery leaves that grows 30 to 40 feet tall. It is a tropical tree native to China. Cinnamon is used as a both food and a medicine. While widely known for adding a pleasing, mellow flavor to desserts and ethnic foods, it is very safe as a medicine for children and adults. As a tea for nausea, vomiting, and motion sickness, it is pleasant and soothing.

Ground cinnamon can reduce diarrhea, especially if mixed in applesauce, because applesauce contains pectin, which helps bind the bowels. Cinnamon also possesses antibacterial properties. Because it is a warming herb, it can be used to increase circulation. Prevention and treatment of peripheral neuropathies (numbness of the fingers and toes common in advanced diabetes) is an appropriate use of this herb. An easy way to take Cinnamon for this purpose is in capsules.

Cayanne *(Capsicum annum)*
FAMILY: Solanaceae
OTHER NAMES: Hot pepper, red pepper
HABITAT: Tender annual can be cultivated in any good garden soil
COMMON USES: Stimulate circulation, aid in nerve pain, anti-inflammatory
PARTS USED: Dry, ground pods without seeds
CAUTION: Do not use the seeds (as they can be too irritating). Use with caution during pregnancy. Do not use on broken or injured skin. Avoid getting capsicum in the eyes. Some individuals may develop sensitivity to both internal and external applications. It is not recommended to take capsicum for more than two days at a time.

Cayenne is popular as a condiment for food, especially in Asian, Mexican, and Indian cuisines. Recently it has gained popularity in contemporary medicine as a topical cream to reduce nerve pain. It has been shown effective in treating mild frostbite, muscle tension, rheumatism, and chronic lumbago (lower back pain) by increasing circulation.

Internal uses include stimulating the appetite and the prevention of atherolosclerosis (plaque buildup in the arteries). Cayenne is available in capsule form, which helps in avoiding its hot, spicy sensation. Many topical ointments are available over the counter. Always follow the manufacturer's directions.

Dandelion *(Taraxacum officinale)*
FAMILY: Compositae
OTHER NAMES: Piss-a-bed, teeth of the lion, *Dent de' Leon*
HABITAT: Lawns, meadows, and roadsides
PARTS USED: Whole plant, leaves, flowers, roots, stem
COMMON USES: Blood tonic, diuretic, digestive bitter, stimulates the liver
CAUTIONS: Do not collect from sprayed lawns or roadsides

This ubiquitous little weed, which is the bane of many homeowners, is indeed, a wonderful tonic and medicine, with every part having uses. The leaves are a rich source of calcium, magnesium, sodium, zinc, manganese, copper, iron, phosphorus, and vitamins C and D. It is so nutritious that it made the top of the list in a Japanese vegetable survey of the world's most nutrient-dense plants! The golden yellow flowers are high in flavonoids and antioxidants and a good way to use them is in savory spring biscuits or salads. The tender young leaves are also good steamed, sautéed, or raw in salads. The leaves as a medicine are a gentle, potassium-sparing (will not deplete the body of vital potassium) diuretic, making it useful in some types of congestive heart failure, high blood pressure, and water retention related to PMS. The stem, if pulled apart, exudes a milky white liquid that when applied directly and consistently 2 to 3 times daily for a couple of weeks can alleviate warts. The root can also be eaten as food in addition to having medicinal uses, which include blood purifier (alterative) and liver remedy. It gently supports and strengthens liver function while reducing liver congestion and enhancing the flow of bile. Furthermore, dandelion's bitter action stimulates digestion, absorption of nutrients, and elimination of wastes. These are some of the reasons why dandelion was usually one of the plants used to make traditional spring tonics. After a long sedentary winter eating heavy foods people took advantage of the freshly sprouting herbs around them to effect their own internal spring cleaning.

NOTE: Seek the advice of your practitioner or medical doctor if your symptoms include pain or the whites of your eyes are yellow.

Dong Quai *(Angelica sinensis)*
FAMILY: Umbelliferae
OTHER NAMES: Tang kwei (there are a variety of spellings and pronunciations)
HABITAT: China

COMMON USES: PMS, menopause, balancing female hormones, anemia, heart and circulatory tonic, antispasmodic

PARTS USED: Root

CAUTION: Individuals who have mid-cycle spotting or menstrual flooding should not take dong quai. Do not take during pregnancy.

This is a small fern-leafed, aromatic plant, which is native to China. Dong quai is a much revered, traditional Chinese tonic herb and can be found in many oriental grocery stores. The roots, which are the parts used, are often sliced and incorporated in soups and stews. In the West, it is used as a circulatory stimulant, and as a laxative in older people. It can help nourish women with long menstrual cycles, bloating, and heavy bleeding with associated weakness, mild anemia (because of its significant iron content), and menopausal symptoms of hot flashes, skin crawling, and vaginal dryness.

Dong quai can be added to any soup by placing the roots in a cheese cloth bag and removing it before serving. This herb can also be taken as a tea or tincture.

Echinacea (Echinacea angustifolia, prupurea, or pallida)

FAMILY: Compositae

OTHER NAMES: Purple coneflower

HABITAT: Prairies, meadows; is easily cultivated

PARTS USED: Root, whole flowering head

COMMON USES: Immune system stimulant, anti-inflammatory, antibacterial

CAUTIONS: Do not use with autoimmune diseases, such as lupus, some forms of arthritis, or AIDS. Because it stimulates the immune system it has the potential of causing a flare up.

Echinacea once grew in abundance on the Great Plains. Native Americans used this plant for medicinal purposes long before white settlers arrived on the shores of North America. It is now grown commercially with tons being exported to Europe annually. It has also become a common garden perennial, growing well in most sunny, dry locations and attracting butterflies.

Many people know echinacea as the immune herb. It has gained popularity for its ability to prevent a cold or flu or shorten the duration and severity of symptoms. A tincture is an effective way to take this herb for this purpose. Be aware that a good quality preparation will make the inside of the mouth tingle for a short period of time. The most appropriate and effective use is on exposure to a bacterial or viral infection or at the first signs of the same. The strategy most people find effective is to use the tincture, taking 1 or 2 droppers full every 2 to 3 hours as long as symptoms exist (or a couple of days), four times a day for another 2 to 3 days.

A less well-known use for echinacea is as a topical treatment for skin infections, such as boils, carbuncles, and bug bites. For this purpose, a strong tea or tincture can be applied as a compress. A tea may also serve as a mouthwash or gargle for gingivitis or inflamed sore throat.

Garlic *(Allium sativium)*

FAMILY: Allium
OTHER NAMES: Stinking rose
HABITAT: Any good garden soil
PARTS USED: Individual cloves from the bulb
COMMON USES: Heart tonic, blood thinner, lung infections, lower cholesterol, lower blood pressure
CAUTIONS: Do not take medicinal amounts of garlic if you are on blood thinners (such as coumadin) or high daily doses of vitamin E without medical advice. Discontinue at least one week before any surgical procedure, to avoid prolonged bleeding.

Garlic was cultivated over 5,000 years ago. It is sometimes know as the stinking rose due to its acrid smell when sliced or chopped. Garlic is rich in germanium, which is a powerful antioxidant, and sulfur, which can reduce the risk of stomach, lung, and bowel cancers. In WWI and WWII, garlic was used as a wound dressing because of its strong antibacterial and antiviral properties.

Garlic is both a food and a medicine as many herbs are—adding to the wisdom "let your medicine be your food and your food be your medicine." Activity of garlic makes it good for preventing atherosclerosis (buildup of plaque in the veins and arteries). It also acts as a mild blood thinner and can help lower blood lipids (cholesterol) and blood pressure.

Garlic possesses potent antimicrobial (antibacterial, antiviral, and antifungal) activity, but it is best used fresh and uncooked for this purpose. Because the medicinal volatile oils are excreted through the lungs, it is useful for respiratory infections, such as colds and bronchitis. The suggested dose is to crush 2 to 3 raw cloves (the small sections of the garlic bulb) four times a day.

Because garlic can be unpleasant if taken straight, mixing it with a little honey, yogurt, or applesauce is very helpful. Or try chopping the clove up and placing it on a spoon, don't chew it, but wash it down with water (like a pill). This method can help reduce the taste and residual odor. Also, raw garlic can be delicious and medicinal eaten when in the form of pesto or grated over pasta. Because of the high levels of volatile oil compounds, garlic can be irritating to the stomach lining despite taking it with food. If irritation occurs, discontinue use for a period of time then restart at a small dose.

There are a great variety of commercial products available, manufactured to minimize the odor and other less desirable effects. Some of these have been the subject of research for their effects on cholesterol and blood pressure and are quite effective. However, for the antimicrobial action and cost effectiveness, fresh organically grown garlic is still the best bet.

Siberian Ginseng *(Elutherococcus senticosus)*
FAMILY: Araliaceae
OTHER NAMES: Ginseng
HABITAT: Siberia, China, Northern Korea
PARTS USED: Root bark
COMMON USES: Normalize body systems, help in adapting to stress (adaptogen)
CAUTIONS: Breast tenderness in some normally menstruating women. Some individuals may develop high blood pressure and should discontinue use. No other side effects have been documented with proper use.

Siberian ginseng is a relative of American and Chinese ginsengs. It was first studied in Russia for its effects on productivity of factory workers, and was shown to increase productivity and reduce the incidence of disease. In studies among athletes, endurance, speed, and stamina were increased, and recovery time was shorter.

Siberian ginseng is used as a tonic remedy for people who are stressed out, over worked, and burning the candle at both ends. It is milder and less stimulating than American ginseng (Panax) and greatly valued for its ability to help the body adapt to and handle stress.

It can be taken as a tea or tincture for up to three months at a time, then take a break, and reevaluate how you are feeling.

Goldenseal *(Hydrastis canadensis)*
FAMILY: Ranunculaceae
OTHER NAMES: Yellow root
HABITAT: Deciduous woodlands (endangered species)
COMMON USES: Antibacterial, anti-inflammatory, antifungal
PART USED: Rhizome and root
CAUTION: Do not use during pregnancy. Do exceed the recommended dose. Not for long-term use.

Goldenseal is native to deciduous woodlands of North America. Overcollection and misuse has made it an endangered species. Although it can be cultivated, it is a slow and tricky process. Therefore, it is best to reserve use for stubborn, resistant infections of the mucous membranes that cannot be eliminated with other herbs or medications. Fortunately, there are other herbs that contain some of the same powerful constituents as goldenseal.

Goldenseal is often misused in remedies for colds and flu. It is not effective, and therefore wasted, on systemic (distributed by the blood stream) diseases. It will not help with general malaise, fever, or aches and pains. It is only useful to the body tissue with which it comes in direct contact. In other words, eyes, mouth, and digestive and urinary tract. For example, if goldenseal is used for a sore throat during a cold or flu, it will help the sore throat, but will not strengthen the general immune system or reduce fever. Other herbs, such as echinacea are better suited for helping to fight the flu or a cold. Suggested and appropriate uses for goldenseal include urinary tract infections, gastritis, and athlete's foot. It is a very strong herb and a little goes a long way.

Use a tea for nasal wash, eyewash (sterile tea solution) for conjunctivitis, and as a mouth rinse for gum disease, infection, or sore throat. When preparing an eyewash, carefully strain the tea through a coffee filter then reheat to sterilize. Cool to room temperature for use.

Milk Thistle *(Silybum marianum)*

FAMILY: Compositae
OTHER NAMES: St. Mary's thistle
HABITAT: Originated in Europe but will grow in any temperate climate (can become a noxious weed)
COMMON USES: Liver tonic, liver protectant, stimulating breast milk production
PARTS USED: Leaves, seeds
CAUTION: Do not take during pregnancy. Can cause mild diarrhea in large doses.

Milk thistle is a stout, hardy, invasive, annual plant. It can grow to up to three-feet-high sporting dark green, scallop-edged spiny leaves with white streaks. The petals of the solitary purple flowers end in sharp spines. While the leaves and seeds both have medicinal value, the seed contains the highest amount of the active component *sylibin*, which is credited with the ability to protect the liver from the damage caused by many drugs, including chemotherapy. It also provides protection from the potentially harmful effects of many environmental pollutants, chemicals, and alcohol.

Milk thistle has been the focus of many scientific investigations using human studies. It is effective in treating some types of liver disease, including cirrhosis, viral hepatitis, and chronic liver degeneration and has been shown to stimulate regeneration of the liver cells. For these purposes standardized extracts (tinctures and freeze-dried extracts) are probably most appropriate, because of the high concentration of active constituents that are most soluble in alcohol.

Silybum marianum was named milk thistle because of the traditional use of a tea from the leaves to stimulate milk production in nursing mothers. The leaves also enhance digestion.

Milk thistle is also good for inflammation of the joints associated with arthritis, sometimes combined with other herbs, such as black cohosh, ginger, and turmeric.

Plantain (Plantago major, lanceolata)

FAMILY: Plantaginacea

OTHER NAMES: White man's foot

HABITAT: Common weed of lawns, gardens, and meadows

COMMON USES: Topical and internal antibacterial, anti-inflammatory, demulcent (soothing) coughs, wound healing, insect bites and stings, seed can be used as a bulk laxative

PARTS USED: Leaves, root, seed

CAUTION: Do not collect plantain from contaminated areas or sprayed lawns. Some individuals may be allergic to plantain.

The American Indians named plantain white man's foot because it appeared to sprout up in the footsteps of the white settlers as they moved west. It is now common throughout most of the United States. The dark green, glossy, ribbed leaves radiate from the ground. Beneath the earth are the short, dense, radiating, brown roots. The flowers and seeds form at the top of tall stalks.

Plantain has extraordinary healing properties. Use a poultice of the leaves for insect or spider bites and bee stings. In an emergency, plantain can be gathered from a lawn or meadow, chewed up, and applied directly onto the bite or sting. Cover and keep it in place for 1 to 2 hours. The pain and swelling will quickly diminish. This remedy often works better than over-the-counter pharmaceuticals. A poultice can also be applied to cuts, scrapes, and burns to aid in healing. Plantain leaf tea or juice (combine with tomato, carrot, or vegetable juice) is an effective way to soothe the symptoms of gastritis, irritable bowel, or colitis, and relieve the discomfort from urinary tract infections. A tea of the leaf or root is also a mild, soothing expectorant (facilitates removal of secretions from the lungs), which makes it useful for treating bronchitis and lung congestion. The seeds are a rich source of zinc and psyllium, which is a popular bulk laxative.

Rosemary (Rosmarinus officinalis)

FAMILY: Labiatae

OTHER NAMES: Dew of the Sea

HABITAT: Native to the Mediterranean region, will grow in any average garden soil.

COMMON USES: Antimicrobial, dyspepsia, rheumatism, moth repellant, some types of headache, memory aid, antioxidant, digestive aid

PARTS USED: Leaves

CAUTION: Do not use in medicinal amounts during pregnancy. Rosemary leaves are quite safe, but the essential oil should be used with caution due to its potency.

Rosemary is a native of the Middle East and around the Mediterranean Sea. From afar, it looks like green sea foam on the face of the cliffs by the sea; hence its name "dew of the sea." It is easy to grow in average garden soil, but is not winter hardy. It can be grown indoors, but it is temperamental and does not like to dry out.

This herb is excellent on roasted potatoes and with lamb and other foods, but as a medicine the crushed leaves possess potent antimicrobial activity (kills bacteria and virus), which is due to the high content of volatile oils. During World War II, rosemary leaves and juniper berries were burned in hospitals as a disinfectant.

For gas, nausea, and biliousness take as a tea or tincture. To stimulate circulation, soothe aches and rheumatic pain, make a strong tea and add it to bath water or make a warm compress and apply over affected areas. This is a good herb to use in steam inhalations for prevention or treatment of colds.

Lemon Balm *(Melissa officinalis)*

FAMILY: Laminacea

OTHER NAMES: Sweet Mary, honey plant, cure-all, dropsy plant, Melissa

HABITAT: Native to the Mediterranean region and western Asia. Lemon balm will grow vigorously in average soil in temperate climates; it is a common garden herb.

COMMON USES: Antibacterial, antiviral, antidepressant, nervine (calms nervousness), insomnia

PARTS USED: Fresh leaves are preferred, dry leaves can be used

CAUTION: Hypothyroidism

Lemon balm is a mild, aromatic, tasty, and effective remedy. It can be safely used for children's colds and stomachaches. It has a mild sedative effect and can be used to reduce melancholy and anxiety. It has been know for centuries as the gladdening herb. Just sniffing fresh lemon balm can lift one's spirits.

For adults, lemon balm can be combined with St. John's Wort for seasonal affective disorder (SAD or winter blues). Add St. John's Wort tincture to lemon balm tea. Because of its antiviral activity it can be an extremely effective treatment for mouth ulcers and canker sores. Just place a poultice of ground or liquefied fresh leaves on the site. Keep in place up to several hours, repeat as needed. A poultice or compress (made by soaking a cloth in a strong tea) can be used to ease the discomfort of herpes lesions or shingles.

For cold sores, mix a few drops of lemon balm essential oil with 2 to 3 tablespoons of glycerin and dab on the sore.

Licorice *(Glycyrrhiza glabra)*

FAMILY: Leguminosae

OTHER NAMES: Sweet root

HABITAT: Southeastern Europe and western Asia

COMMON USES: Gastric irritation, tonic, expectorant (helps remove secretions from the chest), anti-inflammatory

PARTS USED: Root

CAUTION: Licorice should be avoided by individuals with high blood pressure, kidney disease, and edema. Large amounts over time can cause sodium retention and potassium depletion. Avoid during pregnancy.

This perennial member of the pea family has long been cultivated for its flavorful root. Licorice has been a popular ingredient in candy and to disguise the unpleasant taste of other medicine. It is an integral part of traditional Chinese medicine and is used to balance other herbs used in a formula.

Licorice is used to reduce cough and soothe the chest in bronchitis and congestion. It can reduce stomach acid and is therefore, useful for stomach ulcers.

Saw Palmetto *(Seranoa repens)*
FAMILY: Palmaceae
OTHER NAMES: Seronna serrulata, sabal
HABITAT: Subtropical sandy soil
COMMON USES: Tonic for male and female reproductive organs, respiratory system, irritable bladder
PARTS USED: Berry
CAUTION: No known side effects when used as recommended.

Saw palmetto is also known as Spanish sword because its long slender leaves, which radiate from the ground, have sharp serrated edges that can rip clothing and skin. This can make collecting the berries a challenge. Writings suggest that the berries smell and taste like rotten cheese. Due to this and the added fact that many of the activities are not released in water make its use as a tea undesirable.

Saw palmetto has gained recognition as the prostate herb and is beginning to be accepted by many medical doctors for its ability to relieve symptoms associated with an enlarged prostate (also known as benign prosthetic hypertrophy or BPH). Its effectiveness has been born out in modern studies. Additional uses include the treatment of chronic lung disease, upper respiratory tract infections, and stimulation of the immune system. Furthermore, it has been found useful for ovarian pain and cysts, and male and female infertility.

It is best taken as a liquid or powdered alcohol extract as the active properties are not water soluble.

St. John's Wort *(Hypericum perforatum)*
FAMILY: Guttiferae
OTHER NAMES: Hardhay, amber, goatweed, klamath weed, tipton weed
HABITAT: Open fields, roadsides
COMMON USES: Antidepressant, antianxiety

PARTS USED: Flowers and buds

CAUTION: Some individuals may become sensitive to the sun with high doses. There has been much discussion and controversy regarding occurrences of side effects related to combining St. John's Wort with pharmaceutical antidepressants. A common sense approach is to check with your healthcare practitioner before combining any herb and drug.

This stout little plant has come to be known as the depression herb, but its uses are much broader. St. John's Wort has been the subject of substantial research and clinical trials. It is effective in the treatment of peripheral neuropathies (numbness and tingling in the toes and fingers), inflamed nerve endings, brain and spinal cord injuries, and shingles. It has been referred to as "food for the nervous system." Its ability to help in cases of melancholy or mild-to-moderate depression is well documented. The effectiveness of St. John's Wort for treating seasonal affective disorder (SAD) can be enhanced when combined with lemon balm. The remedy should be taken for 4 to 6 weeks before evaluating the effect. If there is no improvement in the condition, reevaluation or another therapy is advocated.

The tea can be useful for menopausal symptoms (along with other herbs) and for inflammation of the digestive system, including gastritis (inflammation of the stomach lining), and peptic ulcer. St. John's Wort oil has been found effective in the topical treatment of wounds and burns.

Thyme (Thymus vulgaris)

FAMILY: Laminacea

OTHER NAMES: Garden Thyme

HABITAT: Native to the Mediterranean region, northern Africa, and parts of Asia. It can be grown in average garden soil in a sunny location.

COMMON USES: Antibacterial, antiviral, expectorant (helping to remove secretions) of colds and bronchitis, antifungal

PARTS USED: Leaves

CAUTION: Avoid large amounts with hypothyroidism

Thyme has been widely used for centuries as both a culinary and medicinal herb. This perennial shrub can be easily grown in a sheltered spot in the garden.

Thyme has powerful antiseptic activity. A strong tea should be considered to help eliminate mucus congestion, coughs, or sore throat associated with a cold or flu. A soothing cough medicine can be made by steeping dried thyme in honey. Tea can also be used as a gargle to ease or prevent a sore throat. Add a strong tea to bath water to soothe and deodorize the skin. A steam inhalation is effective for sinus congestion.

Ginkgo (Ginkgo biloba)
   FAMILY: Ginkgoaceae
   OTHER NAMES: Maidenhair tree
   HABITAT: Native to China
   COMMON USES: Improve circulation
   PARTS USED: Leaves
   CAUTION: Some individuals may have allergic reactions. Ginkgo dilates blood vessels, therefore individuals who have fragile blood vessels and a tendency to bleed easily should not take ginkgo. Those with a history of stroke-related aneurysm (bleeding as opposed to blood clot) should avoid ginkgo as should those on blood-thinning therapies, such as coumadin.

Ginkgo trees are among the oldest living plants in the world. Their survival is partly explained by the fact that they were considered sacred trees by the Chinese and therefore protected. Recently, cultivated trees have proven to be one of the finest specimen trees for inner cities, thriving undeterred by pests and pollution. These are usually the trees you see growing out of cracks in the sidewalk.

Ginkgo is one of the most researched herbs in the world. It has many uses, but most people know ginkgo as the memory herb. It can help if poor memory is due to insufficient blood flow to the brain. Increased circulation to the brain may help dementia (memory loss and confusion often in old age), Alzheimer's disease, vertigo (dizziness, light-headed), disorientation (confusion), and tinnitus (ringing in the ears).

Other circulatory deficiencies can be improved with the use of ginkgo. For example, individuals with poor circulation in their legs my have pain when walking. The pain can be reduced over time with the use of ginkgo. Other indications for ginkgo include macular degeneration (a type of loss of vision), diabetic retinopathy (diabetes-related eye damage), Reynaud's syndrome (decreased circulation in the fingers), some types of headache due to blood vessel constriction, and impotence (if related to decreased blood flow).

Take tinctures as recommended by the manufacturer for up to 2 to 3 months before evaluating improvement. Because of the blood-thinning potential of ginkgo consult your practitioner or herbalist prior to self-treatment.

Sage (Salvia officinalis)
   FAMILY: Laminacea
   HABITAT: Mediterranean region; can be grown in average garden soil
   COMMON USES: Antiseptic, astringent, antispasmodic, antioxidant, antiviral, antibacterial

PARTS USED: Leaves
CAUTION: Do not take during pregnancy.

This beautiful, woody perennial makes a nice addition to any herb garden. It likes a sheltered, sunny location and will withstand moderately cold, snowy winters.

Historically, sage was associated with longevity and mortality. Native Americans used it topically for skin conditions and baths. The astringent, antiseptic qualities of sage make it an ideal gargle for sore throats, gingivitis, or bleeding gums in the form of a tea. A tea is also a good way to make a digestive tonic and to relieve night sweats during menopause, or reduce excessive perspiration.

Brew a strong tea for making a compress to soothe slow healing wounds. Add honey to an infusion for sore throat or cough and take over 1 to 3 days. For colds and sinus congestion, use a steam inhalation to dry up excessive secretions and postnasal drip.

Yarrow (Achillea millefolium)

FAMILY: Compositae
OTHER NAMES: Soldier's wound wort, thousand weed, staunchweed, sanguinary, milfoil
HABITAT: Temperate regions of North America and Europe
COMMON USES: Styptic, anti-inflammatory
PARTS USED: flower heads
CAUTION: Some individual's skin my be sensitive; avoid during pregnancy.

Yarrow is a hardy, rampant grower and easily crowds out more delicate plants. So, you may want to confine it to its own section of the garden. It likes a hot, sunny location and is not fussy about rich soil, but will not tolerate wet roots.

Archeologists have identified fossils of yarrow pollen in Neanderthal burial caves of 60,000 years ago. It was used as a styptic 3,000 years ago to stop bleeding from wounds suffered in the Trojan War. Native American tribes used this herb for skin sores and wounds and it was included in the medical supplies issued during the American Civil War.

Yarrow is best known for its ability to stop bleeding and to reduce inflammation. A tea can be useful for irritable bowel syndrome and gastrointestinal complaints in general. It may be useful in alleviating the symptoms of bladder infections or as an aid to treat hemoptysis (coughing up blood).

A poultice can be placed directly onto bleeding cuts and wounds to stop bleeding.

Chapter Summary

Phytochemicals are chemicals that occur in plants. Herbs can have therapeutic effects in the body, some of which include: tonics, which are nourishing, adaptogens, which help the body regain normal function in the presence of stress, and immune stimulants, which enhance the immune system's ability to fight an illness.

Herbal remedies can be used in the form of an extract, tea, infusion, decoction, tincture, capsule, compress, poultice, liniment, salve, or ointment.

When wildcrafting herbs, caution must be taken to properly identify the plant, assure there is no contamination from pesticides or other chemicals, and to avoid picking endangered species.

Children require lower doses of herbs. Herbs should not be used with infants unless guided by a healthcare practitioner.

Each herb has unique uses and cautions. It is important that individuals become knowledgeable of herbs they intend to use to determine appropriateness for the given condition, dosage, and safety issues.

Suggested Readings

Crawford, M. A. (1997). *Herbal Remedies for Women.* Rocklin, CA: Prima Publishing.

DeBaggio, T. (1995). *Growing Herbs from Seed, Cutting & Root: An Adventure in Small Miracles.* Loveland, CO: Interweave Press.

Duke, J. A. (1997). *The Green Pharmacy.* Emmaus, PA: Rodale Books.

Griggs, B. (1997). *The Green Pharmacy, the History and Evolution of Western Herbal Medicine.* Rochester, VT: Healing Arts Press.

Gruenwald, J., Brendler, T., and Jaenicke, C., eds. (2001). *PDR for Herbal Medicines.* Montvale, NJ: Medical Economics Company.

Hobbs, C. (1998). *Herbal Remedies for Dummies.* Foster City, CA: IDG Books Worldwide, Inc.

Ody, P. (1993). *The Complete Medicinal Herbal.* New York: DK Publishing, Inc.

Winston, D. (1998). *Herbal Therapeutics: Specific Indications for Herbs and Herbal Formulas.* NJ: Herbal Therapeutics Research Library.

Publications

Herbal Gram, PO Box 201660, Austin, TX 78720-1660 (800-373-7105)
Herbs for Health, 201 East Fourth St., Loveland, CO 80401 (800-272-2193)

Organizations

American Botanical Council
PO Box 201660

Austin, TX 78720
515-331-8868; fax 512-331-1924

American Herbalists Guild
PO Box 70
Boulder, CO 80302
Phone 435-722-8434; fax 435-722-8452
www.americanherbalistsguild.com

Herb Research Foundation
1007 Pearl St., Suite 200
Roosevelt, UT 84066
303-449-2265; fax 303-449-7849
www.herbs.org

Resources (mail order)

Herbalist and Alchemist
51 S. Wandling Ave.
Washington, NJ 07882
608-689-9020
Liquid extracts, western and Chinese herbs

Herb Pharm
Box 116
Williams, OR 97544
800-348-4372
Liquid extracts, salves

Jean's Greens
119 Sulfur Springs Rd.
Newport, NY 13416
888-845-8327
Bulk herbs, tea blends, various products

Frontier Herb Co-op
PO Box 299
Norway, IA 52318
800-669-3275
Bulk herbs and variety of products

Seeds of Change
PO Box 15700
Santa Fe, NM 87506-5700
800-957-3337
Organic herb seeds

Shepherd's Garden Seeds
30 Irene St.
Torrington, CT 06790-6658
860-482-3638
Herb seeds

CHAPTER 23

AROMATHERAPY: COMMON SCENTS

Objectives

This chapter should enable you to:

- Define *aromatherapy*
- Describe the method of extraction that makes an essential oil pure
- List the four basic types of aromatherapy
- Describe four methods of using aromatherapy
- Describe the use of aromatherapy for at least five different health problems
- List at least 10 precautions or contraindications with the use of aromatherapy

Aromatherapy refers to the therapeutic use of essential oils. This branch of herbal medicine is often misunderstood and maligned; even its name is a bit of a misnomer. Contrary to popular belief, aromatherapy is not a new therapy, but part of one of the oldest therapies, as herbal medicine dates back 6,000 years. Aromatic plants have been used by many countries, including India, China, North and South America, Greece, the Middle East, Australia, New Zealand, and Europe. According to the World Health Organization, today, more than 85 percent of the world population still relies on herbal medicine, and many of the herbs are aromatic.

The renaissance of modern aromatherapy appeared in France just prior to World War II. (This was around the time the first antibiotics were used.) A physician named Jean Valnet, a chemist named Maurice Gattefosse, and a surgical assistant by the name of Marguerite Maury, were key figures in the rediscovery of this ancient art of healing. What is so fascinating is that they did not use aromatherapy for its nice smell, nor did they use it for stress reduction—two of the most popular ways aromatherapy is used today— instead, they used it clinically, as they would use any natural medicine, to help wounds heal, fight infections, and to improve skin texture. This clinical approach to aromatherapy has survived in France and many physicians still use essential oils as an alternative or enhancement to antibiotics today. In France, as in Germany, the use of plants medicinally (*phytomedicine*), including aromatherapy, is seen as an extension of orthodox medicine.

> ### KEY POINT
>
> Aromatherapy is viewed as such an integral part of medicine in Germany that doctors and nurses there are tested in the use of essential oils in order to become licensed.

Aromatherapy does not just mean using aromas. The real definition of *aromatherapy* is *the therapeutic use of essential oils.* Perhaps we should add the controlled therapeutic use as essential oils are not toys, but powerful tools that can help you stay healthy. Real essential oils are either steam distillates or expressed extracts from aromatic plants. Many of them have familiar smells, such as lavender, rose, and rosemary. However, things are not quite as simple as they seem at first glance.

Essential oils are highly volatile droplets created by a plant itself to help ward off infection (bacterial, fungal, or viral), to regulate growth and hormones, and to mend damaged tissue of the plant. These tiny reservoirs of plant medicine are stored in the plant's veins, glands, or sacs and when they are broken by being crushed or rubbed, the essential oil is released along with the aroma. Lavender has a minimal scent until the flowering head is gently rubbed between two fingers. Some plants store large amounts of essential oils, some store very little. This, along with the difficulty of harvesting the essential oils dictates the price. For example, more than 100 kilograms of fresh rose petals are needed to produce 60 grams of essential oils. (This means that rose is one of the most expensive essential oils on the market today, and also one of the most frequently adulterated!)

There are a few important things to know about essential oils before you start using them for your health and well-being. These are: the method of extraction, the botanical name (for clear identification, see Exhibit 23–1), methods of application, safety, storage, and contraindications.

Extraction

The method of extraction is crucial as only steam-distilled or expressed extracts can legitimately be called essential oils. These two methods produce a pure product

EXHIBIT 23–1 ESSENTIAL OILS MENTIONED IN THIS CHAPTER AND THEIR BOTANICAL NAMES

Aniseed	Pimpinella anisum
Basil	Ocimum basilicum
Chamomile German	Matricaria recutita
Chamomile Roman	Chamomelum nobile
Clary sage	Salvia sclarea
Coriander seed	Coriandrum sativum
Eucalyptus	Eucalyptus globulus
Fennel	Foeniculum vulgare
Geranium	Pelargonium graveolens
Ginger	Zingeber officinale
Hyssop	Hyssopus officinalis
Lavender True	Lavandula officinalis
Lemongrass	Cymbopogon citratus
Neroli	Citrus aurantium var amara
Palmarosa	Cymbopogon martini
Parlsey	Petroselinum sativum
Pennyroyal	Mentha pulegium
Peppermint	Mentha piperita
Rose	Rosa damascena
Rosewood	Aniba rosaeodora
Sage	Salvia officinalis
Sandalwood	Santalum album
Tarragon	Artemesia dracunculus
Wintergreen	Gaultheria procumbens
Ylang ylang	Cananga odorata

with no additional solvent or impurity. A bottle of essential oils should state that the contents are pure essential oils: steam distilled or expressed. (Only the peel from citrus plants, such as mandarin, lime, or lemon produce an expressed oil.)

KEY POINT

Many of the essential oils on the market are solvent extracted using petrochemicals. These hexane-based residues MAY cause allergic or sensitive reactions.

Identification

There can be *many* different species of the same plant. For example the genus (or surname) of thyme is *thymus*, but there are more than 60 different species or varieties of thyme, each with different therapeutic effects. (There are 3 different species of lavender and 600 different species of eucalyptus) It is very important to know the full botanical name of a plant so you can use it correctly. (There is a list of safe essential oils to use at the end of this chapter giving both the botanical name and the common name.) Do not buy anything that is labeled *lavender oil* as you will have no way of knowing what you are buying. Which lavender is it? One lavender is a soothing, calming sedative oil exceptional for burns, but another lavender is a stimulant and expectorant (helps you cough up mucus, and will not help you sleep or sooth your burns). You need to ask the following questions: Is it a true essential oil? How has it been extracted?

The simplest way to ensure you are buying the real thing is to look in one of the professional journals (see Exhibit 23–2) and ask for an order form from one of the advertised suppliers. If they do not list the botanical name, method of extraction, country of origin, and part of the plant you can't be certain what they are selling.

Essential oils are common ingredients in the pharmaceutical, perfume, and food industries and as such, are commonly used by most of the population on a daily basis. Pure essential oils rarely produce an allergic effect, unlike their synthetic cousins. However, many products on the market have been extended with synthetic fragrances and can cause a reaction.

EXHIBIT 23–2 AROMATHERAPY JOURNALS

Aromatherapy Today
PO Box 211
Kellyville, NSW 2155
Australia
02-9894-9933
E-mail: *jkerr@aromatherapytoday.com.* Quarterly

International Journal of Aromatherapy
Aromatherapy Publications
PO Box 945
New York, NY 10159
212-633-3730 or 1800-4ES-INFO
E-mail: *usinfo-f@elsevier.com.* Quarterly

How It Works

As mentioned, the term *aromatherapy* refers to the therapeutic use of essential oils that are the volatile organic constituents of plants. Essential oils are thought to work at psychological, physiological, and cellular levels; this means they can affect our body, our mind, and all the delicate links in between. The effects of aroma can be rapid, and sometimes just thinking about a scent can be as powerful as the actual scent itself. Take a moment to think of your favorite flower. Then think about an odor that makes you feel nauseated. The effects of an aroma can be relaxing or stimulating depending on the previous experience of the individual (called the *learned memory*) as well as the actual chemical makeup of the essential oils used.

KEY POINT

Aromatherapy should not be used as a replacement for medical treatment. It is a complementary therapy and most useful when integrated with conventional medicine.

How Scents Affect You

Olfaction

Essential oils are composed of many different chemical components or molecules. These different chemical components travel via the nose to the olfactory bulb. Nerve impulses travel to the limbic system of the brain, the oldest part of our brain. There the aroma is processed. The limbic part of our brain contains an organ called the *amygdala*. This is the organ that governs your emotional response. Valium is thought to have a calming, sedative effect on the amygdala; lavandula angustifolia (true lavender) has a similar effect. The limbic system also contains another organ called the *hippocampus*. This organ is involved in the formation and retrieval of explicit memories. This is why an aroma can trigger memories that may have lain dormant for years.

Reflection Does the scent of cinnamon buns baking, honeysuckle, or a particular cologne trigger specific memories for you? Can you recall unique scents associated with people or places you have known in the past? What are these?

The effect of scents on the brain has been mapped using computer-generated graphics. These brain electrical activity maps (BEAM) indicate how subjects, linked to an electroencephalogram (EEG), rated different odors presented to them. These maps have shown that scents can have a psychological effect even when the aroma is below the level of human awareness.

There are approximately two million Americans who have lost their sense of smell (1). The loss of the sense of smell is called *anosmia*. However, even in a person who has lost the sense of smell, if the olfactory nerve is intact the chemicals in the aroma will still be able to travel to the limbic part of the brain and have a therapeutic effect.

Absorption Through the Skin

Essential oils are absorbed through the skin through diffusion, in much the same way as medicines administered in patches. The two layers of the skin—the dermis and fat layers—act as a reservoir before the components within the essential oils reach the bloodstream. There is some evidence that massage or hot water enhances the absorption of at least some of the essential oil's components. Essential oils, because they are *lipophyllic* (attracted to fat) can be stored in the fatty areas of the body and can pass through the blood-brain barrier.

Who Uses Aromatherapy?

Aromatherapy is commonly practiced in England, France, Germany, Switzerland, Sweden, Australia, New Zealand, and Japan. It is beginning to grow in use in the U.S. Many nurses and other health professionals are receiving training in aromatherapy to enhance their care. In France, medical doctors and pharmacists use aromatherapy as part of conventional medicine, often for the control of infection.

Types of Aromatherapy

There are four basic types of aromatherapy:

1. Esthetic: Used purely for pleasure, such as in candles and soaps.
2. Holistic: Used for general stress.
3. Environmental fragrancing: Used to manipulate mood or enhance sales.
4. Clinical: Used for specific therapeutic outcomes that are measurable.

Methods of Using Aromatherapy

Essential oils can be absorbed by the body in one of three ways:

1. Inhalation: 1–5 drops undiluted—without touch
2. Through the skin: 1–12 percent diluted in a carrier oil, used with compresses or massage—via touch

3. Orally: 1–2 drops (This is considered aromatic medicine, requiring the training of a primary care provider who has prescribing privileges.)

Inhalation

Direct inhalation means an essential oil is directly targeted to the person: 1–5 drops on a tissue (or floated on hot water in a bowl) and inhaled for 5–10 minutes.

Indirect inhalation includes the use of burners, nebulizers, and vaporizers that can use heat generated by battery or electricity, and may or may not include the use of water. Larger portable aroma systems are available to control the release of essential oils on a commercial scale into rooms up to 1,500 square feet. This is similar to environmental fragrancing (using synthetics), which is common practice in hotels and department stores, and can be useful for mood enhancement and stress reduction.

Baths

Essential oils can be used in baths by dissolving 4–6 drops of essential oil into a teaspoon of milk or salt. Essential oils do not dissolve in water and would float on the top giving an uneven treatment. You then can relax in the bath for 10 minutes.

Compresses

To prepare a compress, add 4–6 drops of essential oil to warm water. Soak a soft cotton cloth in the mixture, wring it out, and apply to the affected area (contusion or abrasion). Cover the external surface with food plastic wrap to maintain moisture, cover with a towel, and keep in place for 4 hours.

Touch

Aromatherapy is often used in a gentle massage or the *m* technique®. Use 1–12 percent essential oils diluted in a teaspoonful (5 ml) of cold-pressed vegetable oil, cream, or gel. Gentle friction and hot water enhances absorption of essential oils through the skin into the blood stream. The amount of essential oils absorbed from an aromatherapy massage will normally be 0.025 ml–0.1 ml: approximately 1/2 to 2 drops.

Aromatherapy and Women's Health

Aromatherapy, which involves the senses of smell and touch, is possibly the most feminine of complementary therapies, and ideally suited to women and their health concerns. (Maybe this is why so many trained aromatherapists are women!)

KEY POINT

As aromatherapy is one of the most nurturing therapies, it is hardly surprising that many nurses throughout the world are learning to use aromatherapy as an enhancement to their nursing care. Aromatherapy began its nursing debut in

England, in geriatric care, when Helen Passant brought it first to the attention of the nursing community in Oxford. She used aromatherapy in the ward and reduced the ward's drug bill by one-third. The hospital immediately responded by reducing her budget by one-third!

Almost every aspect of a woman's life can be enhanced by aromatherapy. It should be noted that although most essential oils have no affect on orthodox medication, some essential oils can augment or diminish the effects of certain medication (1, 2). Following are some women's health problems that can be successfully addressed with aromatherapy.

Problems with the Menstrual Cycle

The menstrual cycle is delicately balanced. Hormones, specifically estrogen, are easily thrown out of balance by stress, illness, poor diet, or overwork. *Pelargonium graveolens* (geranium) has been used for generations to balance the female hormonal system. This species of geranium acts on the adrenal cortex that regulates the endocrine system and, therefore, affects the menstrual cycle (3).

Premenstrual tension, irregular periods, and painful periods can be greatly helped by aromatherapy. Add 3 drops of geranium to a teaspoon of vegetable oil. The vegetable oil should be cold-pressed and not one used for cooking. Gently massage into the lower abdomen and lumbar (lower back) areas. For optimum results, apply morning and evening. For very painful menstrual periods, add 1–2 drops of high altitude *lavandula angustifolia* (true lavender) and *chamaemelum nobile* (Roman chamomile) to enhance the antispasmodic effect. Geranium may also encourage regular ovulation (4).

Menopausal Problems

Pelargonium graveolens (geranium) may be particularly useful during menopause as an adrenal regulator when estrogen supplies begin to dry up. A disruption in the supply of estrogen can lead to irritability, mood swings, and hot flashes. This essential oil is also excellent for mature, dry skin and thread veins that can accompany menopause. Add 3–5 drops of geranium to a teaspoon of evening Primrose oil and rub anywhere on the body, or add 5 drops to a bath and soak for 10 minutes. *Foeniculum vulgare dulce* (sweet fennel), *salvia sclarea* (sage), and *pimpinella anisum* (aniseed) all contain a molecule similar to estradiol—the female hormone—and can be very beneficial at menopause, also.

Hot flashes can be helped with a spritzer of geranium, clary sage, and peppermint. To make a spritzer, add 6 drops of each oil to 10 fluid ounces of water and shake vigorously before spraying the face and neck. Keep eyes closed while spraying.

Infertility

Where there is no physical reason why a woman cannot conceive, often the underlying reason can be one of tension. Trying to become pregnant can be emotionally draining and the longer it takes the more stressful it can become. *Salvia sclaria* (clary sage) related to *salvia officinalis* (common sage), can help a woman relax. Clary sage contains an alcohol (sclareol), which is similar in molecular form to estradiol. As well as having an estrogen-like effect, clary sage is very relaxing and antispasmodic (it contains 75 percent linalyl acetate: an ester).

Morning Sickness

Early morning nausea and vomiting often occurs during the first three months of pregnancy, although it can sometimes last the whole nine months. Nausea can be greatly alleviated with a brief inhalation of *zingiber officinale* (5), (ginger), or *mentha piperita* (6) (peppermint). Always bear in mind that only one or two drops on a handkerchief is necessary, and you can repeat it whenever the need arises. Do not use more than two drops of either essential oil at a time as more may exacerbate the nausea, not alleviate it. The inhalation of either ginger or peppermint for nausea during pregnancy is a soothing and safe practice. Aromatherapy is not particularly advocated during the first three months of pregnancy as essential oils do cross the placenta, however, many expectant mothers like to relax in an aromatic bath and the majority of essential oils will have no detrimental effect when used in this gentle way. Aromatherapy can be used during the remainder of pregnancy, but use caution. Certain essential oils can also be safely used during labor. (Please refer to the books listed in the Resource's list for guidance.)

Breast-Feeding, Engorged Breasts, and Sore Nipples

Foeniculum vulgare (fennel) which mimics estrogen (7), has a good-milk producing action, which can help mothers who breastfeed (8). Fennel also has a soothing decongestant effect on engorged breasts, which will be a relief to those in the early stages of feeding. Apply 1–2 drops diluted in a carrier oil to the breasts, avoiding the nipple area, twice a day. Wash area immediately prior to feeding. As fennel is a gentle laxative, the baby may have looser stools.

KEY POINT

Because of their phytoestrogenic effect, sage, fennel, and aniseed are contraindicated in persons with cancer when the tumor is estrogen dependent.

Both *matricaria recutita* (German chamomile) and *chamaemelum nobile* (Roman chamomile) are used in some European commercial brands of ointment available for sore nipples. Both chamomiles are useful for swelling and congestion (9). Apply a diluted solution in a carrier oil (1 drop per 5 mls) after each feeding and be sure to wash off any residual solution before the next feeding. *Lavandula angustifolia* (true lavender) is another useful essential oil for sore nipples as this lavender has recognized properties that enhance healing.

Postpartum Blues

Postpartum blues or just down in the dumps? Aromatherapy can lift spirits and ease those moments when a mother feels she can't cope with yet another dirty diaper. *Citrus aurantium ssp bergamia* (bergamot) and *Melissa officinalis* (true Melissa) are ideal essential oils to make the day just a little brighter (10, 11). Melissa is difficult to obtain unadulterated, but there are some companies with integrity and the real stuff can work miracles! It is used by putting 1–3 drops on a handkerchief and breathing deeply. Bergamot should not be used topically before sunbathing or using a sunbed as this could result in skin photosensitivity and, in some cases, burns.

Vaginal Infections

Yeast Infection, Anaerobic Vaginitis, and Trichomonas   Vaginal yeast infection, caused by *candida albicans*, is a common nuisance factor in many women's lives. Sometimes the yeast infection may be a side effect of antibiotic treatment and it can occur during pregnancy or after an illness. When it does occur, vaginal yeast infection is messy, uncomfortable, and embarrassing. Some forms are now resistant to many of the conventional preparations (12). However, there is an essential oil that can help eradicate this fungal infection in only a few days and it is called teatree (13). Make sure you have the correct essential oil as teatree is the common name of many different types of plants. The right teatree is called *melaleuca alternifolia CT terpineol*. There is another *melaleuca alternifolia* that contains much higher percentages of terpinerol, an oxide, which can produce discomfort when applied to the skin or mucous membrane. Put a teaspoon of carrier oil onto a saucer. Add 2–3 drops of essential oil and mix with a clean finger. Take a tampon, remove the applicator, and roll the tampon in the mixture until all the mixture has been absorbed. Insert tampon into the vagina.

The tampon should be changed three times a day. Each time soak a new tampon in a fresh dilution of carrier oil with 2–3 drops of teatree. The tampon needs to be kept in the vagina overnight. Commonly, teatree will remove vaginal yeast infection in three days, regardless of how long the person has had the infection. This form of treatment is also very effective against anaerobic vaginitis and trichomonas (14). Incidentally, recent research in both Australia and Great Britain has shown this melaleuca to be effective against methicillin-resistant staphylococcus aureus (MRSA), which is endemic in many hospitals (15).

Cystitis

Inflammation of the bladder can be due to infection, but this is not always the case. Cystitis can plague some unfortunate women for much of their lives, bringing pain and misery and taking a high toll on intimate relationships. Although many factors contribute to cystitis, such as tight clothing, insufficient fluid intake, and a diet of high sugar and refined food, stress does play an important role. There are specific essential oils that can help this condition. Choose an antispasmodic essential oil, which also has a strong antibiotic action, such as *juniperus communis var erecta* (juniper) (16), *cymbopogon citratus* (West Indian lemongrass), which contains myrcene is very effective as a peripheral analgesic or *origanum marjorana* (sweet marjoram) (17). Apply 1–2 drops diluted in a teaspoon of cold-pressed vegetable oil to the lower abdomen and lower back (kidney area). Repeat up to four times a day while the attack lasts, and remember to drink at least two liters of water a day. Drinking cranberry juice can also help in the initial stages of cystitis.

Aromatherapy for Common Complaints

Here are some essential oils that can be used for common complaints that typically are self-medicated. When using essential oils on the skin (topically), use 1–5 drops diluted in a teaspoon of carrier oil. When inhaling the essential oil, inhale 1–2 drops on a cotton ball, or add 1–2 drops to a basin of steaming hot water. (Method of application: I = inhalation. T = topical)

Psychological

Insomnia: lavender, ylang ylang, clary sage, frankincense, neroli (I, T)

Depression: bergamot, basil, lavender, geranium, neroli, angelica, rose, melissa (I, T)

Stress & anxiety: lavender, frankincense, Roman chamomile, mandarin, angelica, rose (I, T)

Anorexia: rose, neroli, lemon, fennel (I, T)

Withdrawal from substance abuse: helichrysum, angelica, rose (T)

Reflection   How do different scents affect your moods? How can you intentionally use this to enhance your health and well-being?

Pain Relief

Migraine: peppermint, lavender (T)

Osteoarthritis: eucalyptus, black pepper, ginger, spike lavender, Roman chamomile, rosemary, myrrh (T)

Rheumatoid arthritis: German chamomile, lavender, peppermint, frankincense (T)

Lower back pain: Roman chamomile, black pepper, eucalyptus, lemongrass, rosemary, lavender, sweet marjoram (T)

Cramps: Roman chamomile, clary sage, lavender, sweet marjoram (T)

General aches and pains: rosemary, lavender, lemongrass, clary sage, black pepper, lemon eucalyptus, spike lavender

Women's Problems

Menopausal symptoms: clary sage, sage, fennel, aniseed, geranium, rose, cypress (I, T)

Menstrual cramping: Roman chamomile, lavender, clary sage (T)

Premenstrual syndrome; infertility with no physiological cause: clary sage, sage, fennel, aniseed, geranium, rose (T)

Blood Pressure

Borderline high blood pressure (not on medication): ylang ylang, true lavender

Low blood pressure (can be caused by some antidepressants): rosemary

Urinary

Cystitis: teatree, palma rosa (T, especially sitz bath)

Water retention: juniper, cypress, fennel (T)

Digestive

Irritable bowel syndrome: Roman chamomile, clary sage, mandarin, cardamom, peppermint, mandarin, fennel, lavender

Constipation: fennel, black pepper (T)

Indigestion: peppermint, ginger (I)

Infections

Bacterial (MRSA, VRSA): teatree (I, T)

Other bacteria (depends on bacteria): eucalyptus, naiouli, sweet marjoram, oregano, tarragon, savory, German chamomile, thyme, manuka (I, T)

Viral: ravansara, palma rosa, lemon, Melissa, rose, bergamot (I, T)

Fungal: lemongrass, black pepper, holy basil, clove, cajuput, caraway (T) geranium: teatree—particularly good for toenail fungus (apply twice daily undiluted for three months to nail bed)

Respiratory

Bronchitis: ravansara, euc globlulus, euc smithi, teatree, spike lavender (I)

Sinusitis: euc globulus, lavender, spike lavender, rosemary (I)

Mild asthma: lavender, clary sage, Roman chamomile (I; patch test on arm first)

Skin Problems

Mild acne: teatree, juniper, cypress, naiouli (T)

Mild psoriasis: lavender, German chamomile (T)
Diabetic ulcers: lavender, frankincense, myrrh (T)

Chemotherapy Side Effects
Nausea: peppermint, ginger, mandarin (I)
Post-radiation burns: lavender, German chamomile with Tamanu carrier oil (T)

Muscular
Sports injuries: spike lavender, rosemary, sweet marjoram, black pepper, lemongrass, frankincense (T)

Children
Irritability: mandarin, lavender, Roman chamomile, rose (I, T)
Colic: Roman chamomile, mandarin (T; gently massed to the abdomen)
Diaper rash: lavender, German chamomile (T)
Sleep problems: lavender, rose, mandarin, ylang ylang
Autism (to aid with social interaction): rose, mandarin, lavender, sweet marjoram, clary sage, pinus sylvestris

Geriatric Care
Memory loss: rosemary, rose, eucalyptus, peppermint, bergamot (T, I)
Dry flaky skin: geranium, frankincense, oil of evening primrose carrier oil (T)
Alzheimer's disease: rosemary, lavender, pine, frankincense, rose (I)

End of Life Care: Pain Relief
Spiritual: rose, angelica, frankincense
Physical: lavender, peppermint, lavender, lemongrass, rosemary
Emotional: geranium, pine, sandalwood
Relaxation: lavender, clary sage, mandarin, frankincense, ylang ylang
Bed sores: lavender, teatree, sweet marjoram, frankincense

Care of the Dying
Rites of passage: choose selection of patient's favorite aromas or frankincense or rose
Bereavement: rose, sandalwood, patchouli, angelica

Actions

The pharmacologically active components in essential oils work at psychological, physical, and cellular levels. Essential oils are absorbed rapidly through the skin—some essential oils are now being used to help the dermal penetration of orthodox medication. Essential oils are lipotrophic and are excreted through respiration, kidneys, and skin.

KEY POINT

Because essential oils can produce physiological and psychological effects, inquiry into their use should be made during every assessment.

Risks and Safety

Most essential oils have been tested by the food and beverage industry as many essential oils are used as flavorings. Other research has been carried out by the perfume industry. Most of the commonly used essential oils in aromatherapy have been given GRAS (generally regarded as safe) status.

Aromatherapy is a very safe complementary therapy if it is used within recognized guidelines. Avoid use with people with atopic eczema. Some essential oils have caused dermal sensitivity—mostly through impure extracts. Generally, essential oils that are high in esters and alcohols tend to be gentle in their action and the most safe to use. Essential oils that are high in phenols tend to be more aggressive and should not be used over long periods of time. There is a list of banned or contraindicated essential oils to guide the novice (See Exhibit 23–3). Do not administer essential oils orally unless trained in this method.

Herbs can interact with medications. Some precautions are listed in Exhibit 23–4. Additional warnings to heed are:

- Sage, clary sage, fennel, and aniseed should be avoided with estrogen-dependent tumors

EXHIBIT 23–3 CONTRAINDICATED ESSENTIAL OILS	
Common Name	*Botanical Name*
BASIL (EXOTIC)	Ocimum basilicum
BIRCH	Betula lenta
BOLDO	Peumus boldus
BUCHU	Agothosma betulina
CADE	Juniperus oxycedrus
CALAMUS	Acorus clamus var angustatus
CAMPHOR (brown)	Cinnamomum camphora
CAMPHOR (yellow)	Cinnamomum camphora
CASSIA	Cinnamomum cassia
CINNAMON BARK	Cinnamomum zeylanicum
COSTUS	Saussurea costus

EXHIBIT 23-3 CONTRAINDICATED ESSENTIAL OILS *(continued)*	
Common Name	*Botanical Name*
ELECAMPANE	Inula helenium
HORSERADISH	Armoracia rusticana
MELALEUCA	Melaleuca bracteata
MUSTARD	Brassica nigra
PENNYROYAL	Mentha pulegium
RAVENSARA	Ravensara anisata
SAGE (Dalmation)	Salvia officinalis
SASSAFRAS	Sassafras albidum
TANSY	Tanacetum vulgare
TARRAGON*	Artemesia dracunculus
THUJA	Thuja occidentalis
VERBENA*	Lippia citriadora (Aloysia triphylla)
WINTERGREEN	Gaultheria procumbens
WORMSEED	Chenopodium ambrosiodes var anthelminticum
WORMWOOD	Artemesia absinthium

* Somewhat controversial. Many aromatherapists use tarragon and verbena.

- Hyssop should be avoided in pregnancy
- Rosemary should be avoided in high blood pressure
- Hyssop should be avoided with those prone to seizures
- Cinnamon may cause dermal irritation
- Bergamot may cause dermal irritation or burns when used with sunbeds or sunshine

Pregnancy and Lactation

Use caution during the first trimester. Although many women do use essential oils successfully and safely during their pregnancies, it is suggested that some essential oils should be avoided altogether, although the data is based on taking the essential oils orally, not inhaling or applying them topically. These include: sage, pennyroyal, camphor, parsley, tarragon, wintergreen, juniper, hyssop, and basil. The following are thought to be safe in pregnancy: cardamom, chamomile (Roman and German), clary sage, coriander seed, geranium, ginger, lavender, neroli, palmarosa, patchouli, petitgrain, rose, rosewood, and sandalwood.

EXHIBIT 23–4 DRUG INTERACTION WITH AROMATHERAPY

1. Avoid when using homeopathic remedies; strong aromas like peppermint and eucalyptus can negate homeopathic remedies.

2. Avoid chamomile if allergic to ragweed.

3. *Eucalyptus globulus* and *cananga odorata* may effect the absorption of 5-fluorouracil—a drug commonly used in chemotherapy.

4. Terpinenol (a component of some essential oils) may decrease the narcotic effect of pentobarbital—mainly when used orally.

5. Cymbopogon citratus (West Indian lemongrass) can increase the effects of morphine (according to studies in rats and when given orally).

6. Peppermint may negate quinidine in atrial fibrillation.

7. Lavender may increase the effect of barbiturates.

8. The effect of tranquilizers, anticonvulsants, and antihistamines may be slightly enhanced by sedative essential oils.

KEY POINT

Warnings/Contraindications/Precautions When Using Essential Oils

- Do not take by mouth (unless guided by a person trained in aromatic medicine and preferably someone with prescriptive license).

- Do not touch your eyes with essential oils. If essential oils get into eyes, rinse out with milk or carrier oil (essential oils do not dissolve in water) then water.

- Store away from fire or naked flame as essential oils are highly volatile and highly flammable.

- Store in a cool place out of sunlight, in colored glass—amber or blue. Store expensive essential oils in refrigerator.

- Many essential oils stain clothing—beware!

- Don't use essential oils undiluted on the skin.

- Keep away from children and pets.

- Only use essential oils from reputable suppliers who can supply the correct botanical name, place of origin, part of plant used, method of extraction, and batch number when possible. *Lavender oil* means absolutely nothing!

- Always close the container immediately.

- Use extra care during early pregnancy.

- Use extra care with people receiving chemotherapy.
- Be aware of which essential oils are photosensitive, e.g., bergamot.
- Avoid use with individuals who have severe asthma or multiple allergies.

Adverse Reactions

There have been some rare cases of adverse skin reactions caused by sensitivity. The majority of cases were from extracts that contained residual petrochemicals. People with multiple allergies are more likely to be sensitive to aromas. Bergamot used in conjunction with sunshine or tanning beds can result in skin damage, ranging from redness to full thickness burns (18).

Administration

Essential oils can be used topically or inhaled. 1–5 drops of essential oils are diluted in 5 ccs (a teaspoon) cold-pressed vegetable oil, such as sweet almond oil for topical application. Some French doctors trained in aromatic medicine give essential oils (diluted in carrier oil) orally in gelatin capsules to treat infections. For topical applications, use every four hours. For inhalation, inhale for 10 minutes as necessary. Use touch methods such as massage or the *m* technique® (19) when appropriate. Simple stress management can be incorporated into the every day regime with the use of baths and foot soaks, vaporizers, and sprays.

Self-Help vs. Professional

Aromatherapy can be self applied for stress management, but for more clinical uses it is better to have some training and knowledge of the chemistry and extraction methods. Many essential oils are sold under their common names. *Origanum marjorana* (sweet marjoram) is an excellent essential oil for insomnia. However, *thymus mastichina* (Spanish marjoram) is frequently sold as marjoram, but it is not a marjoram and certainly won't help insomnia. *Lavandula angustifolia* and *lavandula latifolia* are both sold as lavender. Angustifolia has sedative and anti-spasmodic properties: latifolia is a stimulant and expectorant.

The field of aromatherapy is vast. It can be fun to use essential oils in your home everyday just for the pleasure they give you. They can make your home smell more welcoming, they can help your stress level, calm you down, and many other things as listed above. However, if you wish to use essential oils for clinical conditions, such as a chronic health problem, it is best to visit a professional trained in clinical aromatherapy.

KEY POINT

At present there is no recognized national certification and no governing body for aromatherapy. But the steering committee for Educational Standards in Aromatherapy in the U.S., has established the Aromatherapy Registration Board (ARB), a nonprofit entity that is responsible for administering a national exam. This exam is not clinically based. Graduates have RA (registered aromatherapist) after their names. The largest professional body for aromatherapists is the National Association of Holistic Aromatherapy (NAHA). At present there are no requirements to become certified or accredited, and training can range from one weekend to several years. For a clinical aromatherapist who is also a licensed heath professional, look for CCAP (certified clinical aromatherapy practitioner) after his or her name.

Aromatherapy is misunderstood because it is so broad. However, it encompasses many facets from pleasure through pain to infection, and it is not limited to scented candles and potpourri. Commercial use of the word *aromatherapy* to boost sales of products, such as shampoos, has confused the public. In fact few if any cosmetic or pharmaceutical products currently include essential oils—they use synthetic fragrances as they are much cheaper. However, essential oils have been used safely for thousands of years. Aromatherapy used on a daily basis can be a useful component of healthy living.

Chapter Summary

Aromatherapy implies the therapeutic use of essential oils. Individuals can obtain the therapeutic effects of oils by inhaling them or absorbing them through the skin through baths, compresses or touch; oils can be orally administered, but this must only be done by a trained professional. There are four basic types of aromatherapy: esthetic, holistic, environmental, and clinical. Special precautions must be considered when using aromatherapy. Essential oils are specific in their effects and must be selected based on their therapeutic benefit for the intended use and appropriateness for the specific individual.

References

1. Jori, A., Bianchetti, A., and Prestini, P. E. (1969). Effect of essential oils on drug metabolism, *Biochemical Pharmacology*, 18:2081–2085.

2. Blaschke, T. F. and Bjornsson, T. D. (1995). Pharmacokinetics & pharmacoepidemiology. *Scientific American Interdisc*, 8:1–14.

3. Holmes, P. (1989) *The Energetics of Western Herbs*. Raleigh, NC: Artemis Press, pp. 321–323.

4. Belaiche, P. (1979). Traite de phytotherapie et d'aromatherapie. Vol III: *Gynecologie*. Maloine, Paris.

5. Mowrey, D. B. and Clayson, D. E. (1982). Motion sickness, ginger and psychophysics. *The Lancet*, 1:655.

6. Mason, M. (1996) Aromatherapy and midwifery. *Aromatherapy Quarterly*, 48: 32–34.

7. Albert-Puleo, M. (1980). Fennel and anise as estrogenic agents. *Journal of Ethnopharmacology*, 4:337–344.

8. Marini-Betollo, G. B. (1991). Plants in traditional medicine. *Journal of Ethnopharmacology*, 1:303–306.

9. Grieve, M. (1984). *A Modern Herbal*. New York: Penguin.

10. Gattefosse R. M. and Tisserand, R. B., eds. (1993). *Gattefosse's Aromatherapy: The First Book on Aromatherpy*. Essex, England: C.W. Daniels.

11. Lawless, J. (1995). *The Encyclopedia of Essential Oils*. Shaftsbury, England: Element Books.

12. Goldway, M., Teff, D., Schmidt, R., et al. (1995). Multi-drug resistance in candida albicans. *Antimicrobial Agents and Chemotherapy*, 2:422–426.

13. Belaiche, P. (1985). Treatment of vaginal infections of candida albicans with essential oil of melaleuca alternifolia. *Phytotherapie*, 15:13–15.

14. Pena, E. F. (1962). Melaleuca alternifolia. Its use for trichomonal vaginitis and other vaginal infection. *Obstetrics and Gynecology*, *19*(6):793–795.

15. Carson, C. F., Cookson B. D., Farrelly H. D., and Riley, T. V. (1995). Susceptibility of MRSA to the essential oil of melaleuca alternifolia. *Journal of Antimicrobial Chemotherapy*, *35*(3):421–424.

16. Wren, R. C. (1994). *Potter's New Cyclopedia of Botanical Drugs & Preparations*. Essex, England: C.W. Daniels.

17. Belaiche, P. (1997). Traite de phytotherapie et d'aromatherapie. Vol 111: *Gynecologie*. Maloine, Paris.

18. Buckle, J. (2001). The role of aromatherapy in nursing care. *Nursing Clinics of North America*, *36*(1):57–71.

19. Buckle, J. (2000). The *m* Technique. *Massage and Bodywork*, 2:52–65.

Suggested Readings

Buckle, J. (2003). *Clinical Aromatherapy Essential Oils in Practice.*

Cooksley, V. (1995). *Aromatherapy.* New York: Prentice Hall.

Price, S., Price, L., and Daniel, P. (1999). *Aromatherapy for Health Professionals.* New York: Churchill Livingstone.

Schnaubelt, K. (1998). *Advanced Aromatherapy.* Rochester, VT: Healing Arts Press.

Schnaubelt, K. (1995). *Medical Aromatherapy. Healing with Essential Oils.* Berkeley, CA: Frog, Ltd.

Suskind, P. (1987). *Perfume: The Story of a Murderer.* New York: Penguin.

Tisserand, R. (1977). *The Art of Aromatherapy.* Vermont: Healing Arts Press.

Valnet, J. (1990). *The Practice of Aromatherapy.* Vermont: Healing Arts Press.

Worwood, S. and Worwood, V. A. (2003). *Essential Aromatherapy.* Novato, CA: New World Press.

Worwood, V. A. (2003). *The Complete Book of Essential Oils and Aromatherapy.* Novato, CA: New World Press.

Resources

Recommended Essential Oils Distributors
Nature's Gift Ltd.
40 Cheyenne Blvd
Madison, TN 37115
615-612-4270
marge@naturesgift.com
www.naturesgift.com

Elizabeth Van Buren Aromatherapy Ltd.
303 Potrero St. #33,
Santa Cruz, CA 95060
408-425-8218

Northwest Essence
PO Box 428
Gig Harbor, WA 98335
253-858-0777
northwestessence@earthlink.net
Director: Cheryl Young

Florial France
42 Chemin Des Aubepine
06130 Grasse, France
513-576-9944
US distributor: Lisa Roth
www.florial.com
E-mail: *danannscrossing@yahoo.com*

CHAPTER 24

EFFECTIVE USE OF HOMEOPATHIC REMEDIES

Objectives

This chapter should enable you to:

- Define a homeopathic remedy
- Describe the three laws of cure
- List three recommendations for storing homeopathic remedies
- List five suggestions for handling and administering the remedies
- List at least six substances that can reduce or eliminate the effects of a homeopathic remedy

Consumers are becoming increasingly frustrated with health practitioners' traditional approaches that rely heavily on prescribed medications or allopathic drugs. Taking prescription drugs often leads to the development of undesirable side effects. Reports in the United States indicate that there were more than 100,000 deaths (1) and over 2 million injuries related to adverse reactions from prescription medications that were Food and Drug Agency (FDA) approved drugs (2). In addition to adverse effects, drugs often do little to correct the underlying condition, but instead, merely control symptoms (3). Not surprisingly, people are exploring natural products to manage health conditions and homeopathic remedies are among the more popular products that have caught consumers' attention.

Principles of Homeopathy: Actions of Homeopathic Remedies

The roots of the word *homeopathy* come from two Greek words: *homios*, which means *like*, and *pathos*, which means *suffering*. Homeopathy in modern society, is described as treating *like with like*.

The science of homeopathy was discovered in the early 1800s by Dr. Samuel Hahnemann (1755–1843), a physician and chemist (4, 5), who published, "The Organon of Medicine." It describes in depth the philosophical perspective of homeopathy.

KEY POINT

The basic premise underlying the science of homeopathy is that the body's own healing process is activated to cure illnesses naturally. Specifically the remedies stimulate and increase the vital force (often referred to as the life force) and restore balance to it, facilitating the body's innate healing ability (6). The vital force is the energy responsible for the health status of the body and for coordinating its defense against illness. If this vital force is disturbed due to environmental factors, lifestyle, inadequate nutrition, or lack of exercise, illness or unexpected, undesirable symptoms can occur.

Homeopathy is based on the theory that illness emerges as a result of a disturbance of the body's vital force, causing an imbalance in the energy within a person. The individual reacts emotionally, mentally, and physically (6). Each homeopathic remedy has several characteristics that influence specific symptoms and illnesses due to the imbalance.

The effects of homeopathy on the healing process within the human body was identified by Constantine Hering (1800–1880), who became known as the "Father of Homeopathy" in America and who was also the founder of the first schools and hospitals in which homeopathy was taught throughout the United States. He established the laws of cure, which are often referred to as "Hering's Laws" (Exhibit 24–1). These were based on his observations of how healing occurs.

According to Hering's Laws, a person's health seems to get worse before it improves. In these cases where the individuals may experience an initial worsening of their symptoms, their status will be followed by improvement and relief. This so-called worsening is often known as a *healing crisis* that signals the body's increased activity towards

---

EXHIBIT 24–1 HERING'S LAWS OF CURE

Healing takes place from the top to the bottom. Any symptom or ailment associated with the head area heals first, before the symptoms in the feet. Another illustration is that the symptoms disappear first from the shoulders, then the elbow, and then down the arm.

Healing takes place from inside to outside. This law refers to the fact that the symptoms will be relieved from the more centrally located organs before the extremities are improved.

Healing occurs from the most important organs to the least important organs. The symptoms move from the major or vital organs to the less vital or minor ones. Symptoms associated with any conditions of the heart will disappear first before symptoms associated with the intestines.

Symptoms disappear in reverse order of their appearance, with emotions improving first, then the physical symptoms. An example of this law is the instance in which a person who has been struggling with chronic fatigue for several months develops flu or a cold. The symptoms related to the flu or cold will disappear before the chronic fatigue symptoms clear. The healing process occurs in the reverse order to the onset of the symptoms (7).

---

healing and usually passes quickly (8). The homeopathic practitioner refers to this worsening of symptoms as an aggravation. It is viewed as a sign that the remedy is working and has affected the vital force (9).

In essence, it is essential that a person who uses homeopathic remedies understands the action of the remedies. The homeopathic effects on the body are different than what one expects from the use of traditional medicines, especially prescription drugs.

Homeopathic Remedies

Homeopathic remedies produce a therapeutic effect on symptoms, health conditions, and illnesses. For example, homeotherapeutic remedies are beneficial for a variety of ailments, such as digestive problems, neck stiffness, headaches, ear infections, respiratory problems, flu, motion sickness, women's health, men's health, allergies, emotional upsets, depression, anxiety, and hyperactivity.

Panos, a homeopathic physician, recommended 10 essential remedies for homeopathic first aid, as shown in Exhibit 24–2 (10). The general purpose of homeopathic first aid is to calm the mind, relieve pain, and help the body to heal itself.

EXHIBIT 24–2 HOMEOPATHIC FIRST AID: THE TEN ESSENTIAL/BASIC REMEDIES

Remedy (Official name/common name)	Indications
Aconite (Monkshood) Aconite	• early states of swelling and/or rapid swelling • symptoms of colds—fever, chills
Apis mellifica Apis (Honeybee)	• bee stings and other insect bites • inflammation, rash, allergic reactions • swelling • sore throat
Arnica montana Arnica (Leopard's bane)	• serious or extensive sprains, strains, and bruises • muscle soreness/tiredness • external pain • head scrapes and cuts • itching from insect bites
Arsenicum album Arsenicum (Arsenic)	• shock • upset stomach • vomiting • food poisoning • diarrhea • restlessness, anxiety, exhaustion
Belladonna Belladonna (Deadly nightshade)	• sore throats, coughs, headaches, and earache • colds, flu • high fever • pulsation—labored pulse • redness—red, hot face
Gelsemium sempervirens Gelsemium (Yellow jasmine)	• apprehension • flus, head colds • tension headaches

EXHIBIT 24–2 HOMEOPATHIC FIRST AID: THE TEN ESSENTIAL/BASIC REMEDIES *(continued)*

Remedy	*Indications*
	• apathy
	• visual symptoms
Ipecacuanha	
Ipecacuanha (Ipecac root)	• nausea and vomiting
	• nosebleeds
	• cold, sweaty
	• gasping for air
	• convulsive cough with nausea
Ledum palustre	
Ledum (Marsh tea)	• minor puncture wounds
	• bites and stings
	• eye injuries
	• ankle sprains
Nux vomica	
Nux vomica (Poison nut)	• upset stomach (hangover)
	• irritable
	• impatient
Rhus toxicodendron	
Rhus tox (Poison ivy)	• red swollen, intense itchy
	• blisters
	• stiffness
	• sprains, strains
	• muscle pain
Ruta graveolens	
Ruta (Rue)	• sprains, bruised tendons, and sore bones
	• injuries and trauma

*Source: Panos, M. & Heimlich, J. (1981). *Homeopathic Medicine at Home.* Los Angeles: Jeremy P. Tarcher.

Reflection Do the laws of cure make sense to you? Can you think of illnesses you experienced that followed these laws?

Types, Safety, and Effectiveness of Remedies

Oral homeopathic remedies are available in several forms. The most common ones are pellets (most preferably those formed as tiny beads), tablets of soft consistency, and liquids. Some individuals prefer pellets and tablets to liquids because the dose in the tablets is predetermined and uniform. Other types of homeopathic remedies are suppositories, ointments, creams, and gels.

Homeopathic remedies have a history of effectiveness and safety without side effects. One main characteristic of homeopathic remedies is that they are nontoxic. Toxicity, a vital issue in health care, generally refers to a poisonous substance that causes an unhealthy environment within the person, leading to physiological or psychological problems, i.e., unpleasant, aggravating symptoms or illness. An imbalance in the immune system contributes to toxicity.

KEY POINT

There are no known adverse side effects from using homeopathic remedies and no known drug interaction risks between homeopathic remedies and conventional medications.

For effectiveness, homeopathic remedies must be chosen carefully on the basis of known information, as well as the correct usage and handling of the remedy. If the remedies are used incorrectly or handled improperly, the remedies may have only a superficial effect on the symptoms or illness or no effect at all.

Guidelines for Using Homeopathic Remedies

Whenever the client takes homeopathic remedies, there are certain guidelines that must be followed for effectiveness of these natural products in alleviating symptoms and various health conditions.

Storing the Remedies

It is strongly recommended that the suggestions outlined below be followed for storing homeopathic remedies, because improper storage may interfere with the effectiveness of the substance. If these remedies are properly stored and handled, they maintain their strength for years.

- Keep homeopathic remedies in their original containers. Avoid transferring the remedies to another bottle as this helps prevent any contamination (11).

- Secure the container tops of the remedies tightly; this prevents moisture from forming.

- Keep homeopathic remedies in a cool, dry, dark place away from humidity and out of direct sunlight and extremes of temperature (e.g., higher than 100°F). These factors may cause the remedies to lose their potency.

- Store the remedies away from any strong, pungent-smelling substances, such as perfume, camphor products, mothballs, and strong aromatic compounds found in various products, including mint foods and aromatic oils. It is believed that all of these substances act as an antidote and interfere with the effectiveness of the homeopathic therapy.

- Store homeopathic remedies out of the reach of children.

Handling the Remedies

Careful handling of homeopathic remedies, particularly those in liquid or tablet form, is very important.

- The homeopathic remedies (pellets and tablets) or the bottle dropper of the liquid remedies should be handled as little as possible because this is a source of contamination that may reduce the effectiveness of the product.

- When you pour the remedy, gently tip the pellets or tablets into the lid of the bottle or onto a clean, dry teaspoon. If any of the tablets have fallen out onto the floor or anywhere else or are unused, do not put the tablets back into the container as this will contaminate the stock. Discard the tablets.

Administering the Remedies

Following specific recommendations for taking homeopathic remedies will provide the best results of these natural-healing substances.

- The environment of the mouth should be in its natural condition. That is, the homeopathic remedies should not be taken within 20 minutes before or after eating, brushing one's teeth, or drinking anything other than water. It is important to take the solid dosage forms of homeopathic remedies when the mouth is empty and clear of any food or beverages because these other substances in the mouth may decrease the absorption and effectiveness of the remedy.

- When using homeopathic remedies, it is best to eliminate the use of certain spicy foods and strong smelling foods, including garlic, any form of caffeine, camphor, mints, toiletries, and medications (aspirin, laxatives, etc.) during this time, because these substances may counteract the effects of the homeopathic remedies. (See Exhibit 24–3).

EXHIBIT 24–3 COMMON SUBSTANCES THAT REDUCE THE EFFECTS
OF HOMEOPATHIC REMEDIES

Ingredient	Product
Alcohol	Liquor
Caffeine	Chocolate
	Coffee
	Cola (soda)
	Tea
Camphor	Chapstick®
	Deep-heat ointments (Tiger Balm®)
	Lip salves
Eucalyptus	Candy, cough drops
	Cough mixtures
	Karvol® capsules
	Tiger Balm®
	Vick's® products
Menthol	Candy, cough drops
	Cough mixtures
	Fisherman's Friend®
	Nasal drops
	Tiger Balm®
	Vick's® products
	Mint flavors (peppermint, wintergreen)
	Mouthwash
	Toothpaste
Tobacco	Cigarettes

Compiled from Lockie, A. & Geddes, N. (2000). *Natural Health Complete Guide to Homeopathy*, 2nd ed. New York: Dorling Kindersley. Lockie, A. & Geddes, N. (2000). *Natural Health Complete Guide to Homeopathy*, 2nd ed. New York: Dorling Kindersley

- The use of tobacco should be avoided. Nicotine may alter the response of the body to homeopathic remedies.

- Read the label on the specific homeopathic remedy. Pay attention to what is stated. Note the ingredients and amounts.

- Follow the dosage instructions on the container or as instructed by your health-care practitioner.

- Take the homeopathic dose on an empty stomach. This is essential because gastric juices and digestive processes can destroy or inactivate the remedy.

- Place the solid forms (pellets or tablets) under the tongue (sublingually) and dissolve gradually without chewing or any tongue movement. The remedies are absorbed into the buccal lining of the mouth. This in turn allows the remedies to go directly to the point of action, bypassing the stomach, intestines, and liver.

- Place the drops (liquid) under the tongue in amounts ranging from 1 to 10 drops. (Follow the dosage on the label or as suggested by the healthcare practitioner.)

- A general rule of thumb would be to start with 5 drops and then after one week, increase to 10 drops. However, there is an exception to this rule. In the case of sensitivities, the dosage amount is reduced. The healthcare practitioner may recommend starting with one or two drops and increasing the dosage by a drop each week until 10 drops is reached.

- Finally, the homeopathic remedies should be taken only for as long as one needs them. As soon as positive results are observed, the homeopathic remedies should be discontinued.

Chapter Summary

The main action of homeopathic remedies is to stimulate the vital force that is central to health. They energize the vital force within the body to help eliminate undesirable symptoms or illnesses. Using these natural remedies also helps to maintain a healthy, balanced immune system. Recommendations should be followed regarding storage, handling, and the correct taking of the remedies for their effectiveness and maintaining its potency. Homeopathic remedies are considered extremely safe, effective, nontoxic, and helpful in alleviating symptoms in helping the body heal itself. They can contribute to a greater sense of well-being, energy, and an overall improved resistance to illness.

References

1. Update (2001). Supplements Still Safer. *Delicious Living,* 17(7).
2. Gormley, J. (1998). A holiday message (to the NEHJM). *Better Nutrition,* 60(12):8.
3. Austin, J. (1998). Why patients use alternative medicine: Results of a national study. *Journal of the American Medical Association,* 279(19):1548.
4. Cummings, S. and Ullman, D. (1997). *Everybody's Guide to Homeopathic Medicines.* New York: Jeremy P. Tarcher/Putnam.

5. Trivieri, Jr., L. and Anderson, J., eds. (2002). *Alternative Medicine: The Definitive Guide*. Berkeley, CA: Celestrial Arts.

6. Null, G. (1998). *The Complete Encyclopedia of Natural Healing*. New York: Kensington Publishing Corp.

7. Hardy, M. and Nonman, D. (1994). *The Alchemist's Handbook to Homeopathy*. Allergan, Michigan: Delta K Trust.

8. Kuhn, M. (1999). *Complementary Therapies for Health Care Procedures*. Philadephia, PA: Lippincott Wiliams & Wilkins.

9. Lockie, A. and Geddes, N. (2000). *Natural Health Complete Guide to Homeopathy*, 2nd ed. New York: Dorling Kindersley.

10. Panos, M. and Heimlich, J. (1981). *Homeopathic Medicine at Home*. Los Angeles: Jeremy P. Tarcher.

11. Castro, M. (1996). *Homeopathic Guide to Stress*. New York: St. Martin's Griffin.

Suggested Readings

Gottlieb, W., ed. (1995). *New Choices in Natural Healing*. Emmaus, PA: Rodale Press, Inc.

Hammond, C. (1995). *The Complete Family Guide to Homeopathy*. New York: Penguin Studio.

Herhoff, A. (2000). *Homeopathic Remedies*. Garden City, NY: Avery Publishing Group.

Lockie, A. (1993). *The Family Guide to Homeopathy: Symptoms and Natural Solutions*. New York: Fireside.

Lockie, A. (2001). *Homeopathy Handbook*. New York: Dorling Kindersley.

McCabe, V. (2000). *Practical Homeopathy*. New York: St. Martin's Griffin.

Monte, T. (1997). *The Complete Guide to Natural Healing*. New York: Perigee Book.

Reichenberg-Ullman, J. (2000). *Whole Woman Homeopathy*. Roseville, CA: Prima Health.

Reichenberg-Ullman, J. (1994). *The Patients' Guide to Homeopathic Medicine*. Edmonds, WA: Picnic Point Press.

Reiter, R. (2003). *Healing Without Medication*. North Bergen, NJ: Basic Health Publications, Inc.

Skinner, S. (2001). *An Introduction to Homeopathic Medicine in Primary Care*. Gaithersburg, MD: Aspen Publications.

Spencer, J. and Jacobs, J. (1999). *Complementary/Alternative Medicine: An Evidence-Based Approach*. St. Louis: Mosby, Inc.

Sollars, D. (2001). *The Complete Idiot's Guide to Homeopathy.* Indianapolis, IN: Alpha Books.

Ullman, D. (2002). *The Consumer's Guide to Homeopathy.* New York: Jeremy P. Tarcher/Putnam.

Ullman, D. (1991). *Discovering Homeopathy: Medicine for the 21st Century*, 2nd ed. Berkeley, CA: North Atlantic Books.

Ullman, R. and Reichenberg-Ullman, J. (1997). *Homeopathic Self-Care, The Quick and Easy Guide for the Whole Family.* Rocklin, CA: Prima Publishing.

Vithoulkas, G. (1980). *The Science of Homeopathy.* New York: Grove Press.

CHAPTER 25

MEDICATION WISDOM

Objectives

This chapter should enable you to:

- Describe medication-related information that is significant for healthcare providers to review and discuss with consumers
- Distinguish between medication side effects and adverse drug reaction (ADR)
- List eight common undesirable consumer behaviors with prescription medications
- Describe specific interventions the healthcare provider can use to help patients resolve issues related to obtaining prescription medications

Throughout history, people have exerted self-control over selection and use of healing agents, including medicines. The interest in selection and use of medications continues to be important to consumers. People want to know about the medications they are taking, specifically, how medications work, their potential side effects, possible and potential interactions with other medications, and how the medications will impact their functional status.

There are more than 100,000 nonprescription products purchased over the counter each year in the United States and in addition, more than 40,000 drugs are prescribed each year (1). These data do not include herbal and nontraditional medicines.

Consumer Issues Related to Prescription Medications

The ultimate goal of taking medication is to enhance one's health state or level of functioning. The desired outcome is to obtain the maximum benefit with minimal side effects and little or no toxicity. Each person has a unique and individual body composition. Because of each person's unique biochemical composition, no two individuals will respond to a medication in exactly the same way. Table 25–1 depicts general, essential information the consumer needs to have when taking any medication.

Name of the Medication

Medications have both a generic and a trade name. This information is essential for people to know for each of their prescribed medications. The trade (brand) name of the medication is the drug name as it is available from pharmaceutical manufacturers. Pharmacists, unless otherwise indicated, can substitute an equivalent generic drug without prescriber approval and in many cases this will pass on significant cost savings to

---

TABLE 25–1   ESSENTIAL INFORMATION TO KNOW WHEN USING A MEDICATION

- Name (brand and generic)
- Use
- How to administer
- Side effects
- Adverse reactions
- Storage and handling
- Special precautions
- May lose all other activity, but targeted effect
- Interactions with other medications, foods, and supplements
- What to do if there are missed doses

consumers. In some cases, however, only the trade (brand) name medication can be dispensed if the prescription specifies "Dispense as Written." Consumers need to be educated that although generic products are considered to be pharmaceutically equivalent to the trade (brand) name counterparts, not all are therapeutically the same. This could ultimately result in failed therapy due to ineffectiveness of a medication.

Use of the Medication

Consumers need to know the purpose for each medication they use, (e.g., to treat inner ear infection, lower blood pressure, or eliminate fluids). This can be particularly important as there can be situations where the pharmacist cannot accurately read the handwriting on the prescription. Many medication names are spelled very similarly and there could be serious consequences if the wrong medication is given. (An example of two medications that easily could be confused is Celebrex, used to treat musculoskeltal conditions, and Celexa, used for treatment of depressive disorders.) By knowing the name and purpose of their prescribed drugs, consumers can detect errors and spare themselves complications.

Reflection   Do you know the names, purposes, side effects, and adverse effects for every medication you use?

How to Administer the Medication

Healthcare providers need to educate consumers to know the correct dosage of their medications, routes of administration, and any other important information. There are several routes for administration of prescribed medications. The most common routes for home medication administration are oral, rectal, topical, eardrops (otic), eye drops (opthalmic), subcutaneous injection (sub-Q), intranasal, inhaled, and intramuscular injections (IM). Failure to take prescribed medication via the correct route could result in outcomes ranging from insignificant consequence to death. An example of incorrectly administering a medication could be instilling eye drops in the ear. In this case, the patient outcome will most likely not be life-threatening (although not receiving the needed medication could have effects for the eye). An example of serious potential harm might be administering a medication intended for topical (skin) administration orally.

Administration of the correct dosage at the specified intervals is important. Not taking enough of the drug or skipping doses could reduce the benefit and leave the health problem with inadequate treatment. On the other hand, taking doses that exceed the prescribed amount or taking drugs more frequently than prescribed could cause damage to body organs and serious complications. Consideration also must be given to the existence of conditions, such as liver or kidney disease, that could affect the metabolism and excretion of drugs. Dosage adjustments would be warranted in these situations.

Side Effects of the Medication

Medication side effects are responses that can occur with medications. While side effects result in patient discomfort or cause concern they usually are not life threatening. An example of a side effect would be the onset of nausea after taking an antibiotic on an empty stomach.

Side effects may or may not require that a medication be stopped. The consumer must be educated in awareness and recognition of potential and actual side effects in the event that they occur. Healthcare providers need to inform consumers of the side effects that should be reported. Together, the healthcare provider and consumer can discuss the situation and make an informed decision about whether or not to stop the medication and whether or not the side effects warrant intervention.

Adverse Reactions to the Medication

In addition to medication side effects, consumers must be aware of potential adverse drug reactions (ADRs). ADRs have been studied in hospitalized patients and it has been estimated that there are approximately 2 million ADRs annually in the U.S., resulting in ADRs being the fourth leading cause of death (2). ADRs can be severe adverse reactions and toxic effects that can result in loss of life or permanent impairment and loss of functioning. ADRs require prompt intervention by healthcare providers, because without emergent care, some ADRs could result in death within minutes.

KEY POINT

Adverse drug reactions demand speedy attention. A person taking a new medication who develops tightness in the throat or difficulty breathing, indicative of a life-threatening ADR known as anaphylaxis, could die within a short time without intervention.

Storage and Handling of the Medication

Consumers require specific information on medication storage and handling. Improper storage or handling decomposition of biochemical ingredients can result in decreased potency or efficacy. Detailed, specific medication storage and handling instructions should be provided with each medication prescribed. Examples of frequently asked questions regarding storage and handling are: "Does this medication need to be refrigerated?" "Can I travel with this medication?" "How long is the medication good if I store it?" Medication labels contain specific details on storage and handling, but can be difficult to read for some elderly or sight-impaired persons.

Special considerations would be in order in these situations to assist consumers with needed storage and handling information.

Special Medication Precautions

Nearly every prescription medication has some unique precautions making it essential for consumers to be aware of times when a medication should or should not be used. These special precautions also help to alert the healthcare provider that the consumer should be under close surveillance when using the drug. Healthcare providers need to discuss risk and benefit of taking a medication with consumers prior to prescribing any medication.

The elderly, young children, and pregnant women are at increased risk for harmful medication effects as a result of their physiological differences. Children's medication dosages must be carefully and accurately calculated according to age, weight, level of growth and development, and height. Elderly people have an increased risk of ADRs because they do not metabolize nor excrete medications as easily as younger people because of age-related changes. Pregnant women are at increased risk of teratogenicity or harm to the unborn fetus with many medications. Healthcare providers should discuss risks and benefits of medications prescribed during pregnancy with the obstetrician and document the outcome of the conversation in the health record.

Interactions with Other Medications

Drug-to-drug interactions are a significant concern for consumers and healthcare providers. Consumers are using more and more over-the-counter medications, as well as herbal and nontraditional medicinal products. There can be interactions with or contraindications for certain foods with over-the-counter medications, herbal, and nontraditional therapies they may be using. The likelihood of drug-to-drug interaction occurrence is increased because of the complex biochemical composition of the many products now available. As the number of medications a person takes increases, there is a commensurate increase in the likelihood of an interaction. Drug-to-drug interactions can range from relatively benign or not harmful to life threatening. An example of a possible food contraindication would be that when taking coumadin, a blood thinner, green, leafy vegetables, such as lettuce, cabbage, or brussel sprouts should be avoided as these vegetables counter the desired effects of the drug.

Missed Dose of Medication

It is always advisable for the consumer to call the healthcare provider if a dose of medication is missed. This is a situation that may occur because the consumer simply forgot to take their medicine or perhaps he or she was too ill to take it. An example would be a person with diabetes who has intractable nausea and vomiting and does not know whether or not to take their morning insulin. The healthcare provider can review the situation and advise accordingly.

Common Consumer Medication Mistakes and How to Avoid Them

Healthcare providers must emphasize to consumers the need to take medications precisely as prescribed. Consumers can increase medication safety and efficacy by following five fundamental principles of medication administration each time a medication is taken:

1. Right drug
2. Right dose
3. Right route
4. Right time
5. Right person

There are several common undesirable behaviors consumers often engage in with respect to medications. These behaviors are quite common and need to be addressed by the healthcare provider on each patient encounter. Table 25-2 depicts eight common undesirable consumer behaviors that frequently occur with prescribed medications.

TABLE 25–2   COMMON UNDESIRABLE BEHAVIORS TO AVOID WHEN TAKING MEDICATIONS

1. Saving unused medication for oneself or others for future illness
2. Forgetting to get the prescription refilled
3. Not finishing medications as prescribed because symptoms are relieved
4. Forgetting to take the medicine at the prescribed times
5. Not taking the medication as directed
6. Stopping or not filling the prescription because of cost
7. Sharing medications
8. Taking over-the-counter or nonconventional remedies without informing the healthcare provider

Saving Unused Medication for Oneself or Others for Future Illness

Using medications leftover from other times or that have been prescribed for someone else is never advised because the medication prescribed was the amount necessary to treat one specific condition for a particular person at the given time. Prescriptions for the treatment of acute conditions, like infections, need to be fully consumed until the condition is completely resolved. People can develop a flare up of an inadequately treated infection or resistance to certain pathogens by not completing the medication as prescribed, subjecting themselves to new risks.

Forgetting to Get the Prescription Refilled

It has become common for people to get medications filled via direct mail order. This can add to the problem of forgetting to refill a prescription or to refill it in time to avoid missed medication doses. It is never advisable to miss even one medication dose as this can cause potentially serious or life-threatening harm. Many medications are used for the control of long term, chronic conditions, such as heart disease, hypertension, or diabetes, and missing even one dose can result in undesirable or harmful effects. An example would be a person who takes the medication, lanoxin (digoxin). Digoxin affects the contractility of the heart. Missing even one dose of digoxin can result in heart failure, a potentially life-threatening situation.

KEY POINT

When using mail-order services to fill prescriptions, people need to be careful to allow adequate time for ordering refills to assure they do not run out of their existing supply before the new supply arrives.

It is especially important to give the pharmacy where one mails prescriptions ample time to process the order. In the event that a person runs out of a drug, it could prove useful to check with the healthcare provider to see if the provider has any medication samples available to use until the shipment arrives. If the provider does not have samples, then the person must request a written prescription for a few doses, enough to last until their shipment arrives. In the majority of cases, the individual will most likely have to pay for these interim prescriptions as many insurers do not. It is also important to note that many third-party insurers often will not pay for more than 90 days on a prescription, requiring the consumer to return to the primary healthcare practitioner to get a new prescription.

Not Finishing Medications as Prescribed Because a Person Feels Better

Prematurely discontinuing a medication is a common behavior that can result in potentially life-threatening situations later on. For example, in the case of *beta hemolytic strepococcus*, the most frequent cause of strep throat, the bacteria may not be completely eradicated even though a person feels better and the symptoms are essentially resolved. These medications are usually prescribed for a full 10 days of therapy in order to completely eradicate the causative organism. When antibiotic therapy is suboptimal, the organism can become resistant to the treatment for future events or the organism can grow in other areas of the body, such as the heart valves. This organism could then harm the heart valves resulting in abnormal leaking of blood back into the heart chambers and result in impaired circulation or damaged heart valve leaflets.

Forgetting to Take the Medication at Designated Times

Frequently a person forgets to take a dose of medication. In some cases, the dose may be taken as soon as one remembers, if there are no special indications, such as taking it with or between meals. If the missed dose is close to the time of the next scheduled dose, the healthcare provider most likely will advise the person to take the missed dose and resume the usual schedule. The consumer should be educated not to double up or take an extra dose as this can result in a variety of potential outcomes depending on the medication and potential side effects. An example is a missed a dose of penicillin; attempting to double the dose to make up the missed dose often results in gastrointestinal upset, such as nausea, diarrhea, or severe stomach cramping.

Not Taking the Medication as Directed

Medications need to be taken specifically as prescribed. This is a very important consideration, because many medications are designed biochemically to work in certain environments. For example, if the medication is to be taken one hour before meals and is consumed with a meal, its absorption could be affected and the drug may not achieve its intended purpose. Many medications should not be taken with milk or other dairy products. If this is the situation, it will be specified on the medication administration sheet and on the label of the medication container. There can be quite serious, even life-threatening consequences if directions are not adhered to as specified.

Stopping or Not Filling a Medication Prescription Because a Person Cannot Pay for It

There are reasons for medications to be prescribed, therefore, not filling prescriptions has consequences. When the healthcare practitioner prescribes the medication, it is always helpful for people to ask for an estimate of what the prescription will cost. While the provider may not be able to give exact figures, some information regarding the approximate cost of the medication should be available. In other cases, the healthcare provider may ask that a pharmacy be called to obtain the price. If this is a prescription for a new medication and the consumer is just starting it, especially if it is a very new and expensive medication where there is no generic, less expensive equivalent, it is useful to ask the healthcare practitioner if she or he has samples available; this can spare the cost of filling the full prescription only to discover that one cannot tolerate the drug. There is nothing more frustrating than spending a large amount of money on a medication that does not agree with the consumer and produces so many side effects the person cannot take it. If the provider wants the consumer to have the medication, has no samples, and the consumer cannot afford the medication, the consumer can try to contact a hospital social worker or community resource person for assistance. There may be a community agency that assists in these purchases—and there are also some medication programs for those who cannot pay through some of the pharmaceutical companies that cover some medication prescriptions.

The bottom line is that consumers should *never do without a medication if they cannot afford it.* Healthcare providers need to consider this issue when recommending medications.

Reflection   Some people complain about the cost of medications and other healthcare expenses while not hesitating to spend money on expensive restaurant dinners, manicures, theater tickets, and other nonessentials. Why do you think they hold such attitudes?

Sharing Medications

Giving medication to anyone other than the person for whom it was prescribed, unfortunately does occur and this practice carries many significant risks. Using someone else's medications can mask symptoms, resulting in improper diagnosis and treatment of life-threatening disorders. It also can result in microbial resistance to organisms.

Taking Over-the-Counter or Nonconventional Medicines without Informing the Healthcare Provider

As previously stated, there can be potentially lethal or life-threatening interactions between medications and food substances. It is crucial that people share all information regarding over-the-counter, herbal, or nonconventional (complementary or alternative) therapies with their healthcare providers at each visit. In turn, providers need to make a practice of inquiring about the addition of an over-the-counter or nontraditional treatment with each client visit. Health records should reflect this information to provide continuity of care by all providers. An example of the importance of sharing this information involves the use of green tea preparations, which can enhance the potency of coumadin, an agent used to thin the blood. If the herbal substance enhances the effect of the medication, the person may experience a life-threatening hemorrhage, such as in the brain, and die as a result of cerebral hemorrhage.

Suggested Times for Taking Scheduled Medications

All prescribed medications include specificity regarding the frequency of administration. Table 25–3 depicts common abbreviations and meanings for medication administration, suggested times for the common medication administration schedules, and special considerations. These abbreviations are of Latin origin.

TABLE 25–3 COMMON ABBREVIATIONS AND RELATED INFORMATION FOR MEDICATIONS

Common Abbreviation	Meaning of the Abbreviation	Suggested Times for Taking the Medication	Special Considerations
ac	Must be taken before meals in order for it to be effective and to do what it is supposed to do.	• Take the medication 30 minutes prior to the scheduled or planned mealtime.	• If the medication is skipped, take it 30 minutes prior to the meal; wait at least two hours after the meal to take the medication.
bid	Must be taken 2 times a day	• Suggested times for taking the medication should reflect a person's lifestyle for ease of compliance. For example, if one arises at 6 A.M., the medication can be taken at 7 A.M. and 4 P.M. • The two times a day dosing is usually spaced approximately 8 hours apart.	• If one dose is forgotten, take it as soon as remembered and resume the regular schedule the following day. • Do not double up and take two doses at one time.
tid	Must be taken 3 times a day	• Try to incorporate these three times into individual lifestyle if possible to take the medication on time. • Space the medications across the day so doses are not taken close together. For example, if one awakens at 6 A.M., the drug could be taken at 7 A.M., 3 P.M., and 10 P.M. (These sample times are approximately 8 hours apart.	• If one dose is forgotten, take it as soon as remembered and resume the regular schedule the following day. • Do not double up and take two doses at one time.
qid	Must be taken 4 times a day	• Suggested times for a four-times-a-day dosing would be 9 A.M., 1 P.M., 6 P.M., and 9 P.M. • There can be individual variance and adjustment of this suggested schedule to fit individual lifestyles. • It is not recommended to double doses to catch up in the event of a missed dose.	• If one dose is forgotten, take it as soon as remembered and resume the regular schedule the following day. • Do not double up and take two doses at one time.
hs	Must be taken at bedtime	• The suggested time for a bedtime dose is 9 or 10 P.M.; however, if one retires earlier or later individual adjustment can be made.	• None
qd	Must be taken once a day	• This dosing regimen is usually flexible and accommodates the the person's individual lifestyle. • Most persons take the medication for daily dosing at 8 or 9 A.M.	• It is important to take the medication at the same time each day in order not to forget to take it or to mistakenly repeat administration. • Choose a consistent time that will increase the likelihood of remembering, such as with breakfast.

Strategies to Assess Medications' Effectiveness

Most pharmacies now provide informational pamphlets with prescriptions. This information usually provides detailed written information ranging from medication dosing to potential side effects. Consumers should be certain to obtain this information on any prescription that is filled. In addition, many pharmacists now provide individual counseling for each consumer. If consumers opt not to have medication counseling, they may be asked to sign a waiver to that effect. Medication information provided with each prescription includes medication purpose; potential side effects and adverse drug reactions; special precautions when taking the medication; and food/drug interactions. Medication information provided by pharmacies also includes specific tips to insure the prescription medication will be effective (Table 25–4).

Chapter Summary

There are more than 100,000 nonprescription, over-the-counter drugs purchased and 40,000 prescriptions written annually. All of these products, although beneficial in many ways, can carry serious risks if used improperly. Consumers and their healthcare providers need to be in partnership in assuring safe drug use.

TABLE 25–4   SPECIFIC TIPS TO INSURE MEDICATION EFFECTIVENESS AND OPTIMIZE THERAPEUTIC EFFECTS

- Always take medication specifically as prescribed
- Take the medication at the time it is prescribed
- Take the medication in the dose that is prescribed
- Do not skip medication doses
- Do not double up on the medication if a dose is missed
- Notify the primary care provider who prescribed the medication of any symptoms experienced whether they are suspected or known to be related to the medication
- Immediately report to the healthcare provider any unusual feelings or events immediately, such as swelling in any part of the body, joint aching, heart palpitations, or unusual fatigue

Consumers need to be informed users of all medications to assure safety. They need to be knowledgeable about the generic and brand names, intended use, administration, side effects, adverse reactions, storage, handling, precautions, and interactions related to each drug they use.

Common mistakes that must be avoided include saving unused medications for future use, using someone else's drugs, running out of medications due to failure to get refills in time, discontinuing the medication prematurely, forgetting to take the drug, not taking the drug as directed, and using other drugs or over-the-counter remedies without the healthcare provider's knowledge.

Informed medication use is an important part of self-care. Consumers can seek information from pharmacists who fill prescriptions to enhance their knowledge.

References

1. Murray, L. (2001). *Physician's Desk Reference*, 54 ed. New Jersey: Medical Economics Company, Inc.
2. Gurwitz, J. H., Field, T. S., Avon, M., McCormick, D., Jain, S., and Eckler, M. (2000). Incidence and preventability of adverse drug events in nursing homes. *American Journal of Medicine, 10*(2):87–94.

Suggested Readings

Adelman, A. (2001). "Managing Chronic Illness." In A. M. Adelman, & M. P. Daly, eds., *20 Common Problems in Geriatrics*. New York: McGraw Hill.

Brody, T. M. (1998). "Introductions and Definitions." In J. Larner & K. P. Minneman, eds., *Human Pharmacology: Molecular to Clinical*, 3rd ed. St. Louis: Mosby.

Committee on Quality of Health Care in America: Institute of Medicine (2000). *To Err is Human: Building a Safer Health System*. Washington, DC: National Academy Press.

Joyce, E. V. and Villanueva, M. E. (2000). *Say It In Spanish: A Guide for Health Care Professionals*, 2nd ed. Philadelphia: W.B. Saunders.

Karch, A. M. (2000). *Lippincott's Nursing Drug Guide*. Philadelphia: Lippincott. Medwatch, *http://www.drugintel.com/public/medwatch/*.

Patton, C. M. (1999). Preoperative Nursing Assessment of the Adult Patient. *Seminars in Perioperative Nursing*, 8:42–47.

Patton, C. M. (2000). Traditional Pharmacological Approaches to Women's Wellness. In E. Olshansky, ed., *Integrated Women's Health: Holistic Approaches for Comprehensive Care*. Maryland: Aspen Publishers, Inc.

Patton, C. M. (2000). Diagnostic tests. In J. Nagelkirk, ed., *Diagnostic Reasoning*. St. Louis: Mosby.

United Health Foundation (2003). *Clinical Evidence*, 6th ed. London: BMJ Publishing Group.

CHAPTER 26

SURVIVING CAREGIVING

Objectives

This chapter should enable you to:

- Define the terms *sandwich generation* and *club sandwiches*
- Discuss the many roles caregivers can fill
- List at least two major instructions provided in an advance directive
- Discuss the difference between a delirium and a dementia
- Describe at least two ways that caregivers' burdens can be relieved

There has been a tremendous increase in the number of aging Americans causing a graying of the population. The fact that growing numbers of people can expect to live longer lives than their grandparents is wonderful news, but it does create major challenges. These challenges can affect people very directly, either in terms of the human and financial resources needed to meet their own needs as they age, or the care they'll have to provide to the older adults in their lives.

In the early 1900s life expectancy was age 47 and only about 4 percent of the population lived to age 65 or older. In the early years of the 21st century, life expectancy will be 75 years, with 12 percent of the population 65 years or older. The fastest growing segment within the elder group are those over the age of 85. It will become more commonplace to see people reaching their 100th birthday.

Sandwich Generation

In the early 90s the term *sandwich generation* was coined. This term appropriately described the way that it feels to be caught in the middle: responsible for the care of both parents and children at the same period of time. For centuries, family members took care of each other, so this certainly is not a recent development. The important differences now, however, are that so many more people are surviving much longer, primarily due to new medications and advances of technology in health care; rather than a few years, care of an elder relative can span several decades. Also noteworthy is the fact that few families have the luxury of having a stay-at-home parent as most women are employed outside the home. The combined stressors, both internal and external, often contribute to feelings of alienation within families instead of enjoyment in relationships.

Increasingly, what can be termed *club sandwiches* is being added to the menu of family profiles. That is a caregiver who is providing support and assistance to a parent, a child, as well as a grandchild. There are, however, a variety of club sandwiches. Sometimes the grandparent may become the primary care provider. The reasons for this are many. With approximately 50 to 60 percent of marriages ending in divorce, some grandparents are faced with assisting their single-parent children with the demands of raising children. Others are handed their new obligations because their adult children became involved in drugs, alcohol abuse, or other unhealthy lifestyles that prevented them from raising their own children. Whatever the forerunner, the fact remains that many families are struggling with caregiver issues and need information and assistance.

Caregiving wears many faces and includes a variety of tasks and responsibilities.

Many Faces of Caregiving

Providing daily personal care or supervision to a parent can be demanding and overwhelming. However, caregiving often entails more than physical care. One's presence—being there for a parent—can be a significant factor in preserving emotional well-being.

An example of a situation that may require intervention is the vulnerable time when one's parents are attempting to make a sometimes difficult adjustment to retirement. The opportunities of retirement, although perhaps envied by many, are often accompanied by loss and role confusion.

> **KEY POINT**
>
> If you consider the fact that a person may have worked in a job for decades and then one day is no longer required to perform that role, it is easy to understand how emotional upheaval may occur in retirement, especially if the individual has not prepared for this change.

Adult children may assist their parents to recognize their continued value during the time of transition to retirement. It is also a time when children can be instrumental in assisting their parents to navigate the healthcare system. Older parents may be very concerned about their ability to pay for their health care with a limited income. The complexity of Medicare billing is also worrisome to many. There have been so many changes in the healthcare delivery system that clarification and advocacy are often the most supportive activities that children can provide for their parents. Being available to accompany them to doctors' visits and helping them to make some very difficult healthcare decisions can be valuable ways children can help their parents in late life.

As one ages, chronic health problems become more common. These chronic conditions (e.g., hypertension and other cardiac diseases, arthritis, diabetes, and gastrointestinal disturbances) can interfere with the quality of life and ultimately disrupt a person's function. Often, these conditions may necessitate more frequent visits to healthcare providers. Many older people have never challenged a physician's diagnosis or requested a second opinion. They may be fearful of offending their doctors by asking questions. Adult children can help their parents to be assertive in this most important aspect of decision making. Frequently, making the right choice means preventing unnecessary discomfort and decline in function, which could accompany inappropriate treatments.

> **KEY POINT**
>
> Any declines in function that can be prevented will help to preserve independence and enhance quality of life, as well as reduce caregiving responsibilities.

Advance Directives

To help assure appropriate care is provided and that informed decisions are made, discussions and thoughtful planning should be done well in advance of when needed. These issues can be addressed in a document called an *Advanced Directive* or *Living Will*.

> **KEY POINT**
>
> An Advance Directive provides specific instructions on the treatment people want or do not want to have in the event they are not capable of expressing their opinions. This document also names a person who is authorized to make healthcare decisions for matters not specifically described in the document.

Preparation of an Advanced Directive is extremely beneficial. This is frequently a topic of discussion at senior meetings and senior centers, however, if one's parents have not yet completed this document, he or she should encourage or assist them in this process. A copy of an Advanced Directive is usually available from a healthcare provider or area agency on aging office.

The decision of naming a healthcare representative—someone who can make decisions regarding treatments if an individual is unable to do for himself/herself—is sometimes a difficult one for an older adult to make. It is vital that permission be obtained from the person who will be named as proxy healthcare representative. Also, the physician, hospital, perhaps an attorney, and other interested family members should have a copy of the Advance Directive, in addition to the named representative. The original should remain in a safe place with important papers.

Financial Considerations

Assisting parents or other older relatives to establish a financial system and help them to prevent financial chaos or hardship is another useful action. Often, the elderly are the victims of scams. In their attempt to handle situation independently they frequently become easy prey to unscrupulous predators. Once they have sustained significant loss, they may conceal the facts and bear their shame with a mask of depression. They may be fearful that they will be considered incompetent, therefore, they may never come forward or even share the information with people who could assist them to recoup their losses. Putting some financial safety checks in place early on, often helps to prevent loss and provides a good record keeping mechanism for a future accounting. These records may be necessary to justify financial eligibility for a state or federal assistance program or to verify appropriate distribution of funds, which sometimes becomes a significant issue even within close-knit families.

> **KEY POINT**
>
> It is possible that early caregiving interventions can be so natural and subtle that you may not even realize that you are doing anything that resembles taking care of another.

Financial issues that may be difficult to discuss should not be avoided, but rather brought to awareness and addressed before a crisis or disability occurs. Critical topics, those of financial consequence as well as those of advanced directives, end-of-life issues, healthcare proxy, and guardianships are too important to wait until a court makes the decisions for individuals and their loved ones.

Reflection   Have you and your older relatives discussed issues pertaining to their finances and health care in the event that they are incapacitated by illness or disability? If you have, what were some of the emotional issues that you had to confront? If you haven't, what are the issues preventing this discussion and how can you address them?

Age-Related Changes

Many changes occur with age. People develop into more complex physical, psychological, and spiritual beings with a greater understanding of life, having experienced many unique situations. On the down side, aging usually brings negative changes in all of the senses. Vision is frequently compromised by such conditions as aging, macular degeneration, cataracts, or *presbyopia* (blurring of vision up close due to changes in the lens). Hearing may deteriorate and limit the tones that can be heard, with the lower tones being the most audible. This condition, known as *presbycusis*, causes people to miss large portions of conversation because certain letters sound muffled. Often older adults hesitate to obtain or use hearing aids because the aids can be distracting, difficult to adjust to, or emphasize the fact that they are getting old.

KEY POINT

Sometimes presbycusis can cause people to give inappropriate responses because they misinterpret speech. Others mistakenly may view them as being confused or having early dementia.

Diminished sense of smell and taste may lead to nutritional problems, social isolation, and unsafe conditions in the home. Common reasons for visits to the emergency room for older adults are dehydration, electrolyte imbalance, malnutrition, and falls. These conditions sometimes can be prevented by frequent contact with family, friends, and others who can make visits and identify problems early. In some communities, a friendly visitor service is provided by church groups or gatekeeper programs. The postal service as well as utility companies (gas/electric/telephone/cable) often train their employees to look for signs that indicate a customer may need assistance. In many communities the elderly can receive Meals on Wheels or daily lunches through senior centers.

With funding from the Older Americans Act, seniors can be transported to local sites where nutritious meals, social stimulation, and interaction await them. Coordinators of these programs are usually aware of significant changes in their members and can intervene before unsafe conditions develop or provide rapid assistance through Adult Protective Services personnel if a senior becomes unable to make independent decisions any longer.

Changes in tactile (touch) sensations cause difficulty feeling heat, cold, pain, and pressure, which increases the risk of personal injury. Sometimes, fear of being injured by temperature extremes, the discomfort of feeling chilled, as well as fear of falling in the bathtub or shower interferes with bathing and personal care needs. This can be most distressing to family or others who attempt to provide care. It should be noted, however, that in the older person, there is a process where their skin becomes drier than when they were younger. Unless there is incontinence or it is necessary to remove other irritants from the skin, a shower or bath twice a week will suffice for hygienic needs.

Perhaps the most distressing alterations are the cognitive changes, which are increasingly common with advanced age. Age-related changes in cerebral function can result in slower reaction time and increased time to learn new information, as well as greater potential for attention to be distracted. These events, coupled with the sensory changes already mentioned, and the stress of every day living can create memory difficulties. Memory loss, significant personality changes, confusion, or changes in intellectual abilities are not normal consequences of aging. If an older adult is experiencing what is thought to be unusual changes in cognitive function, a comprehensive geriatric assessment is a wonderful means to identify the source of the problem. Some causes of memory problems that can be detected in a comprehensive geriatric assessment include delirium, depression, and dementia.

KEY POINT

A *delirium* is a change in mental function with a rapid onset that usually can be treated and corrected. Some possible causes are infections, low blood pressure, dehydration, and side effects from medications.

A *dementia* is a deterioration in mental function that has a slow, subtle onset. Some possible causes include Alzheimer's disease, AIDS, and alcoholism. The losses sustained cannot be regained.

Although a dementia is not able to be reversed there have been tremendous strides in new medications that delay further impairment. These medications are most successful when begun at an early stage of the disease. The longer function can be maintained, the longer one will be able to remain independent. When memory impairment or other cognitive changes are present, it is essential that the individual obtain a comprehensive assessment. Typically, this assessment consists of a series of visits to a geriatrician, an advanced practice geriatric nurse, and a geriatric social worker. Included in the examination are blood tests that assess complete blood count, folic acid, thyroid function, and electrolyte imbalances. There also is radiological imaging of the brain. Sufficient testing is done to assure that the memory changes are not the result of a severe depression. After all other disease processes are ruled out, a diagnosis can be established and appropriate treatment prescribed. The goal of this therapy is to help the individual maintain function as long as possible.

Reflection How would your life be affected if a parent developed a dementia? What plans for that person would you believe to be necessary?

Function vs. Diagnosis

Despite having their diagnoses, most people with chronic conditions are able to do quite well. Function is a key indicator for a caregiver to use to assess how the person is doing, which includes the present state of wellness/illness and the potential for the person to increase or decrease independence. Changes in function can be clues of changes in the status of a disease or the presence of new factors that require intervention. For example, if your mother was walking 100 feet unassisted last week and today she is huffing and puffing at 20 feet, something has occurred that should be addressed with her healthcare provider immediately.

Because of the numerous changes that take place throughout the body with age, physical diseases are more difficult to detect. It is very common for an older person to have an unusual response to illness. Signs and symptoms may be diminished, absent, or vary significantly from what one would observe in a younger individual. An example of this is delirium (acute onset of confusion) which may occur in older persons when they develop infections, such as urinary tract infections. In younger persons there usually are signs and symptoms that would indicate the urinary tract infection, such as pain on urination, fever, frequent urination, etc. These symptoms may be absent in older adults and instead, they may experience an acute episode of or a general feeling of being run down.

KEY POINT

It is important for older adults and their caregivers to establish relationships with healthcare providers who are knowledgeable about geriatric medicine, sensitive to the elderly, and aware of caregiver issues.

Medications

Medications afford many people not only more years to their lives, but add a higher quality of life to those years. However, medications can create a new host of problems. Every drug carries a risk of side effects and interactions with other drugs, herbs, and food. There is the chance that a medication may be indiscriminately used to manage a symptom when a nonpharmacologic approach could suffice. Side effects of drugs can be missed or attributed to another problem; worse still, another drug can be ordered to manage the side effects of the drug.

KEY POINT

Drug toxicity is an important consideration in caregiving to older adults. Because medications are absorbed, metabolized, and excreted very differently in the older person, a skilled geriatric professional is needed to assure safe drug prescription and management.

It is beneficial for caregivers to maintain a list of all prescriptions, over-the-counter medications, and dietary supplements that the individual is using. This list should accompany the individual to all visits to healthcare providers.

To assist the individual with self-administration of medications, the caregiver can develop a charting system whereby the person checks off the times medications are taken or use a multiday container in which several days' supply of medications can be pre-poured (these are available at pharmacies or medical supply stores).

Becoming a Caregiver

Families have their own unique manner of selecting who will be the designated caregiver. Statistically, it will be a women (about 75 percent)—a wife, daughter, or daughter-in-law.

KEY POINT

Despite the difficulties and complexities of family life today, most older adults are cared for in the home by family and friends.

Although many people perceive a caregiving responsibility as a burden, it can prove to be a special experience. Much can be discovered through the caregiving process when it is manifested as an act of love. It allows the caregiver the opportunity for intimacy and to heal relationships. Caregivers also can learn much about themselves—their talents, strengths, and weaknesses. Sometimes they can gain new direction in their lives or at least awareness of the relationship between themselves and others, especially those in their families. Positive family relationships and traditions can be strengthened. The act of caregiving can serve as an important lesson on values to younger members of the family.

This is not to minimize the stress and sacrifice involved with caregiving. There is usually significant effort and frustrations that may be endured while providing care. Caregiving can result in financial strain, fewer social opportunities, inconvenience in living arrangements, and reduced personal space. Career opportunities are frequently lost by caregivers and this can have great impact on someone who is torn between climbing that corporate ladder and being the dutiful daughter or son. If a caregiver attempts to perform all caregiving responsibilities unassisted, it can be a very trying and difficult road.

Finding Help

When care is needed for a short time, as with a terminal illness, there may be sufficient help available among family and friends. However, when an illness is chronic and the need for caregiving extends for years, support and assistance may wane. Alternative arrangements for help from outside the family become crucial. There are organizations that assist people who are in need of caregiving and their caregivers that can be found through local information and referral services. Churches often have ministries that can provide assistance; a network of interfaith volunteer caregivers is available to assist those who desire help through faith communities (see Resources listing). Nonprofit organizations that assist people with specific conditions (e.g., Alzheimer's Disease and Related Disorders Association, Multiple Sclerosis Society) can provide valuable assistance, also.

KEY POINT

The local office of the Area Agency on Aging can provide assistance in locating resources within your community. You can contact your local library for information and referral assistance.

Support Groups

A wonderful resource available for caregivers is special support groups that address issues of people dealing with caregiving. Information as well as successful techniques in handling complex situations are often shared at these informal meetings. There is a special bond that develops between members who share their unique stories that hold aspects to which many others in the group can relate.

An important message that surfaces in support groups is that caregivers have rights, too. Some caregivers need to be given permission to take care of themselves. Somewhere along the road they may have put their own self-care needs on the back burner. They may need to be encouraged to maintain their self-esteem and emotional balance.

There can be valuable exchanges between those who are experiencing the daily challenges of caring for loved ones who may be difficult or deteriorating very rapidly. Suggestions on the most workable method of handling a situation can save another group member hours of aggravation and frustration.

KEY POINT

There sometimes is the problem of who will stay with the dependent individual while the caregiver goes to a support group meeting. The facilitator may have suggestions to help with this.

Caregiver support groups are an efficient, economical, user-friendly way of gaining access to a very complicated social and healthcare services maze. To obtain information about a local caregiver support group, meeting time, and place, call a nearby hospital's Community Education Department or the local Agency on Aging. If they do not host the meetings themselves, they will be able to offer assistance in finding them. Searching the Internet by using the condition a person has (e.g., Alzheimer's disease, multiple sclerosis) often leads to information about local support groups and resources. (See Resources at the end of this chapter.)

Planning

To provide caregiving duties efficiently a plan should be established with the input of the person who is receiving the care when possible. The plan will identify what the person needs and details on the caregiving arrangements (who will do what and when). Sometimes the person who is the recipient of the care may be a very private person or very demanding and have a specific idea of the assistance desired; the desired conditions may be unrealistic or unreasonable. The caregiver needs to be kind yet firm about setting limits. Too often, guilt or fear of displeasing the sick person leaves the caregiver a victim of never saying "no," which can lead to caregiver burnout.

Caregiving can be a full-time job, yet often it must be combined with many other household responsibilities and/or a paid job. It is important that the caregiver doesn't exceed realistic limits, but reaches for help to family, friends, professionals, or community resources. If other family members are unable to provide hands-on assistance, they can be asked to contribute financially to the purchase of services that can ease the caregiving burden. Respite from caregiving responsibilities is something that should be incorporated into the plan. Often a professional can assist the caregiver in obtaining respite services.

Respite is a break from caregiving duties. It can be for several hours a week or several weeks a year. Respite can be achieved from a home health aide companion coming into the home, or the ill person attending adult day care services or briefly staying at an assisted-living residence, nursing facility, or with a another relative. The important point is that the caregiver receives a break from daily caregiving or duties and is able to return to responsibilities refreshed, renewed, healthy, and in good spirits. When burnout is not addressed and respite care is not arranged, the caregiver is at risk for illness.

Stresses of Caregiving

Caregiver stress is not only something that one experiences in the day-to-day, hands-on care of a loved one. This stress can exceed all boundaries and distance. Long distance caregiving can be extremely difficult and challenging. With many families spread across the nation and around the world, caregiving has taken on a whole new appearance. Previously, families remained in close proximity and there were family members who did not work outside the home. The care of young children and the aged was considered a normal family responsibility. There were few "old peoples' homes," as they were called, in which to place an elderly person. The conditions of most of those facilities were very poor, causing them to be the dread of the elderly. Many families committed never to put their loved ones in such a place. Although the conditions of today's long-term care facilities are significantly improved over those of the past, many families continue to be reluctant to seek institutional care for a loved one and experience tremendous guilt when there is no alternative but to do so.

Long Distance Caregiving

Family lifestyles have changed and often both parents work outside the home. With some families separated by thousands of miles, family visits may be rare. Telephone calls, pictures, and even e-mails have taken the place of Sunday and holiday gatherings for many extended families. Although only about 5 percent of the senior population live in nursing facilities, many older adults have moved to a more supportive environment. Assisted-living residences, continuing care retirement communities, and adult communities have become increasingly common residences for elders. Most older adults no longer expect their children to provide for their daily care.

Many adult children who do not live in close proximity to their parents may not know that there is a problem with their parents until they receive a crisis telephone call; they may be ill prepared to handle that emergency. They may have never discussed advanced directives, healthcare proxy, and other important issues with their parents, yet they may be facing some difficult decisions that have to be made. Decisions may need to be based on secondhand information (e.g., what a parent's friend recalls her desires to be regarding life-sustaining treatments).

KEY POINT

Every state has local Area Agency on Aging (AAA) offices provided under the Older American Act, Title III. They frequently are excellent providers of information and referral, and are able to make the task of long distance caregiving easier. In some states the AAA is the center for one-stop shopping for all issues that involve the older adult.

There is another group of professionals who have assisted many long distance caregivers: geriatric care managers. This group of professionals are located throughout the United States. Their role is complex and varied. They are advocates for their clients, liaisons to clients' families, and supporters of their client's well-being. They perform assessments, develop care plans, arrange for services, supervise auxiliary personnel, and serve as surrogate families. An additional function that is provided by many geriatric care managers is that of family or individual counseling. Many geriatric care managers are self-employed professionals, usually nurses or social workers. Some of them are part of larger corporations or affiliations, such as hospitals, Catholic Charities, or Jewish Family Services. There is a fee for their services, usually determined on an hourly basis. The cost of services vary and can be quite expensive, but these care managers are able to deliver high quality service and peace of mind that can be invaluable for long distance caregivers. More information about care managers can be obtained from their national office: National Association of Geriatric Care Managers, *www.caremanager.org*.

KEY POINT

The Family Medical Leave Act entitles employees to as much as 12 weeks of unpaid leave for the care of a family member.

Being Proactive

Caregivers can face significant change and loss. There is an alteration of roles and frequently their entire lives are greatly affected. They may find themselves in the position of parenting their parents. Such lifestyle changes may result in them, as the caregivers, displaying adaptive behaviors that could include denial, excessive physical complaints, rigidity or stubbornness, an overly critical attitude, selective memory, or regression. They also could experience exhaustion, loneliness, depression, anger, or guilt. These behavioral manifestation sometimes cause them to experience the additional loss of friends, co-workers, and other support systems at a time when they most need this support. It is important for caregivers to recognize negative feelings toward their responsibilities and perhaps toward the individuals for whom they are providing care. It could prove very helpful for them to ask themselves the questions shown in Exhibit 26–1 to help identify red flags for problems.

EXHIBIT 26–1 SELF-ASSESSMENT OF CAREGIVER STRESS

_____ There are many days that I wonder if my life is worth living

_____ The care recipient requires care and attention that exceed my abilities

_____ I'm often overwhelmed by my responsibilities

_____ My spouse and children feel that I am neglecting their needs

_____ I often don't sleep or eat properly

_____ There is little-to-no opportunity for me to exercise or engage in recreation

_____ I have postponed taking care of my own health needs due to the caregiving demands

_____ I often argue or have conflicts with the care recipient

_____ Sometimes I have thoughts of harming the care recipient

_____ I worry about what will happen to the care recipient if something happens to me

_____ My health is suffering

_____ There is little time or space for me to have personal private time

_____ It has become difficult for me to have a social life

_____ I have become resentful of other family members who do not provide assistance

_____ The care recipient takes me for granted

_____ Caregiving is creating financial hardship for me and/or my family

_____ I'm feeling guilty that my best doesn't seem good enough

After answering the questions in Exhibit 26–1, caregivers should consider discussing the "yes" responses with family and friends who form their support system and asking for advice and assistance in finding ways to change the situation. Options could include:

- Calling a family meeting to assign or encourage additional family support
- Negotiating expectations and limitations with the care recipient
- Contacting outside community resources to come into the home and assist with care
- Finding someone to listen
- Scheduling time off
- Joining a support group
- Seeking counseling
- Exploring assisted living or nursing home care

It is far wiser to develop strategies to avoid having caregiver stress lead to negative consequences for all parties involved.

Chapter Summary

As more people are reaching their senior years and living longer once they do, their risk of becoming disabled and dependent on others increases. For most of these people, care will be provided by family members. This can present many challenges for the care recipients and the caregivers.

Caregivers can fill many roles, such as providing supervision, personal care, guidance in navigating the healthcare system, assistance with decision making, and support.

Often, caregivers have to juggle caregiving responsibilities with other family and work demands. Many people are caught between the care of their children and the care of their parents, leading to them being referred to as the *sandwich generation*. The term *club sandwich* is being added to family profiles to include caregivers who are providing care to their parents, children, and grandchildren.

It is important for caregivers to help their family members consider financial and health plans in the event that the dependent family members are incapable of making decisions and performing functions independently. An advance directive is one means to plan for future events; it provides instructions on treatment desired in the event people cannot express their opinions at a later date, and the person authorized to make healthcare decisions for them.

A variety of age-related changes can affect elders' abilities to function independently and engage in self-care. Further, aging changes can alter the presentation of symptoms.

It is important for caregivers to understand age-related changes to differentiate normal from abnormal findings.

Caregivers can lighten their burdens by planning care, seeking help with caregiving, participating in support group, and preventing and managing stress.

Suggested Readings

Acton, G. J. and Miller, E. W. (2003). Spirituality in caregivers of family members with dementia. *Journal of Holistic Nursing, 21*(2):117–130.

Astor, B. (1998). *Baby Boomers' Guide to Caring for Aging Parents.* New York: Macmillan.

Brandt, A. L. (1998). *Caregivers' Reprieve: A Guide to Emotional Survival When You're Caring for Someone You Love.* San Luis Obispo, CA: Impact Publishers.

Davidhizar, R., Bechtel, G. A., and Woodring, B. C. (2000). The changing role of grandparenthood. *Journal of Gerontological Nursing, 26*(1):24–29.

Eliopoulos, C. (1997). Chronic care coaches. *Home Healthcare Nursing, 15*(3): 185–188.

Eliopoulos, C. (1999). *Integrating Conventional and Alternative Therapies: Holistic Care for Chronic Conditions.* St. Louis: Mosby.

Farran, C. J. (2001). Family caregiver intervention research: Where have we been? Where are we going? *Journal of Gerontological Nursing, 27*(7):38–45.

Grollman, E. A. and Grollman, S. H. (1997). *Your Aging Parents: Reflections for Caregivers.* Boston: Beacon Press.

Kelley, L. S. and Specht, J. K. P. (2000). Family involvement in care for individuals with dementia protocol. *Journal of Gerontological Nursing, 26*(2):13–21.

Larrimore, K. L. (2003). Alzheimer disease support group characteristics: A comparison of caregivers. *Geriatric Nursing, 24*(1):32–35.

Lerner, H. (2002). *The Dance of Connection.* New York: Quill.

Levin, N. J. (1997). *How to Care for Your Parents: A Practical Guide to Eldercare.* New York: Norton.

Li, H. (2002). Family caregivers preferences in caring for their hospitalized elderly relatives. *Geriatric Nursing, 23*(2):204–207.

Li, Y. (1999). The graying of American and Chinese societies: Young adults' attitudes toward the care of their elderly parents. *Geriatric Nursing, 20*(1):45–47.

Lilly, M. L., Richards, B. S., and Buckwater, K. C. (2003). Friends and social support in dementia caregiving: Assessment and intervention. *Journal of Gerontological Nursing, 29*(1):29–36.

Logue, R. M. (2003). Maintaining family connectedness in long-term care: An advanced practice approach to family-centered nursing homes. *Journal of Gerontological Nursing,* 29(6):24–31.

McCall, J. B. (1999). *Grief Education for Caregivers of the Elderly.* New York: Haworth Pastoral Press.

Meyer, M. M. and Derr, P. (1998). *The Comfort of Home: An Illustrated Step-by-step Guide for Caregivers.* Portland, OR: CareTrust Publications LLC.

Moore, S. L., Metcalf, B., & Schow, E. (2000). Aging and meaning in life: Examining the concept. *Geriatric Nursing,* 21(1), 27–29.

Morse, S. and Robbins, D. Q. (1998). *Moving Mom and Dad: Why, Where, How, and When to Help Your Parents Relocate,* 2nd ed. Berkeley, CA: Lanier Publishing International.

National Family Caregivers Association. (1996). *The Resourceful Caregiver: Helping Caregivers Help Themselves.* St. Louis: Mosby Lifeline.

Ostwald, S. K., Hepburn, K. W., and Burns, T. (2003). Training family caregivers of patients with dementia: A structured workshop approach. *Journal of Gerontological Nursing,* 29(1):37–44.

Ruppert, R. A. (1996). Caring for the lay caregiver. *American Journal of Nursing,* 96(3):40–45.

Schomp, V. (1997). *The Aging Parent Handbook.* New York: Harper Paperbacks.

Stocker, S. (1996). Six tips for caring for aging parents. *American Journal of Nursing,* 96(9):32–33.

Stokes, S. A. and Gordon, S. E. (2003). Common stressors experienced by the well elderly: Clinical implications. *Journal of Gerontological Nursing,* 29(5):38–46.

Winters, S. (2003). Alzheimer disease from a child's perspective. *Geriatric Nursing,* 24(1):36–39.

Resources

Family Caregiver Alliance
690 Market Street, Dept. P, Suite 600
San Francisco, CA 94104
www.caregiver.org/factsheets/out_of_home_care.html

National Council on Family Relations
3989 Central Avenue NE, Suite 550
Minneapolis, MN 55420
612-781-9331
www.ncfr.com

National Eldercare Locator
1112 16th Street NW, Suite 100
Washington, DC 20036
800-677-1116
www.eldercare.gov

National Federation of Interfaith Volunteer Caregivers
800-350-7438
www.NFIVC.org

RESOURCES

A variety of resources exist to provide guidance and assistance in living a healthy, balanced life and the savvy consumer needs to be equipped to use them. Some tips for developing a personal resource list; state, national, and international resources; and important Internet sites, which address both conventional, and complementary/alternative therapies are offered in this chapter.

Tips for Developing a Personal Resource File

There is wisdom in having resources on hand before they're needed. This is similar to preparing for the proverbial rainy day, or buying the hurricane shutters before the storm hits. Resources help people find information, and information offers more control of one's life. Here are some hints that can be beneficial to healthcare professionals and their clients.

- Purchase an accordion file that offers plenty of room for expansion. You can organize your resource file in any way that makes sense to you. One idea would be to divide the file into four sections: 1) local; 2) state; 3) national, and 4) international. This Personal Resource File can help to organize information you may need and enhance your self-care ability. There is value in having information when you face an actual health challenge or even before a challenge to your health occurs.

- Remember that information can come from a variety of places. The trick is to be able to collect the information as soon as it is found and save it for when it is needed. Some places that you can find information are: a) friends who have had positive experiences with healthcare providers (KEEPER LIST), as well as less than adequate experiences (I'LL HAVE TO THINK ABOUT IT); b) local newspapers; c) special TV programs that offer current information about a variety of topics (be sure to jot down the highlights of what was said); d) your local library; e) workshops and seminars in your community; f) books; g) journals, and h) the Internet.

Special Guidelines for the Internet

- Don't assume that just because it is labeled "medical advice" that it is "good advice." It is wise to check with a trusted healthcare provider before you take any remedies or discontinue prescribed medications or treatments.

- Always tab down to the end of the Web page to see if the Web site is updated on a monthly basis. This will at least let you know that the information is current. Try more than one Web site pertaining to the topic.

- Recognize that commercial sites are just that. They are on the Web to capture your business. A more reliable source of information would come from a medical center, a university hospital, a college of: nursing, medicine, physical therapy, social work, pharmacy, chiropractic, naturopathy, TCM (traditional Chinese medicine), or Ayurvedic, etc., or a Government Health Agency. A simple rule of thumb is: certification and accreditation = highest standards.

- It is necessary to ask yourself these questions when visiting sites:
  - Is there any chance that the information I am downloading is biased?
  - Is the information being shared for the greater good of all individuals?
  - Whose benefit does it serve?
  - Is the information based on opinion only and not referenced from current professional (nursing, medical, social work, pharmacological, complementary, and naturopathic) resources?

- Know that it is important for people to make sense of the information gathered so they can discuss it with their healthcare providers for clarification. Clients can be guided to form questions, such as:
  - "Dr., [Nurse, etc.] "I found this on the Internet, it's about my condition and I want to know more about how this can help me."

- ° "This condition is being helped by _____, what is being done in our area?"

- ° "I'd like to try _____. How does this effect the medicine I am taking now?"

- ° "I trust the treatment you and I agreed upon, but have an interest in trying something different as well. Can I use both of these approaches together?"

Local Resources
Tips For Finding Local Resources

- The American Holistic Nurses' Association (AHNA) has networks throughout the country. Call the national number: 800-278-AHNA for information. This would be a valuable resource and well worth your effort to find out about what is happening at your local level. Meetings are open to members of the community who value holism in their lives.

- Always consider local healthcare information talent. Most communities have a community college or university that has a college or school of nursing, medicine, social work, physical therapy, dentistry, massage, acupuncture, or allied health, etc., whose faculty may be excellent resources. These potentially valuable resources can be tapped by doing the following:

  1. Call the main number of the area you need e.g., department of nursing.
  2. Identify yourself as an individual in the community.
  3. State your need, e.g., "I am interested in talking to someone on your faculty who knows about _____. I'd appreciate his or her ideas."
  4. Leave a message so that faculty can get in touch with you.

- Don't be intimidated if you have had little involvement with a college or university. The faculty often is eager to assist and enjoy the opportunity to put their knowledge to good use.

- There are many individuals in the community who experience similar issues/concerns who come together in support groups. Check local newspapers for health sections or community meeting announcements that list support group meetings. Even if you are not in need of a support group at present, it could be helpful to cut this information out and place it in your Personal Resource File for future reference.

  - ° Don't forget the weekly columns on "You and Your Health" or "Pharmacology News." Become a resource finder.

- Libraries are rich resources not only for the books and journals they contain, but also for the workshops and printed material that are made available to the general public. Librarians can be a valuable guide to resources on the Internet, as well as reference material in their holdings and in other libraries.
  - ○ Don't forget that videos are available on health-related content.
- You probably have great resources at your fingertips that you may be overlooking: telephone directories. Directories typically have listings for "Community Resources." Also, depending on your interest, simply look for a local agency e.g., American Cancer Society® or American Heart Association®. Let the agency know specifically what your needs are (e.g., literature, schedule of classes).

Tips For Finding Local Resources on the Internet

- Go to your favorite search engine, e.g., Google, Search.com, Mama.com, Metacrawler®, Dogpile, Healthfinder.gov®, etc. and type in the query that best describes your needs. An example would be *Palm Beach County, Arthritis Resources*, or *Bucks County, Area Agency on Aging*.
- Any time you are looking for resources at the local level try typing in the county where you live. This provides a more specific, local search. The reverse also may hold true. If you are not able to locate your needs at the local level you may need to start more globally and then work your way to the local level. An example might be looking for resources for *American Cancer Society* and then linking until you find local resources.
- Please be patient! Consider yourself a detective who is looking for clues for resources to help you. It's worth the effort!

State Resources

Tips for Finding State Resources

- Check the state health department for your area of interest (e.g., AIDS Administration, Department of Mental Health, Nursing Home Licensing and Certification. State health departments also have divisions that license and monitor the practice of various professionals, such as nursing, medicine, nursing home administrators, dentists, acupuncturists, and massage therapists.

Tips for Finding State Resources on the Internet

- Go to your favorite search engine as you did in your local search, e.g., Dogpile, Google, Mama, Metacrawler®, Healthfinder.gov®, etc. and type in the query that best describes what it is you are looking for. An example would be: *New York State, Licensed Acupuncturists*, or *Oregon, Naturopaths*. This should lead you to information pertinent to your state.

- Also consider the various state agencies that may lead you to the information that you need. An example would be: *Michigan, Department of Health*, or *Florida, AIDS resources*.

- Think about the hospitals in your state that are major medical centers. An example of this would be: *Texas, Baylor University*, or *Philadelphia, Jefferson University*. This may open up information for you that you never suspected were available to the consumer. Another way of getting information about your major medical centers would be to type in the state and the term: *Arizona, medical centers* or *Alabama, health resources*.

- Keep trying and with patience you will find that the Internet can offer rich resources.

National Resources

- *National Institutes/Centers:*

National Institutes of Health (NIH)
http://www.nih.gov/health
A large resource for government agencies. This site has valuable publications that are free (usually for less than 25 cents a copy).

National Cancer Institute
Building 31, Room 10A18
Bethesda, MD 20205
800-492-6600
www.nci.nih.gov

National Center for Complementary & Alternative Medicine of NIH (NCCAM)
http://nccam.nih.gov
Valuable clearinghouse for information

National Heart, Lung, and Blood Institute (NHLBI)
http://www.nhlbi.nih.gov/
PO Box 30105
Bethesda, MD 20824-0105
301-592-8573
fax: 301-592-8563

National Dissemination Center for Children with Disabilities
PO Box 1492
Washington, DC 20013
800-695-0285
www.nichcy.org

National Institute on Aging (NIA)
Building 31, Room 5C27
31 Center Drive, MSC 2292
Bethesda, MD 20892
301-496-1752
www.nia.nih.gov/
Note: A resource directory is available for $11.00 (prepaid) #0106200145-1800

National Institute on Alcohol Abuse & Alcoholism (NIAAA)
301-443-3860
www.niaaa.nih.gov/

National Institute of Arthritis & Musculoskeletal and Skin Diseases (NIAMS)
301-495-4484
www.niams.nih.gov

National Institute of Child Health & Human Development (NICHD)
PO Box 3006
Rockville, MD 20847
800-370-2943
fax: 301-984-1473
www.nichd.nih.gov/

National Institute of Dental & Craniofacial Research (NIDCR)
Building 45, Room 4AS19
45 Center Drive
Bethesda, MD 20892-6400
301-496-4261
fax: 301-496-9988
http://www.nidcr.nih.gov

National Institute of Diabetes & Digestive & Kidney Diseases (NIDDK)
Building 31, Room 9A04
31 Center Drive, MSC 2560
Bethesda, MD 20892-2560

301-654-3327
fax: 301-907-8906
ndic@info.niddk.nih.gov
www.niddk.nih.gov/
US Center for Disease Control & Prevention
www.cdc.gov
US Environmental Protection Agency
Ariel Rios Building
1200 Pennsylvania Avenue, NW
Washington, DC 20460
www.epa.gov
Warren Grant Magnuson Clinical Center
Clinical Center, NIH
Building 10, Room B1S234
Bethesda, MD 20892-1078
301-496-3311
fax: 301-496-0622
www.cc.nih.gov/
Requests can be made for Clinical Center nutrition education materials
- *National & Professional Organizations:*
Academy for Guided Imagery
P.O. Box 2070
Mill Valley, CA 94942
800-726-2070
www.interactiveimagery.com
Alzheimer's Disease & Related Disorders Association (ADRDA)
225 North Michigan Ave., Suite 1700
Chicago, IL 60601-7633
800-272-3900
www.alz.org
American Academy of Pain Management
13947 Mono Way #A
Sonora, CA 95370
209-533-9744
www.aapainmanage.org
American Association of Acupuncture & Oriental Medicine
1925 West County Road B2

Roseville, MN 55113
651-631-0204
www.aaaom.org
American Association of Critical Care Nurses (AACN)
www.aacn.org
American Heart Association
800-242-8721
www.americanheart.org
American Association of Kidney Patients
3505 E. Frontage Rd Ste 315
Tampa, FL 33607
800-749-2257
www.aakp.org
American Association of Naturopathic Physicians
3201 New Mexico Ave., NW Ste 350
Washington, DC 20016
800-538-2267
www.naturopathic.org
American Botanical Council
6200 Manor Rd.
Austin, TX 78723
512-926-4900
www.herbalgram.org
American Chiropractic Association
1701 Clarendon Blvd.
Arlington, VA 22209
703-276-8800
www.amerchiro.org
American College of Hyperbaric Medicine
2476 Bolsover Box 130
Houston, TX 77005
713-528-0657
www.hyperbaricmedicine.org
American Council on Exercise
4851 Paramount Dr.
San Diego, CA 92123
858-279-8227
www.acefitness.org

American Diabetes Association
National Call Center
1701 North Beauregard St.
Alexandria, VA 22311
800-342-2383
www.diabetes.org
*American Holistic Nurses' Association
PO Box 2130
Flagstaff, AZ 86003
800-278-AHNA
www.ahna.org
*American Holistic Medical Association
12101 Menaul Blvd. NE, Suite C
Alburquerque, NM 87112
505-292-7788
www.holisticmedicine.org
*Gateway to complementary/alternative health information
American Liver Foundation
75 Maiden Lane, Suite 603
New York, NY 10038
800-465-4837
www.liverfoundation.org
American Lung Association
61 Broadway, 6th floor
New York, NY 10006
212-315-8700
www.lungusa.org
American Massage Therapy Association
820 Davis Street, Suite 100
Evanston, IL 60201-4444
847-684-0123
www.amtamassage.org
American Sleep Disorders Association
1610 14th Street NW, Suite 300
Rochester, MN 55901
507-287-6006
Arthritis Foundation
1314 Spring Street NW

Atlanta, GA 30309
800-283-7800
www.arthritis.org

Asthma Hotline
800-222-LUNG

Ayurvedic Institute
11311 Menaul NE
Albuquerque, NM 87112
505-291-9698
www.ayurveda.com

Colorado Center for Healing Touch
12477 W. Cedar Dr., Suite 206
Lakewood, CO 80228
303-989-0581
fax: 303-985-9702
ccheal@aol.com
www.healingtouch.net/ccht.shtml

Lighthouse National Center for Vision & Aging
111 East 59th Street
New York, NY 10022
800-829-0500
www.lighthouse.org

Multiple Sclerosis Association of America
706 Haddonfield Road
Cherry Hill, NJ 08002
800-532-7667
fax: 856-661-9797
www.msaa.com

National Association for the Deaf
814 Thayer Avenue
Silver Spring, MD 20910
301-587-1789
www.nad.org

National Center for Homeopathy
801 North Fairfax, Suite 306

Alexandria, VA 22314
703-548-7790
www.homeopathic.org

National Hospice and Palliative Care Organization
1700 Diagonal Rd., Suite 625
Alexandria, VA 22314
703-837-1500
fax: 703-837-1233
www.nho.org

National Osteoporosis Foundation
1232 22nd Street NW
Washington, DC 20037-1292
202-223-2226
www.nof.org

National Parkinson's Disease Foundation
1501 NW 9th Avenue
Bob Hope Road
Miami, FL 33136
800-327-4545
www.parkinson.org

National Stroke Association
9707 E. Easter Lane
Englewood, CO 80112
800-STROKES
www.stroke.org

North American Vegetarian Society
PO Box 72
Dolgeville, NY 13329
518-568-7970
www.navs-online.org

Nurse Healers Professional Associates, Inc.
3760 South Highland Drive, Suite 429
Salt Lake City, UT 84106
801-273-3399
fax: 509-693-3537
www.therapeutic-touch.org

United Ostomy Association
19772 MacArthur Blvd., #200
Irvine, CA 92612-2405
800-826-0826
www.uoa.org

- *Web Sites Related to Healthcare Information:*
ACTIS (Clinical Trials for HIV/AIDS)
800-TRIALS-A
www.actis.org

Adult Children of Alcoholics Worldwide Services Organization
www.recovery.org/acoa/acoa.html

A J N Online (American Journal of Nursing)
www.ajnonline.com
Has articles and general information

Al-Anon Family Group Headquarters
www.Al-Anon-Alateen.org

American Holistic Nurses' Association
www.ahna.org

American Nurses Association
www.nursingworld.org

Anxiety Disorders Association of America
www.adaa.org

Association for Applied Psychophysiology & Biofeedback
www.aapb.org

Bioport
http://bioport.com
Links to medical news sites, research sites, medical universities

CenterWatch
www.centerwatch.com
A resource for clinical trials on various diseases, a summary of research, and numbers of whom to contact.

Health on the Net
www.hon.ch/home.html
Searches available for information/resources

*Healthfinder
www.healthfinder.gov
*A gateway site sponsored by the government with links to more than
  1,400 health sites

Healthy People 2010
www.health.gov/healthypeople/
A national health initiative coordinated by the Office of Disease Prevention
and Health Promotion & US Department of Health & Human Services
Looks at health issues for the next decade

JAMA (*the Journal of the American Medical Association*)
www.jama-assn.org
Valuable resource for consumers—access to the "patient page"

Medhunt
www.hon.ch/medhunt
A medical search engine

Medscape
www.medscape.com
A gateway to reviewed information from reputable medical journals

National Council on Family Relations
www.ncfr.com

National Library of Medicine
www.nlm.nih.gov
Offers access to the world's largest biomedical library.

Pharm Info Net
www.pharminfo.com
Information about medications

Prostate Cancer Resource Network
www.hmri.com

Self-Help Group Sourcebook Online
http://mentalhelp.net/selfhelp/
An online directory of thousands of medical and mental health support
organizations around the world

The NIH Office of Dietary Supplements
dietary-supplements.info.nih.gov/

Provides a list of scientific publications. There are 250,000 citations and abstracts on dietary supplements, botanicals, vitamins, and minerals

International Resources

International Organizations:

Global Alliance for Women's Health
www.gawh.org

International Association of Yoga Therapists
PO Box 426
Manton, CA 96059
530-474-5700
www.iayt.org

MEL: International Health Resources
http://mel.lib.us/health/healthinternational.html

World Health Organization (W.H.O.)
www.who.int
Resource for issues around the globe

U.C. Berkeley, Public Health Library
International Health Resources
www.lib.berkeley.edu/PUBL/Inthealth.html

UN Aids Organization
www.unaids.org/
Global source of HIV/AIDS information

INDEX